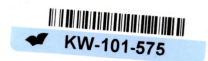

Pearls and Pitfalls in
MUSCULOSKELETAL
IMAGING
Variants and Other
Difficult Diagnoses

Pearls and Pitfalls in
MUSCULOSKELETAL IMAGING

Variants and Other Difficult Diagnoses

Edited by

D. Lee Bennett, MD, MA, FACR

Vice Chair for Clinical Operations in the Department of Radiology
at the University of Iowa, Roy J. and Lucille A. Carver College of
Medicine at the University of Iowa, Iowa City, IA, USA

Georges Y. El-Khoury, MD, FACR

Section Director for Musculoskeletal Imaging, and a Professor of
Radiology at the University of Iowa, Iowa City, IA, USA

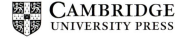

CAMBRIDGE UNIVERSITY PRESS
Cambridge, New York, Melbourne, Madrid, Cape Town,
Singapore, São Paulo, Delhi, Mexico City

Cambridge University Press
The Edinburgh Building, Cambridge CB2 8RU, UK

Published in the United States of America by Cambridge University Press, New York

www.cambridge.org
Information on this title: www.cambridge.org/9780521196321

First published 2013

Printed and bound by Grafos SA, Arte sobre papel, Barcelona, Spain

A catalog record for this publication is available from the British Library

Library of Congress Cataloging in Publication data

Pearls and pitfalls in musculoskeletal imaging : variants and other difficult diagnoses /
edited by D. Lee Bennett, Georges El-Khoury.
    p. ;   cm.
Includes bibliographical references and index.
ISBN 978-0-521-19632-1 (Hardback)
I. Bennett, D. Lee.   II. El-Khoury, Georges Y.
[DNLM: 1. Musculoskeletal Diseases–diagnosis.   2. Diagnosis, Differential.
3. Diagnostic Imaging–methods.   WE 141]
616.7075–dc23   2012041310

ISBN 9780-521-19632-1 Hardback

Contents

v

Contributors

Joong Mo Ahn, MD, PhD
Department of Radiology
University of Pittsburgh Medical Center
Pittsburgh PA, USA

D. Lee Bennett, MD, MA, FACR
Department of Radiology
University of Iowa Roy J and Lucille A Carver College
of Medicine, University of Iowa
Iowa City IA, USA

Georges Y. El-Khoury, MD, FACR
Department of Radiology
University of Iowa Roy J and Lucille A Carver College
of Medicine, University of Iowa
Iowa City IA, USA

Kenjirou Ohashi, MD, PhD
Department of Radiology
University of Iowa Roy J and Lucille A Carver College
of Medicine, University of Iowa
Iowa City IA, USA

Foreword

It is my honor and pleasure to write a foreword for the newest publication from Drs. Bennett and El-Khoury. My affiliation with the authors for the past 15 years has proven to be one of my most meaningful professional relationships. Through their work in the Department of Musculoskeletal Radiology at the University of Iowa Hospitals and Clinics, hundreds of radiology residents, fellows, and visiting fellows have benefitted from formal musculoskeletal training. Thousands more "learners" at all stages of training have benefitted from their books, presentations, and scholarly articles, which have enriched our profession as a whole.

The cases found in these pages reflect some of the most frequent decision points in musculoskeletal radiology. Nevertheless, these cases remain challenging. The authors have spent their lives finding a balance between simplicity and complexity when teaching others about these troublesome cases, and have now distilled the best of their ideas into this text. The result is a simple, straightforward collection of cases we can quickly refer to when faced with these common, yet vexing situations.

The distilled wisdom contained herein attests to the depth and breadth of the authors' knowledge and the variety of the casework available to them. The quality of the book reflects the joy they have in teaching. I hope you enjoy and profit from their teachings as I have for so many years!

Scott M. Truhlar, MD
President, Radiologic Medical Services, PC
Corridor Radiology

Preface

This book focuses on musculoskeletal diseases encountered in the shoulder, upper extremity, pelvis, and lower extremity that are problematic because they are less common, relatively recently described, or can mimic more common pathology leading to a misdiagnosis. This work demonstrates succinct imaging findings that differentiate these less common findings or normal variant mimickers from the more common similar-appearing diseases so as to prevent misdiagnosis. This text will function as a useful resource to both residents and general practicing radiologists when they encounter problematic imaging findings that resemble a common disease, and yet the imaging findings just don't quite seem like the common disease. The collection of diseases in this book has been drawn from the literature (text) as well as the substantial teaching and clinical experience of the authors (images). The final chapter of the text functions as a succinct review of musculoskeletal tumors and tumor-like lesions encountered in a general radiology practice.

Pseudocyst of the humeral head

Imaging description

The area of rarefaction, located in the lateral aspect of the proximal humerus, may be a prominent radiographic finding in young individuals (Figures 1.1 and 1.2). In older individuals, with loss of trabecular bone in the proximal portion of the humerus, a less obvious rarefaction is present.

Importance

It is important to recognize the humeral pseudocyst and avoid performing a biopsy of it. Other pseudolesions that produce areas of radiolucency may be encountered at the femoral neck (Ward's triangle) and body of the calcaneus.

Typical clinical scenario

Radiographs may reveal an area of rarefaction in the humeral head. This rarefaction may mimic a lytic lesion.

Differential diagnosis

Although disease processes such as myeloma, giant cell tumor, chondroblastoma, and metastatic disease can occur in the humeral head and mimic a pseudocyst, these pathologic processes can usually be differentiated by criteria such as cortical break-through, periosteal new bone formation, more extensive involvement than the pseudocyst, and poorly defined margins.

Teaching point

When there is a question of whether this area of radiolucency is a true lesion or pseudocyst, magnetic resonance imaging can be of value, because it will show whether the area consists of normal marrow rather than tissue supportive of a neoplasm.

READING LIST

Helms CA. Pseudocysts of the humerus. *AJR Am J Roentgenol* 1978;**131**:287–288.

Peh WC. Humeral pseudocyst. *Am J Orthop* 2003;**32**:569.

Resnick D, Cone RO III. The nature of humeral pseudocysts. *Radiology* 1984;**150**:27–28.

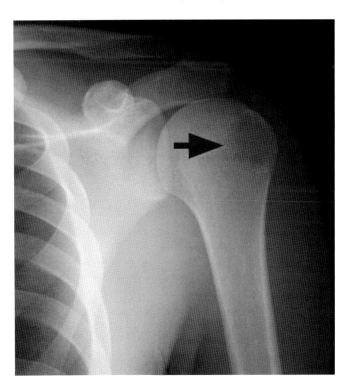

Figure 1.1 Pseudocyst of the humeral head. Anteroposterior view of the shoulder shows an area of rarefaction (arrow), located in the lateral aspect of the proximal humerus.

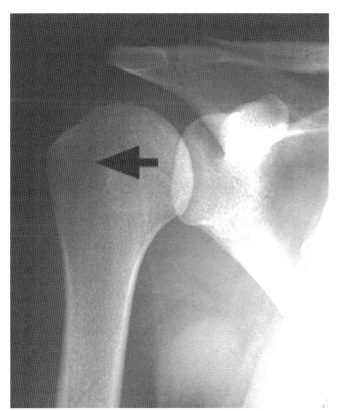

Figure 1.2 Pseudocyst of the humeral head. Anteroposterior view of the shoulder shows an area of rarefaction (arrow), located in the lateral aspect of the proximal humerus.

Pearls and Pitfalls in Musculoskeletal Imaging, ed. D. Lee Bennett and Georges Y. El-Khoury. Published by Cambridge University Press. © Cambridge University Press 2013.

SLAP tear versus sublabral foramen/recess

Imaging description

SLAP (superior labral anteroposterior) lesions are a tear of the superior labrum usually centered on the attachment of the long head of the biceps tendon (Figure 2.1). Sublabral foramen is located anterior to the biceps tendon attachment and involves the anterior labrum (Figure 2.2). Sublabral recess (Figure 2.3) is a sulcus between the capsuloligamentous complex and the superior glenoid cartilage.

Importance

Radiologists should perform a dedicated approach to these lesions with the description of the biceps-labral complex abnormality, extension of lesions, and associated lesions in ligament, adjacent cartilage, and tendons.

Typical clinical scenario

The clinical diagnosis of a SLAP lesion is difficult. Nonspecific shoulder pain, particularly with overhead or cross-body motion, is the most common clinical presentation. Additional symptoms include popping, clicking, catching, weakness, stiffness, and instability.

Differential diagnosis

Sublabral foramen and recess can simulate a SLAP lesion. The sublabral foramen shows medial slip which courses medially and posteriorly towards the glenoid and attaches to the anterior labrum more inferiorly. Sublabral recess has smooth edges and usually measures less than 2 mm in width. Conventionally, the sublabral recess does not extend behind the biceps anchor. Additionally, articular cartilage interface can simulate a SLAP lesion on oblique coronal MR images. In general, SLAP lesions are oriented laterally, whereas the cartilage interface is oriented parallel to the glenoid cortex.

Teaching point

Magnetic resonance (MR) imaging analysis in multiple planes and close attention to clinical history and mechanisms of injury are strongly recommended. When appropriate, radiologists should describe the lesion as indeterminate for sublabral recess versus SLAP lesion and suggest clinical correlation or MR arthrography for better delineation of the labral abnormality.

READING LIST

Beltran J, Bencardino J, Mellado J, Rosenberg ZS, Irish RD. MR arthrography of the shoulder: variants and pitfalls. *Radiographics* 1997;**17**:1403–1412.

Chang D, Mohana-Borges A, Borso M, Chung CB. SLAP lesions: anatomy, clinical presentation, MR imaging diagnosis and characterization. *Eur J Radiol* 2008;**68**:72–87.

Mohana-Borges AV, Chung CB, Resnick D. Superior labral anteroposterior tear: classification and diagnosis on MRI and MR arthrography. *AJR Am J Roentgenol* 2003;**181**:1449–1462.

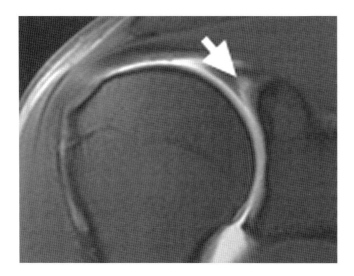

Figure 2.1 SLAP (superior labral anteroposterior) lesion. Fat-suppressed T1-weighted coronal MR arthrogram shows a superior labral tear with contrast extending into the labral substance (arrow).

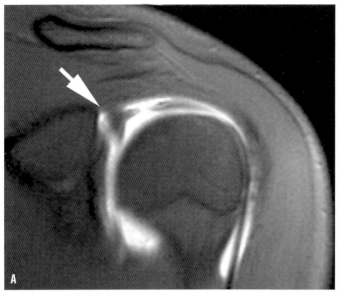
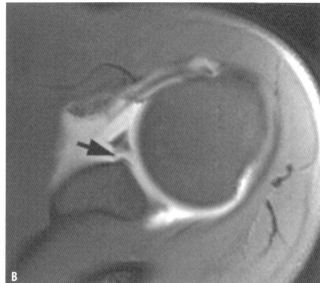
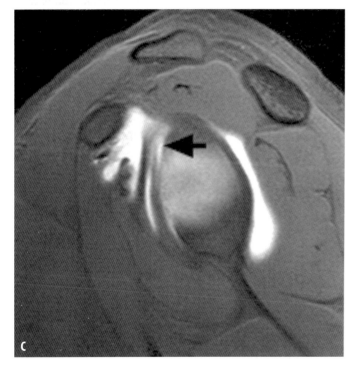

Figure 2.2 Sublabral foramen. Fat-suppressed T1-weighted coronal MR arthrogram (**A**) shows absence of anterosuperior labrum (arrow). Fat-suppressed T1-weighted axial MR arthrogram (**B**), obtained in the same patient as in A, shows separation of anterosuperior labrum (arrow) from glenoid cartilage. Fat-suppressed T1-weighted sagittal MR arthrogram (**C**), obtained in the same patient as in B, shows absence of anterosuperior labrum (arrow).

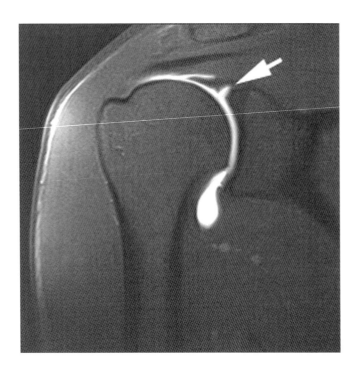

Figure 2.3 Sublabral recess. Fat-suppressed T1-weighted coronal MR arthrogram demonstrates a linear space (arrow) between the superior labrum and the adjacent glenoid.

3 SLAP tear versus normal variant of biceps labral complex

Imaging description

The diagnosis of SLAP (superior labral anteroposterior) lesions is based on abnormalities in signal intensity and morphology. MR imaging findings reported to be characteristics of SLAP lesions include increased signal intensity in the labrum, with or without extension to the biceps anchor, and cleavage of the superior labrum (Figure 3.1). Pseudo-SLAP is a small sulcus between the superior labrum and the origins of the biceps tendon. It is a small contrast-filled sulcus with variable depth observed on oblique coronal MR images (Figure 3.2).

Importance

Pitfalls in standard MR imaging are related to the presence of increased intralabral signal intensity without surface irregularity or definite labral tear.

Typical clinical scenario

The majority of patients present with concurrent shoulder injuries.

Differential diagnosis

A deep sulcus between the superior labrum and the biceps tendon may simulate a SLAP lesion. Increased intralabral signal intensity is a common finding and may be associated with magic angle phenomena or intrasubstance labral degeneration. Partial volume averaging with the glenohumeral ligaments is also a common finding.

> ## Teaching point
>
> Careful evaluation of the whole extension of structures usually allows differentiation of a normal structure from a tear.

READING LIST

Beltran J, Bencardino J, Mellado J, Rosenberg ZS, Irish RD. MR arthrography of the shoulder: variants and pitfalls. *Radiographics* 1997;**17**:1403–1412.

Chang D, Mohana-Borges A, Borso M, Chung CB. SLAP lesions: anatomy, clinical presentation, MR imaging diagnosis and characterization. *Eur J Radiol* 2008;**68**:72–87.

Mohana-Borges AV, Chung CB, Resnick D. Superior labral anteroposterior tear: classification and diagnosis on MRI and MR arthrography. *AJR Am J Roentgenol* 2003;**181**:1449–1462.

Monu JU, Pope TL Jr, Chabon SJ, Vanarthos WJ. MR diagnosis of superior labral anterior posterior (SLAP) injuries of the glenoid labrum: value of routine imaging without intraarticular injection of contrast material. *AJR Am J Roentgenol* 1994;**163**:1425–1429.

Pearls and Pitfalls in Musculoskeletal Imaging, ed. D. Lee Bennett and Georges Y. El-Khoury. Published by Cambridge University Press. © Cambridge University Press 2013.

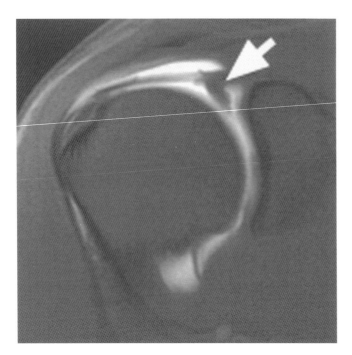 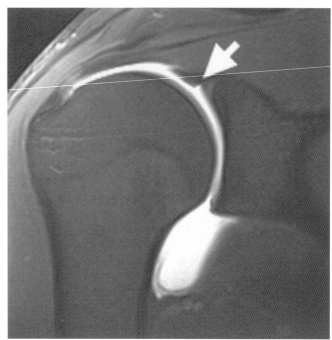

Figure 3.1 SLAP (superior labral anteroposterior) lesion. Fat-suppressed T1-weighted coronal MR arthrogram shows cleavage of the superior labrum (arrow).

Figure 3.2 Pseudo-SLAP. Fat-suppressed T1-weighted coronal MR arthrogram shows a small sulcus (arrow) between the superior labrum and the origins of the biceps tendon.

Labral tear versus hyaline cartilage undercutting

Imaging description

To identify labral tears, morphologic criteria such as absence, fraying, detachment, displacement, or deformity, can be used. Fluid or contrast within the labral substance is also an indication of a labral tear (Figure 4.1). Labral tears occasionally present on MR imaging as focal or diffuse increase in signal intensity extending to the surface on all imaging sequences, but this is less reliable. In standard MR images, higher signal intensity is present between the labrum and the glenoid cartilage in short-TE sequences, occurring in the transition zone between two histologic structures. Areas of the transitional zone do not fill with contrast material in arthrographic images.

Importance

Pitfalls in standard MR imaging are related to the presence of transitional zones. The transitional zone is the area located between the fibrocartilage of the labrum and the hyaline cartilage of the glenoid.

Typical clinical scenario

Tears of the labrum are common in athletes with instability, especially those in sports that require forceful and repetitive adduction and overhead rotation of the humerus.

Differential diagnosis

Articular cartilage is frequently present between the labrum and the glenoid cortex, predominantly in the superior half of the joint. This interface can simulate a labral tear on axial MR images (Figure 4.2).

> ## Teaching point
>
> The most common variants and pitfalls are related to labral lesions in the anterior-superior aspect.

READING LIST

Beltran J, Bencardino J, Mellado J, Rosenberg ZS, Irish RD. MR arthrography of the shoulder: variants and pitfalls. *Radiographics* 1997;**17**:1403–1412.

Mohana-Borges AV, Chung CB, Resnick D. Superior labral anteroposterior tear: classification and diagnosis on MRI and MR arthrography. *AJR Am J Roentgenol* 2003;**181**:1449–1462.

Monu JU, Pope TL Jr, Chabon SJ, Vanarthos WJ. MR diagnosis of superior labral anterior posterior (SLAP) injuries of the glenoid labrum: value of routine imaging without intraarticular injection of contrast material. *AJR Am J Roentgenol* 1994;**163**:1425–1429.

Rudez J, Zanetti M. Normal anatomy, variants and pitfalls on shoulder MRI. *Eur J Radiol* 2008;**68**:25–35.

Steinbach LS. MRI of shoulder instability. *Eur J Radiol* 2008;**68**:57–71.

Pearls and Pitfalls in Musculoskeletal Imaging, ed. D. Lee Bennett and Georges Y. El-Khoury. Published by Cambridge University Press. © Cambridge University Press 2013.

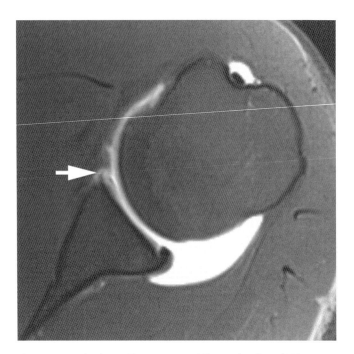

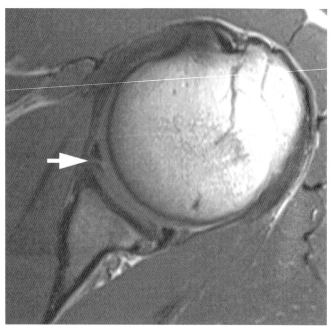

Figure 4.1 Labral tear. Fat-suppressed T1-weighted axial MR arthrogram shows contrast extension (arrow).

Figure 4.2 Normal interface. Intermediate-weighted axial MR image shows the area (arrow) located between the fibrocartilage of the labrum and the hyaline cartilage of the glenoid. This interface can simulate a labral tear.

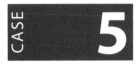

CASE 5

Buford complex of the shoulder

Imaging description

A Buford complex, found in 1.5% of individuals, is the absence of the anterior superior labrum in conjunction with a thickened cord-like middle glenohumeral ligament. The thick middle glenohumeral ligament attaches directly to the anterosuperior glenoid. In cases of Buford complex, axial MR images at the level of the superior half of the glenoid cavity show a thickened middle glenohumeral ligament close to the glenoid margin with an absent labrum (Figure 5.1), simulating labral tear.

Importance

If the Buford complex is mistakenly surgically reattached to the neck of the glenoid cartilage, severe painful restriction of humeral rotation and elevation can occur.

Typical clinical scenario

Buford complex can be identified in patients who were examined by MR imaging, MR arthrography, or arthroscopy to evaluate shoulder instability.

Differential diagnosis

A Buford complex can be confused with a sublabral foramen or pathologic labral detachment.

Teaching point

Identification of a thick middle glenohumeral ligament on oblique sagittal MR images helps one avoid this pitfall. The Buford complex should be suspected if the contiguous superior labrum and anterior inferior labrum appear normal.

READING LIST

Beltran J, Bencardino J, Mellado J, Rosenberg ZS, Irish RD. MR arthrography of the shoulder: variants and pitfalls. *Radiographics* 1997;**17**:1403–1412.

Chang D, Mohana-Borges A, Borso M, Chung CB. SLAP lesions: anatomy, clinical presentation, MR imaging diagnosis and characterization. *Eur J Radiol* 2008;**68**:72–87.

Tirman PF, Feller JF, Palmer WE, *et al*. The Buford complex is a variation of normal shoulder anatomy: MR arthrographic imaging features. *AJR Am J Roentgenol* 1996;**166**: 869–873.

Williams MM, Snyder SJ, Buford D Jr. The Buford complex – the "cord-like" middle glenohumeral ligament and absent anterosuperior labrum complex: a normal anatomic capsulolabral variant. *Arthroscopy* 1994;**10**:241–247.

Pearls and Pitfalls in Musculoskeletal Imaging, ed. D. Lee Bennett and Georges Y. El-Khoury. Published by Cambridge University Press. © Cambridge University Press 2013.

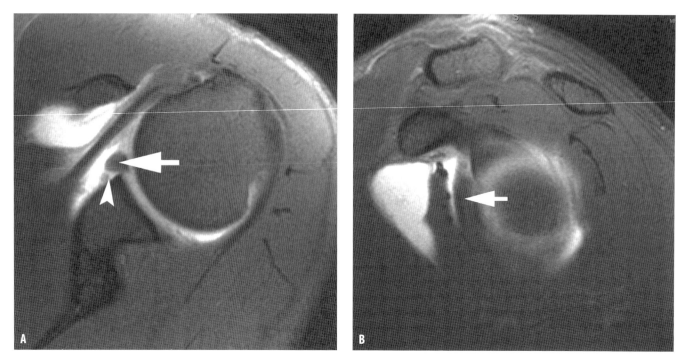

Figure 5.1 Buford complex of the shoulder. Fat-suppressed T1-weighted axial MR arthrogram (**A**) at the level of the superior half of the glenoid cavity shows a thickened middle glenohumeral ligament (arrow) close to the glenoid margin with an absent labrum (arrowhead). Fat-suppressed T1-weighted sagittal MR arthrogram (**B**), obtained in the same patient as in A, shows cord-like middle glenohumeral ligament (arrow).

Pseudosubluxation of the shoulder

Imaging description

The humeral head appears subluxed inferiorly (Figure 6.1).

Importance

The recognition of the inferior subluxation of the humeral head, also known as the drooping shoulder, is of extreme importance to the orthopedic surgeon. Whereas true fracture dislocations of the shoulder are serious injuries often requiring surgical correction, inferior subluxations associated with fractures are relatively benign lesions which respond to a few simple measures, namely support of the arm and joint arthrocentesis. The pathophysiology of inferior shoulder subluxation in hemiplegia is due to muscular flaccidity.

Typical clinical scenario

Inferior subluxation of the humeral head occurs following fracture of the surgical neck of the humerus and may be secondary to hemarthrosis or injury to the joint capsule or surrounding musculoligamentous structures (Figure 6.2).

Additionally, there are non-traumatic causes of the drooping shoulder which are associated with shoulder pain. Erect radiographs of the shoulder are necessary to demonstrate the inferior subluxation of the humeral head in patients with stroke or brachial plexus involvement by tumor.

Differential diagnosis

Differential diagnosis includes shoulder dislocation.

Teaching point

If any doubt arises as to the diagnosis, repeat radiographs with the arm elevated in a sling and after joint aspiration will prove beneficial.

READING LIST

Laskin RS, Schreiber S. Inferior subluxation of the humeral head: the drooping shoulder. *Radiology* 1971;**98**:585–586.

Lev-Toaff AS, Karasick D, Rao VM. "Drooping shoulder" – nontraumatic causes of glenohumeral subluxation. *Skeletal Radiol* 1984;**12**:34–36.

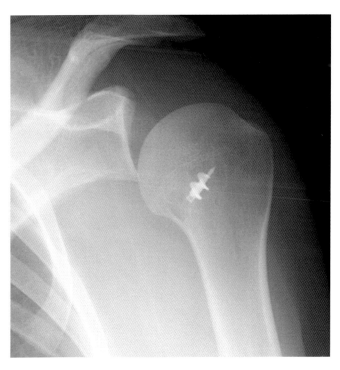

Figure 6.1 Pseudosubluxation of the shoulder. Anteroposterior view of the shoulder shows inferior subluxation of the humeral head.

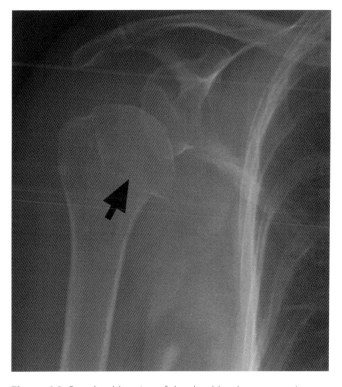

Figure 6.2 Pseudosubluxation of the shoulder. Anteroposterior view of the shoulder shows inferior subluxation of the humeral head. Note the fracture of the proximal humerus (arrow).

Pearls and Pitfalls in Musculoskeletal Imaging, ed. D. Lee Bennett and Georges Y. El-Khoury. Published by Cambridge University Press. © Cambridge University Press 2013.

Posterior dislocation of the shoulder

Imaging description

When the humeral head is dislocated posteriorly, it is also displaced laterally by the posterior glenoid rim; therefore the shoulder joint may appear widened on frontal projection (Figure 7.1). In many patients with posterior shoulder dislocation, two parallel lines of cortical bone may be identified on the superomedial aspect of the humeral head (Figure 7.1). One line represents the articular cortex of the humeral head and the other denotes the margin of a trough-like impaction fracture. Reverse Hill–Sachs fracture is an impaction fracture of the anteromedial humeral head after a posterior humeral dislocation (Figures 7.1 and 7.2). Reverse osseous Bankart fracture is a fracture of the posteroinferior rim of the glenoid that may occur after posterior glenohumeral dislocation.

Importance

The primary problem with posterior dislocation of the shoulder is in making the diagnosis. More than 50% of cases are missed at the initial examination.

Typical clinical scenario

Seizures are the most common cause of posterior shoulder dislocation. Injury to the dynamic posterior shoulder stabilizers after posterior dislocation is often seen in young patients presenting with shoulder pain or posterior glenohumeral instability.

Differential diagnosis

Hemarthrosis or lymphedema of the extremity may lead to some confusion with posterior dislocation by the widened joint space on the frontal radiographs.

Teaching point

The trough sign may be the only indication of posterior shoulder dislocation on frontal radiographs. Although anterior instability is the most common type of glenohumeral instability, a recent increase in the diagnosis of posterior instability after athletic injuries can be attributed to growing awareness.

READING LIST

Cisternino SJ, Rogers LF, Stufflebam BC, Kruglik GD. The trough line: a radiographic sign of posterior shoulder dislocation. *AJR Am J Roentgenol* 1978;**130**:951–954.

Lenchik L. The shoulder and humeral shaft. In Rogers LF, ed. *Radiology of Skeletal Trauma*. 3rd edn. Philadelphia, PA: Churchill Livingstone, 2002;662–669.

Shah N, Tung GA. Imaging signs of posterior glenohumeral instability. *AJR Am J Roentgenol* 2009;**192**:730–735.

Pearls and Pitfalls in Musculoskeletal Imaging, ed. D. Lee Bennett and Georges Y. El-Khoury. Published by Cambridge University Press. © Cambridge University Press 2013.

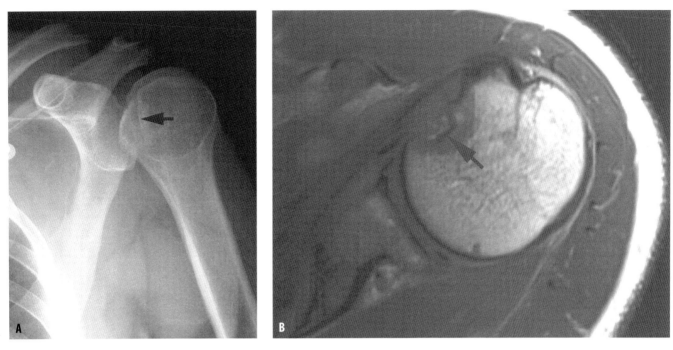

Figure 7.1 Posterior dislocation of the shoulder. Anteroposterior view of the shoulder (**A**) demonstrates trough line (arrow), indicating impaction fracture. Axial T1-weighted MR image (**B**), obtained in the same patient as in A, shows a reverse Hill–Sachs fracture (arrow) of the anteromedial humeral head after posterior humeral dislocation.

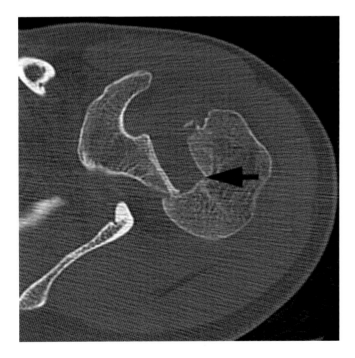

Figure 7.2 Posterior dislocation of the shoulder. CT scan of the shoulder obtained in a different patient, shows a reverse Hill–Sachs fracture (arrow) of the anteromedial humeral head after the posterior humeral dislocation.

13

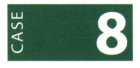

CASE 8

Avulsion fracture of the greater tuberosity

Imaging description

Radiographs may show the non-displaced or displaced fractures with cortical step-off in the greater tuberosity (Figure 8.1).

Importance

The greater tuberosity is the attachment site of the supraspinatus, infraspinatus, and teres minor tendons. Isolated fractures of the greater tuberosity are uncommon. It is difficult to distinguish between isolated humeral avulsion fractures of the greater tuberosity and rotator cuff tears at clinical examination. However, the distinction is crucial because treatment of the two injuries is different. Non-displaced fractures of the greater tuberosity are particularly common in association with fractures of the surgical neck of the humerus and anterior shoulder dislocation.

Typical clinical scenario

Patients present with a history of falling on an outstretched hand with the elbow extended and often with anterior dislocation.

Differential diagnosis

Occasionally, a grooved defect, Hill–Sachs lesion, in the humeral head may be confused with a fracture of the greater tuberosity.

Teaching point

At radiography, the avulsion fracture of the greater tuberosity may not be readily apparent and may be seen only on delayed images. MR imaging is often requested in cases of suspected rotator cuff tear in which marrow edema is incidentally seen surrounding the greater tuberosity and denoting the margins of the occult avulsion fracture.

READING LIST

El-Khoury GY, Daniel WW, Kathol MH. Acute and chronic avulsive injuries. *Radiol Clin North Am* 1997;**35**:747–766.

Hill HA, Sachs MD. The grooved defect of the humeral head. *Radiology* 1940;**35**:690–700.

Lenchik L. The shoulder and humeral shaft. In Rogers LF, ed. *Radiology of Skeletal Trauma*. 3rd edn. Philadelphia, PA: Churchill Livingstone, 2002;637–638.

Stevens MA, El-Khoury GY, Kathol MH, Brandser EA, Chow S. Imaging features of avulsion injuries. *Radiographics* 1999;**19**: 655–672.

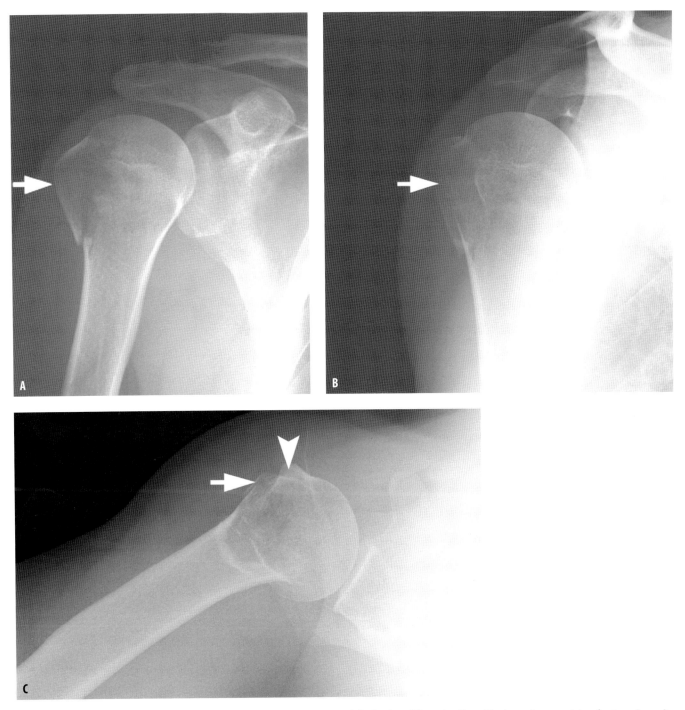

Figure 8.1 Avulsion fracture of the greater tuberosity. Anteroposterior (**A**), Grashey (**B**), and axillary (**C**) views show avulsion fracture (arrow) of the greater tuberosity. Note the lesser tuberosity (arrowhead) on the axillary view.

Imaging description

The earliest detectable changes in denervated muscles in patients with Parsonage–Turner syndrome are diffusely increased signal on fluid-sensitive sequences such as short tau inversion recovery (STIR) or T2-weighted sequences and normal signal on T1-weighted images. After a few weeks in the subacute to chronic phase, the denervated muscle atrophies, seen as a reduction in muscle bulk and increased T1 signal due to fatty infiltration (Figure 9.1). MR imaging findings of quadrilateral space syndrome include atrophy of the teres minor and, less commonly, of the deltoid, which is seen as a reduction in muscle bulk and fatty infiltration with chronic compression.

Importance

No test is specific for the diagnosis of Parsonage–Turner syndrome and MR imaging must be interpreted in light of the patient's clinical history. In patients with quadrilateral space syndrome, MR imaging commonly shows no structural abnormality within the quadrilateral space but may reveal secondary features of denervation myopathy.

Typical clinical scenario

Parsonage–Turner syndrome is an uncommon, self-limiting disorder characterized by sudden onset of non-traumatic shoulder pain associated with progressive weakness of the shoulder girdle musculature. Quadrilateral space syndrome is characterized clinically by poorly localized anterolateral shoulder pain and is exacerbated by forward flexion, abduction, and external rotation of the humerus.

Differential diagnosis

Differential diagnosis includes intrinsic shoulder abnormalities such as rotator cuff tears, impingement syndrome, and labral tears.

Teaching point

MR imaging is the technique of choice in patients with shoulder pain and weakness, and it is sensitive for the detection of signal abnormalities in the shoulder girdle musculature related to denervation injury.

READING LIST

Kamath S, Venkatanarasimha N, Walsh MA, Hughes PM. MRI appearance of muscle denervation. *Skeletal Radiol* 2008;**37**:397–404.

Sanders TG, Tirman PF. Paralabral cyst: an unusual cause of quadrilateral space syndrome. *Arthroscopy* 1999;**15**:632–637.

Scalf RE, Wenger DE, Frick MA, Mandrekar JN, Adkins MC. MRI findings of 26 patients with Parsonage–Turner syndrome. *AJR Am J Roentgenol* 2007;**189**:W39–44.

Yanny S, Toms AP. MR patterns of denervation around the shoulder. *AJR Am J Roentgenol* 2010;**195**:W157–163.

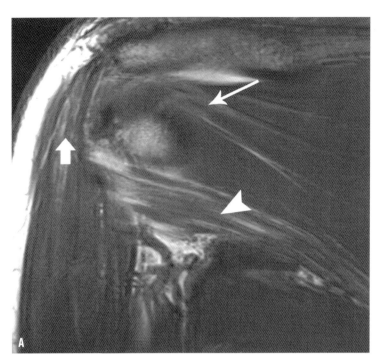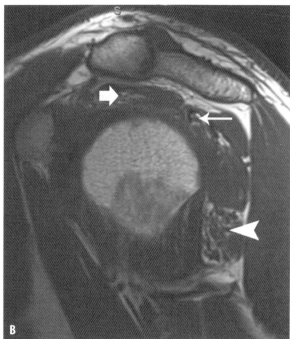

Figure 9.1 Parsonage–Turner syndrome. T1-weighted coronal MR image (**A**) shows fatty infiltration and atrophy of the deltoid (thick arrow), infraspinatus (slender arrow), and teres minor (arrowhead). T1-weighted sagittal MR image (**B**), obtained in the same patient as in A, shows fatty infiltration and atrophy of the supraspinatus (thick arrow), infraspinatus (slender arrow), and teres minor (arrowhead).

ABER positioning during MR arthrogram: anterior labral tears

Imaging description

Abduction and external rotation (ABER) of the shoulder (Figure 10.1), when used with MR arthrography, may result in greater sensitivity than conventional positioning in detecting partial thickness tears (Figures 10.2 and 10.3) of the rotator cuff as well as some types of labral tears (Figures 10.1 and 10.3). The most sensitive sign of detachment of the anterior inferior glenoid labrum after ABER positioning of the shoulder in MR arthrography may be the presence of a contrast material-filled gap between the labrum and glenoid.

Importance

ABER positioning increases the sensitivity of MR arthrography in detecting anterior labral tears, particularly non-detached ones found at or near the insertion of the inferior glenohumeral ligament.

Typical clinical scenario

Patients with anterior glenoid labrum tears may present with shoulder pain or anterior instability.

Differential diagnosis

In non-detached anterior glenoid labrum tears, defined as tears that spare the deep fibers of the inferior glenohumeral ligament and anterior scapular periosteum, contrast material fills a gap at the base of the anterior glenoid labrum but stops short of rounding at the corner of the glenoid. Findings suggestive of a Bankart lesion on ABER MR arthrograms include contrast material in a gap at the base of the anterior glenoid labrum, which is characteristically wider and deeper than that of non-detached tears, and less commonly, the presence of contrast material rounding the corner of the glenoid.

Teaching point

Tension on the anterior labral-ligamentous complex created by the ABER position facilitates characterization of the anterior glenoid labrum tear.

READING LIST

Cvitanic O, Tirman PF, Feller JF et al. Using abduction and external rotation of the shoulder to increase the sensitivity of MR arthrography in revealing tears of the anterior glenoid labrum. *AJR Am J Roentgenol* 1997;**169**:837–844.

Neviaser TJ. The GLAD lesion: another cause of anterior shoulder pain. *Arthroscopy* 1993;**9**:22–23.

Tirman PF, Bost FW, Steinbach LS et al. MR arthrographic depiction of tears of the rotator cuff: benefit of abduction and external rotation of the arm. *Radiology* 1994;**192**:851–856.

Tirman PF, Bost FW, Garvin GJ et al. Posterosuperior glenoid impingement of the shoulder: findings at MR imaging and MR arthrography with arthroscopic correlation. *Radiology* 1994;**193**:431–436.

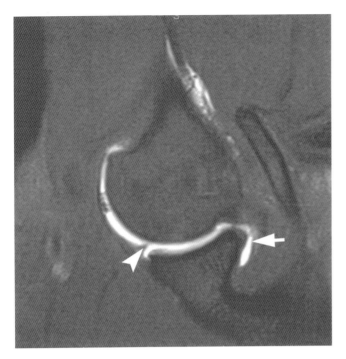

Figure 10.1 Abduction and external rotation (ABER) of the shoulder. Fat-suppressed T1-weighted MR arthrogram with abduction and external rotation of the shoulder demonstrates torn anteroinferior labrum (arrowhead) and supraspinatus tendon (arrow).

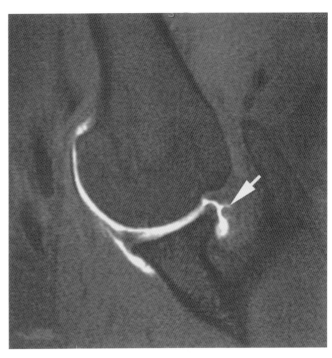

Figure 10.2 Abduction and external rotation (ABER) of the shoulder. Fat-suppressed T1-weighted MR arthrogram with abduction and external rotation of the shoulder demonstrates articular-sided partial thickness tear of the supraspinatus tendon (arrow).

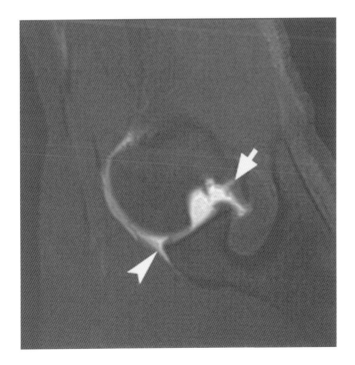

Figure 10.3 Abduction and external rotation (ABER) of the shoulder. Fat-suppressed T1-weighted MR arthrogram with abduction and external rotation of the shoulder demonstrates anteroinferior labral detachment (arrowhead) and articular-sided partial thickness tear of the supraspinatus tendon (arrow).

Os acromiale

Imaging description

The os acromiale is an accessory bone that is found in 7–15% healthy subjects. This acromial bone is formed when there is a non-union of ossification centers during development. Os acromiale is easy to detect on an axillary view of the shoulder on plain radiographs but is difficult to see on a standard anteroposterior view.

Importance

The os acromiale (Figure 11.1) – optimally seen on axial MR images – is connected to the basiacromion via a diarthrosis or synchondrosis and should not be diagnosed as fracture. The acromion is normally formed by the fusion of several ossification centers, which is generally complete by the age of 25. The discovery of os acromiale on plain radiographs in a symptomatic patient should prompt a search for rotator cuff tendon disease. Its recognition in patients with rotator cuff disease may help the surgeon select an appropriate therapy.

Typical clinical scenario

Presence of os acromiale may be associated with rotator cuff impingement.

Differential diagnosis

The presence of an os acromiale may be confused with a fracture of the acromion distally.

Teaching point

Os acromiale, which can predispose to rotator cuff impingement, can be detected on routine shoulder MR imaging.

READING LIST

Morag Y, Jacobson JA, Miller B *et al.* MR imaging of rotator cuff injury: what the clinician needs to know. *Radiographics* 2006;**26**:1045–1065.

Park JG, Lee JK, Phelps CT. Os acromiale associated with rotator cuff impingement: MR imaging of the shoulder. *Radiology* 1994;**193**:255–257.

Prescher A. Anatomical basics, variations, and degenerative changes of the shoulder joint and shoulder girdle. *Eur J Radiol* 2000;**35**:88–102.

Rudez J, Zanetti M. Normal anatomy, variants and pitfalls on shoulder MRI. *Eur J Radiol* 2008;**68**:25–35.

Swain RA, Wilson FD, Harsha DM. The os acromiale: another cause of impingement. *Med Sci Sports Exerc* 1996;**28**:1459–1462.

Pearls and Pitfalls in Musculoskeletal Imaging, ed. D. Lee Bennett and Georges Y. El-Khoury. Published by Cambridge University Press. © Cambridge University Press 2013.

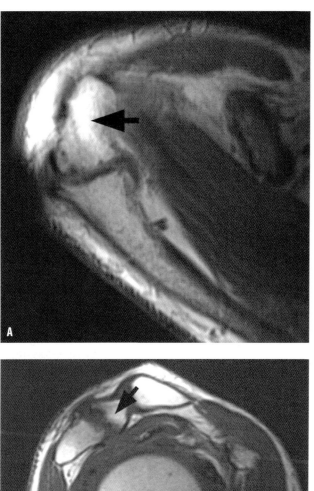

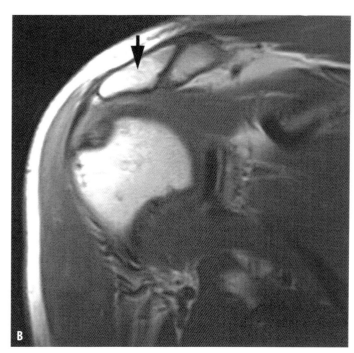

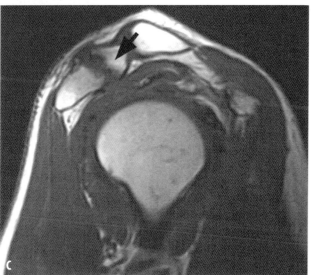

Figure 11.1 Os acromiale. Intermediate-weighted axial (**A**), coronal (**B**), and sagittal (**C**) MR images show unfused ossification center (arrow).

Hill–Sachs injury versus normal flattening of posterolateral humeral head

Imaging description

In cases of anterior dislocation of the glenohumeral joint, the posterolateral portion of the humeral head becomes lodged against the anterior glenoid rim. This often causes a compression fracture of this area of the humeral head, commonly known as a Hill–Sachs lesion (Figure 12.1).

Importance

The proximal humerus includes the head, which is round and slightly flattened postero-inferiorly, the greater and lesser tuberosities, as well as the anatomical and surgical neck. An anatomical indentation (Figure 12.2) in the posterolateral portion of the proximal humerus may simulate Hill–Sachs lesion. One way to distinguish the normal anatomy from pathologic finding is that the Hill–Sachs lesion is found at or above the level of the coracoid process.

Typical clinical scenario

The majority of patients present with anterior glenohumeral joint dislocation.

Differential diagnosis

Physiologic humeral neck is seen on an axial MR image below the level of the coracoid. This should not be confused with a Hill–Sachs lesion. Occasionally, a grooved defect, Hill–Sachs lesion, in the humeral head may be confused with a fracture of the greater tuberosity.

Teaching point

A Hill–Sachs lesion is best differentiated from the anatomic groove by means of its more cephalic position along the longitudinal humeral axis.

READING LIST

Hill HA, Sachs MD. The grooved defect of the humeral head. *Radiology* 1940;**35**:690–700.

Richards RD, Sartoris DJ, Pathria MN, Resnick D . Hill–Sachs lesion and normal humeral groove: MR imaging features allowing their differentiation. *Radiology* 1994;**190**:665–668.

Rudez J, Zanetti M. Normal anatomy, variants and pitfalls on shoulder MRI. *Eur J Radiol* 2008;**68**:25–35.

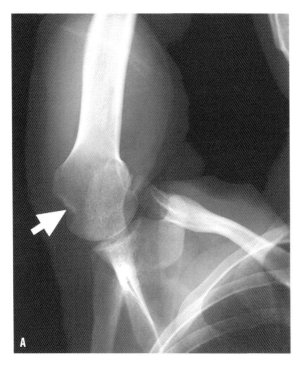 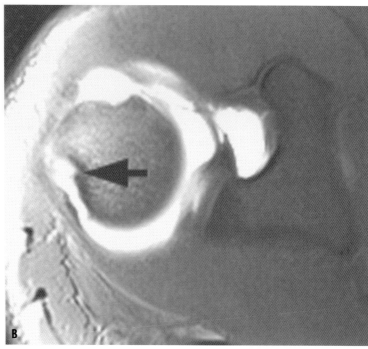

Figure 12.1 Hill–Sachs lesion. Stryker notch view (**A**) shows Hill–Sachs lesion (arrow). Fat-suppressed T1-weighted axial MR arthrogram (**B**), obtained in the same patient as in A, shows a Hill–Sachs lesion (arrow) above the level of the coracoid process.

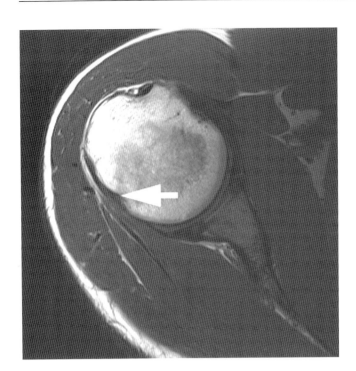

Figure 12.2 Normal flattening of posterolateral humeral head. T1-weighted axial MR image shows normal anatomical indentation (arrow) in the posterolateral aspect of the proximal humerus below the level of the coracoid process.

Red marrow versus tumor in the proximal humeral shaft

Imaging description

In the adult, it is widely recognized that residual hematopoietic marrow is present throughout the axial skeleton. In addition, hematopoietic marrow is usually present within the proximal metaphyseal areas of the femur and humerus. Residual hematopoietic marrow may be observed within the proximal humeral epiphyseal area in normal adults. Hematopoietic marrow does not result in significant hyperintensity on images acquired with T2-weighted, fat-suppressed T2-weighted, or STIR sequences (Figure 13.1). Hematopoietic marrow is not associated with cortical destruction or an adjacent soft tissue mass. Hematopoietic marrow usually demonstrates bilateral symmetry, and evaluation of the contralateral extremity may be useful in problematic cases. The MR imaging characteristics of infiltrative lesions vary. All demonstrate some decreased signal intensity on T1-weighted images (Figure 13.2). Their appearance on T2-weighted sequences varies depending on tissue type, cellularity, water content, and the presence of fibrosis, necrosis, hematoma, or inflammatory debris.

Importance

Awareness of the normal physiologic variations of hematopoietic and fatty marrow distribution is important because these normal patterns can mimic marrow-based disease.

Differential diagnosis

Differential diagnosis includes marrow reconversion, marrow infiltration or replacement, myeloid depletion, and marrow edema.

Teaching point

When signal intensity variations are observed, the possibility of residual or reconverted hematopoietic marrow should be considered.

READING LIST

Daffner RH, Lupetin AR, Dash N et al. MRI in the detection of malignant infiltration of bone marrow. AJR Am J Roentgenol 1986;146:353–358.

Deutsch AL, Mink JH, Rosenfelt FP, Waxman AD. Incidental detection of hematopoietic hyperplasia on routine knee MR imaging. AJR Am J Roentgenol 1989;152:333–336.

Mirowitz SA. Hematopoietic bone marrow within the proximal humeral epiphysis in normal adults: investigation with MR imaging. Radiology 1993;188:689–693.

Richardson ML, Patten RM. Age-related changes in marrow distribution in the shoulder: MR imaging findings. Radiology 1994;192:209–215.

Vogler JB 3rd, Murphy WA. Bone marrow imaging. Radiology 1988;168:679–693.

Weinreb JC. MR imaging of bone marrow: a map could help. Radiology 1990;177:23–24.

Zimmer WD, Berquist TH, McLeod RA et al. Bone tumors: magnetic resonance imaging versus computed tomography. Radiology 1985;155:709–718.

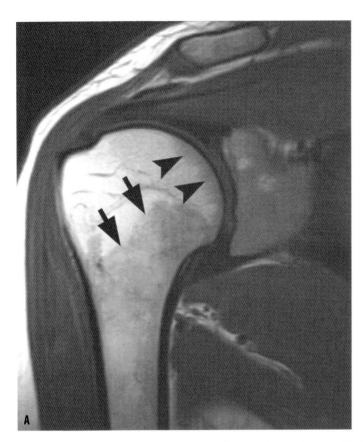 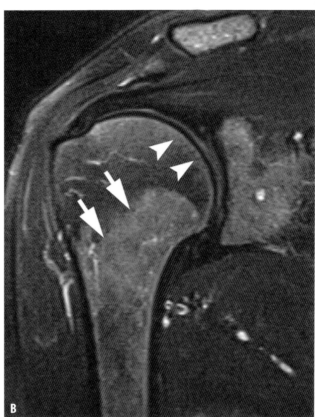

Figure 13.1 Hematopoietic marrow. Coronal T1-weighted MR image (**A**) shows areas of slightly decreased signal intensity in the epiphyseal (arrowheads) and metaphyseal (arrows) location. Coronal fat-suppressed T2-weighted MR image (**B**), obtained in the same patient as in A, demonstrates the epiphyseal (arrowheads) and metaphyseal (arrows) areas which do not show significant fat-suppression.

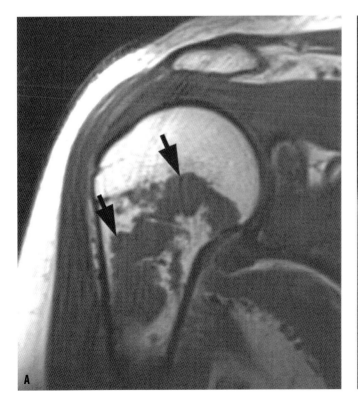 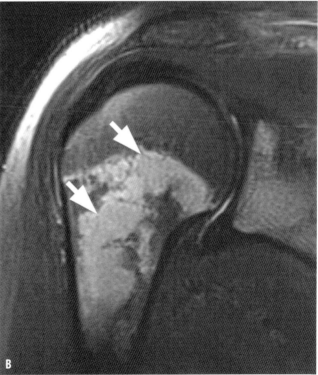

Figure 13.2 Leukemic infiltration. Coronal T1-weighted MR image (**A**) shows areas of markedly decreased signal intensity in the metaphyseal (arrows) location. Coronal fat-suppressed T2-weighted MR image (**B**), obtained in the same patient as in A, demonstrates areas of hyperintensity (arrows).

25

Kim's lesion

Imaging description

Signs of Kim's lesion on MR arthrography include incomplete avulsion or flattening of the posteroinferior labrum, chondrolabral retroversion, and preserved relationship between the glenoid cartilage and labrum (Figures 14.1 and 14.2).

Importance

The posteroinferiorly directed forces exerted on the posteroinferior labrum initiate labral tears from the deep portion. The tear may not extend to involve the superficial portion of the chondrolabral junction initially and, hence, could be missed arthroscopically if the deep portion is not probed. MR imaging helps the detection of these deep-portion tears of the labrum.

Typical clinical scenario

Patients present with unidirectional posterior instability or multidirectional posteroinferior instability.

Differential diagnosis

In the reverse Bankart lesion, the posteroinferior labrum is detached from its glenoid attachment and there is an avulsive tear of the posterior scapular periosteum. With posterior labrocapsular periosteal sleeve avulsion (POLPSA), the posterior labrum and the intact posterior scapular periosteum are stripped from the glenoid.

Teaching point

A recently reported lesion associated with posterior glenohumeral instability is Kim's lesion, a superficial tear between the posteroinferior labrum and the glenoid articular cartilage without complete detachment of the labrum.

READING LIST

Harish S, Nagar A, Moro J *et al.* Imaging findings in posterior instability of the shoulder. *Skeletal Radiol* 2008;**37**:693–707.

Kim SH, Ha KI, Yoo JC, Noh KC. Kim's lesion: an incomplete and concealed avulsion of the posteroinferior labrum in posterior or multidirectional posteroinferior instability of the shoulder. *Arthroscopy* 2004;**20**:712–720.

Shah N, Tung GA. Imaging signs of posterior glenohumeral instability. *AJR Am J Roentgenol* 2009;**192**:730–735.

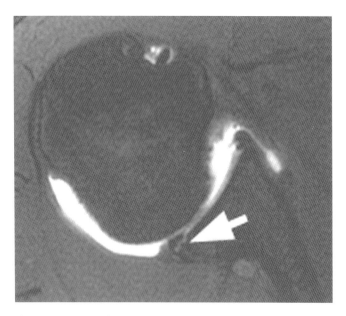

Figure 14.1 Kim's lesion. Fat-suppressed T1-weighted axial MR arthrogram shows flattening of the posteroinferior labrum (arrow).

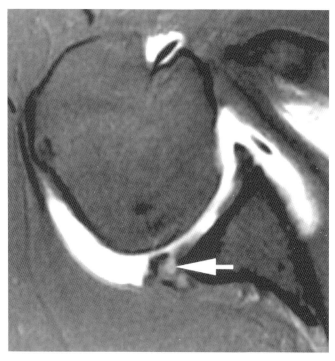

Figure 14.2 Kim's lesion. Fat-suppressed T1-weighted axial MR arthrogram shows incomplete avulsion of the posteroinferior labrum with increased retroversion of the labrum (arrow).

Pearls and Pitfalls in Musculoskeletal Imaging, ed. D. Lee Bennett and Georges Y. El-Khoury. Published by Cambridge University Press. © Cambridge University Press 2013.

Internal impingement of the shoulder

Imaging description

The constellation of findings of undersurface tears of the supraspinatus or infraspinatus tendon and cystic changes in the posterior aspect of the humeral head associated with posterosuperior labral pathology is a consistent finding diagnostic of internal impingement (Figures 15.1 and 15.2).

Importance

Internal impingement, also known as posterosuperior impingement, is a condition that occurs in athletes in which the shoulder is put in extreme abduction and external rotation during overhead movements.

Typical clinical scenario

Impingement of the rotator cuff on the posterosuperior glenoid labrum is a cause of posterior shoulder pain in athletes who throw. Patients present with posterosuperior shoulder pain that is sometimes associated with anterior instability.

Differential diagnosis

Cystic lesions are commonly visible in the posterosuperior portions of the humeral heads, the bare areas, just posterior to the greater tuberosity on shoulder MR images. Posterior cyst-like changes along with the changes in the rotator cuff and posterosuperior labrum should suggest internal impingement. Intraosseous humeral cysts in the posterior aspect of the greater tuberosity that communicate with the joint would appear to be incidental findings.

> ## Teaching point
>
> MR arthrography may allow detection of abnormalities associated with internal impingement.

READING LIST

Giaroli EL, Major NM, Higgins LD. MRI of internal impingement of the shoulder. *AJR Am J Roentgenol* 2005;**185**:925–929.

Opsha O, Malik A, Baltazar R *et al*. MRI of the rotator cuff and internal derangement. *Eur J Radiol* 2008;**68**:36–56.

Tirman PF, Bost FW, Garvin GJ *et al*. Posterosuperior glenoid impingement of the shoulder: findings at MR imaging and MR arthrography with arthroscopic correlation. *Radiology* 1994;**193**:431–436.

Williams M, Lambert RG, Jhangri GS *et al*. Humeral head cysts and rotator cuff tears: an MR arthrographic study. *Skeletal Radiol* 2006;**35**:909–914.

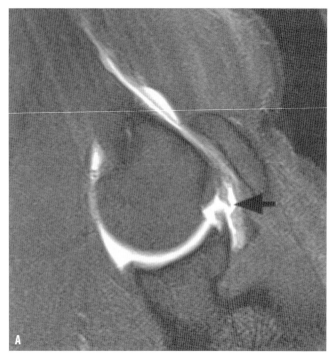

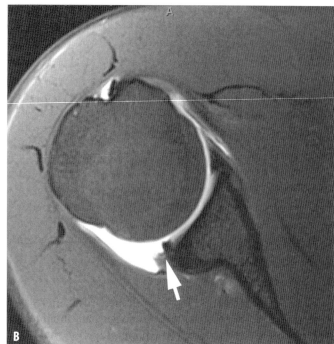

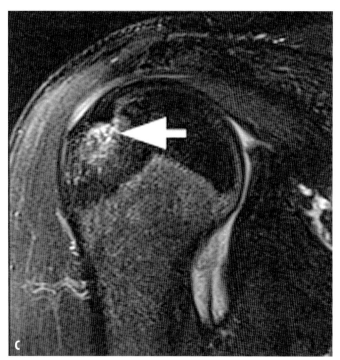

Figure 15.1 Internal impingement of the shoulder. Fat-suppressed T1-weighted MR arthrogram (**A**) with abduction and external rotation of the shoulder demonstrates articular-sided partial thickness tear of the supraspinatus (arrow). Axial fat-suppressed T1-weighted MR arthrogram (**B**), obtained in the same patient as in A, demonstrates blunting of the posterior labrum with scar tissue formation (arrow). Coronal fat-suppressed T2-weighted MR arthrogram (**C**), obtained in the same patient as in A, demonstrates bone marrow edema (arrow) in the posterior aspect of the humeral head.

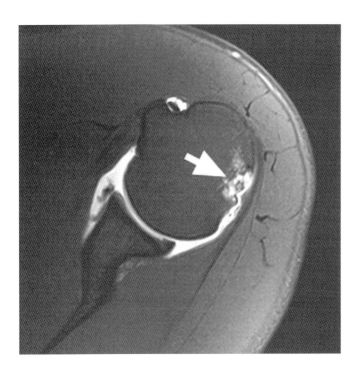

Figure 15.2 Internal impingement of the shoulder. Axial fat-suppressed T1-weighted MR arthrogram shows cystic changes (arrow) in the posterior aspect of the humeral head.

Supracondylar process: ligament of Struthers

Imaging description

Supracondylar process of the humerus is an osseous anatomic variation protruding on the anteromedial surface of the distal humerus 4 to 8 cm proximal from the medial epicondyle (Figure 16.1). The process extends inferiorly to the direction of the medial epicondyle. The process is usually about 1 cm long, but it may take the form of tubercle. Ligament of Struthers variably presents and extends from the apex of the supracondylar process to the medial epicondyle. These structures create a fibro-osseous tunnel, in which the median nerve (rarely ulnar nerve) and the brachial (or ulnar) vessels pass through.

Importance

Supracondylar process is found in 0.4–2.7% of Whites. The individuals with this anomaly are usually asymptomatic. However, symptoms have been reported with a fracture of the supracondylar process or entrapment of the nerve or vessel in the fibro-osseous tunnel. Associated anatomic variants include high division of the brachial artery, high origin of the anterior interosseous nerve branch, and high origin of the pronator teres. These anatomical variations need to be considered clinically as the presenting symptoms may vary and surgical treatment may need to be modified.

Typical clinical scenario

Supracondylar process is more prevalent in Whites than in Blacks, Native Americans, and Asians. It is more commonly found on the left and in males. There have been variable clinical presentations associated with supracondylar process in the sporadic case reports. Median nerve entrapment is most frequently seen and is designated as "supracondylar process syndrome," associated with numbness and paresthesia of the radial and palmar skin. The symptoms are commonly related to or exacerbated by certain postures of the elbow and forearm. The supracondylar process may be palpable as a firm mass in its anatomical location. Following conservative treatment, resection of the process with the Struthers' ligament and the periosteum may be indicated.

Differential diagnosis

Differential diagnosis of the supracondylar process includes osteochondroma and myositis ossificans, for which characteristic imaging features are diagnostic. Diagnosis of median nerve entrapment is challenging because symptoms and signs are often similar, electrodiagnostic studies are frequently normal, and the sites of compression are numerous. Therefore, other causes including carpal tunnel syndrome and pronator syndrome should be considered when the symptoms are related to median nerve. Hypercoagulopathy and vascular injury may be considered when complicated with digital embolization, which has been reported in a softball player associated with supracondylar process.

Teaching point

Radiography is diagnostic for supracondylar process. Anteroposterior view with a slight internal rotation may best visualize the process. Radiologists need to be familiar with associated variations of the nerve, artery, and muscle, which would be related to a variety of presenting symptoms. MRI and ultrasound may be helpful to evaluate these associated anomalies, and therefore, responsible pathology.

READING LIST

Camerlinck M, Vanhoenacker FM, Kiekens G. Ultrasound demonstration of Struthers' ligament. *J Clin Ultrasound* 2010;**38**:499–502.

Horak BT, Kuz JE. An unusual case of pronator syndrome with ipsilateral supracondylar process and abnormal muscle mass. *J Hand Surg Am* 2008;**33**:79–82.

Lordan J, Rauh P, Spinner RJ. The clinical anatomy of the supracondylar spur and the ligament of Struthers. *Clin Anat* 2005;**18**:548–551.

Natsis K. Supracondylar process of the humerus: study on 375 Caucasian subjects in Cologne, Germany. *Clin Anat* 2008;**21**:138–141 .

Thompson JK, Edwards JD. Supracondylar process of the humerus causing brachial artery compression and digital embolization in a fast-pitch softball player. A case report. *Vasc Endovascular Surg* 2005; **39**:445–448 .

Pearls and Pitfalls in Musculoskeletal Imaging, ed. D. Lee Bennett and Georges Y. El-Khoury. Published by Cambridge University Press. © Cambridge University Press 2013.

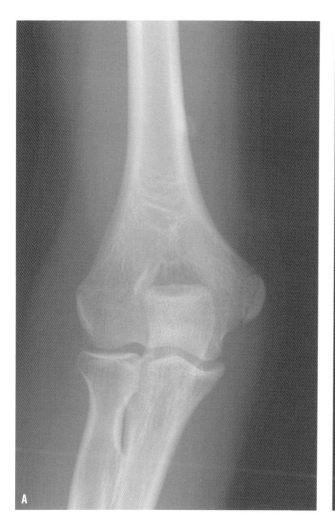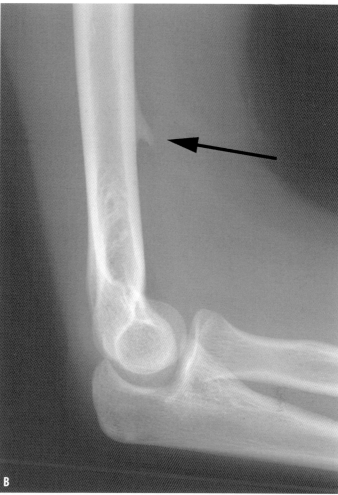

Figure 16.1 Anteroposterior (A) and lateral (B) radiographs of the humerus of a 12-year-old girl show supracondylar process (arrow) on the anterior medial surface of the distal humerus. A small palpable mass was noted with tenderness on physical exam, but neurovascularly intact. She had a symptomatic contralateral supracondylar process excised 5 years before.

Ball-thrower's fracture: not a pathological fracture

Imaging description

The radiographs show a comminuted spinal fracture in the distal half of the humerus with a butterfly fragment (Figure 17.1). The butterfly fragment is typically seen medially. No underlying lesion is seen to suggest a pathological fracture.

Importance

Distal humerus fracture can be caused by severe muscular pulling from throwing action without direct trauma and is called ball-thrower's fracture. Because the lack of history of trauma may prompt the search for underlying pathology, knowledge of this entity is important to preclude unnecessary imaging studies or biopsy.

Typical clinical scenario

Ball-thrower's fractures commonly affect recreational athletes who are involved in throwing actions. The average age of patients was 25 and 36 years from two large series. It can occur in teenagers and rarely affects professional players. The majority of the patients are male. The patient is trying to perform a hard throw, during which a closed, external rotation spiral fracture occurs in the distal humerus. The sound of the fracture may be heard by the patient and/or others. The fracture is considered to occur during the acceleration phase before ball release. The throwing objects vary and include a stone, snowball, handball, softball, baseball, and hand grenade. Ball-thrower's fracture has uneventful prognosis with conservative treatment with a hanging cast for 6–8 weeks.

Differential diagnosis

Little League shoulder (physeal stress fracture), medial epicondyle injury, and stress fracture of the proximal ulna may be suspected clinically as sports-related injuries. Radiographic study is diagnostic for ball-thrower's fracture. MRI may be helpful for subtle physeal stress fractures, stress fractures, and medial epicondyle injuries.

> ## Teaching point
>
> Radiologist should be aware of clinical and radiographic features of ball-thrower's fractures to avoid unnecessary imaging studies or clinical work-up.

READING LIST

Callaghan EB, Bennett DL, El-Khoury GY, Ohashi K. Ball-thrower's fracture of the humerus. *Skeletal Radiol* 2004;**33**:355–358 .

Ogawa K, Yoshida A. Throwing fracture of the humeral shaft. An analysis of 90 patients. *Am J Sports Med* 1998;**26**:242–246 .

Pearls and Pitfalls in Musculoskeletal Imaging, ed. D. Lee Bennett and Georges Y. El-Khoury. Published by Cambridge University Press. © Cambridge University Press 2013.

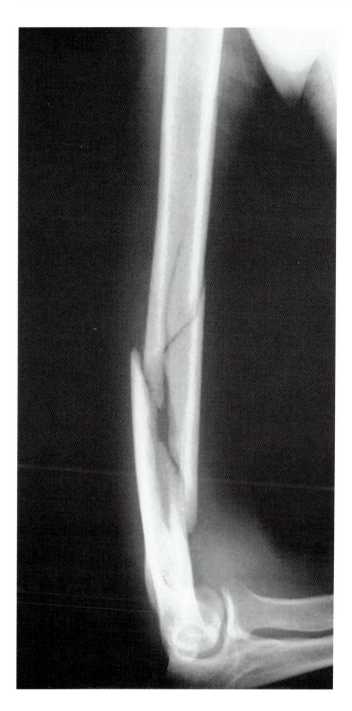

Figure 17.1 Lateral radiograph of the humerus of a 28-year-old male shows a comminuted fracture of the distal humeral diaphysis with a large butterfly fragment. A recreational athlete, he injured his right arm during a softball game. He heard a "pop" when he was releasing the ball from his hand. Initially, he did not feel pain, but his range of motion was severely limited.

Imaging description

The radiographs may show focal cortical irregularities in the proximal humerus at various tendon insertion sites. Cortical thickening and lucency may be seen at the deltoid tuberosity (pseudotumor deltoideus) (Figure 18.1). Cortical irregularity may be seen at the anterolateral aspect of the proximal humerus corresponding to the pectoralis major tendon insertion site among gymnasts (ringman's shoulder lesion) (Figure 18.2). Similar radiographic findings may be seen in the proximal humerus anteromedially at the insertion site of the latissimus dorsi and teres major muscles. MR imaging shows signal changes in the corresponding cortex, tendon, and adjacent soft tissue and bone marrow.

Importance

Most of these cortical changes are explained by chronic or subacute avulsive injuries based on clinical history, imaging studies, and follow-up. When symptomatic, because of aggressive radiographic features, a malignant neoplastic lesion may be suspected and the focus may present as a pseudotumor.

Typical clinical scenario

Focal cortical irregularities of the proximal humerus may be asymptomatic, but may become a clinical issue when incidentally found. Symptomatic lesions affect both young and old patients, who usually present with chronic or subacute shoulder pain of insidious onset. History of vigorous exercise may be found in cases of chronic avulsive injuries in young patients. Physical examination may show tenderness to palpation and limited range of motion because of pain. The conditions may be confused with aggressive lesions such as infection and tumor. However, MR imaging is diagnostic for pseudotumor, avoiding biopsy and surgical intervention.

Differential diagnosis

Differential diagnosis of focal cortical thickening of the humerus includes osteoid osteoma and infection. Irregular lucency or erosion of the cortex may be seen in infection (cortical abscess) or calcific tendinitis. History and physical examination are generally helpful especially for the diagnosis of chronic avulsive injury. Other considerations include non-ossifying fibroma and normal anatomic variants. It is important to know that the normal (asymptomatic) deltoid tuberosity has a variable radiographic appearance.

Teaching point

Focal cortical changes of the proximal humerus from benign etiologies may mimic aggressive lesions such as tumor or infection radiographically. Working knowledge of tendon insertions of the proximal humerus and benign etiologies associated with focal cortical changes is important to avoid unnecessary imaging study and biopsy.

READING LIST

Anderson SE, Hertel R, Johnston JO et al. Latissimus dorsi tendinosis and tear: imaging features of a pseudotumor of the upper limb in five patients. *AJR Am J Roentgenol* 2005;**185**:1145–1151.

Donnelly LF, Helms CA, Bisset GS, 3rd. Chronic avulsive injury of the deltoid insertion in adolescents: imaging findings in three cases. *Radiology* 1999;**211**:233–236.

Fulton MN, Albright JP, El-Khoury GY. Cortical desmoid-like lesion of the proximal humerus and its occurrence in gymnasts (ringman's shoulder lesion). *Am J Sports Med* 1979;**7**:57–61.

Morgan H, Damron T, Cohen H, Allen M. Pseudotumor deltoideus: a previously undescribed anatomic variant at the deltoid insertion site. *Skeletal Radiol* 2001;**30**:512–518.

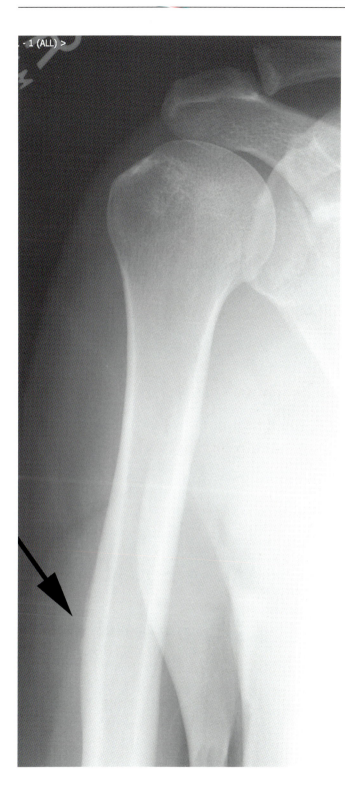

- 1 (ALL) >

Figure 18.1 Anteroposterior radiograph of a 38-year-old male. There is prominence and irregularity to the humeral cortex at the deltoid insertion (arrow). This is a normal finding and should not be confused with abnormal periosteal reaction.

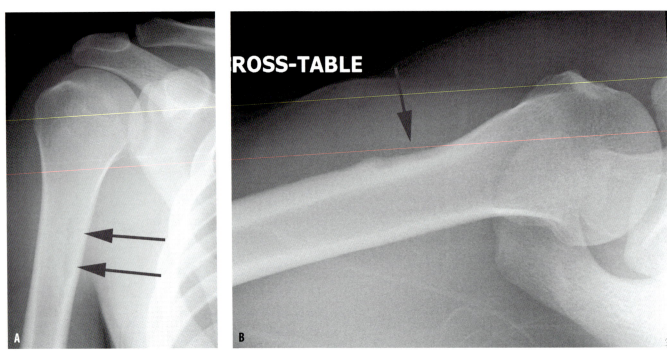

Figure 18.2 Anteroposterior (A) and axillary (B) radiographs of the shoulder demonstrate cortical irregularity and a scooped-out appearance in this incidental ringman's shoulder lesion (arrows).

Pseudodefect of the capitellum versus osteochondral defect

Imaging description

The capitellum is a rounded protuberance that projects off the distal end of the humerus both medial and anterior to the longitudinal axis of the humerus. The width of the articular surface of the capitellum is not uniform. The width tapers as the capitellum curves inferiorly and posteriorly, with the width of the posterior aspect of the capitellum being only half as wide as the anterior aspect. Therefore, when one looks at the capitellum from below, it appears roughly twice as wide anteriorly as posteriorly (Figure 19.1).

Additionally, the lateral edge of the smooth articular surface of the capitellum demonstrates a sharp contrast to the adjacent rough non-articular surface of the lateral epicondyle of the humerus. This articular margin overhangs this adjacent rough bone. This overhanging edge with smooth bone and articular cartilage with the rough lateral epicondylar bone being subjacent gives the false appearance of a defect or notch on MR images (Figure 19.2). This pseudodefect is even more pronounced by the typical positioning of the elbow in extension on MR imaging. The radial head is positioned slightly lateral and posterior to the central articular surface of the capitellum when the elbow is extended. That is, in extension, the anteromedial aspect of the radial head appears to articulate with the smooth surface capitellum; however, the posterolateral aspect of the radial head projects by the rough non-articular surface of the distal humerus. This tends to accentuate the pseudodefect on the capitellum (Figure 19.3).

Importance

When the elbow is imaged by MRI (especially in extension) the pseudodefect can be mistakenly diagnosed as an osteochondral injury resulting in unnecessary and frustrating surgery in an attempt to find the osteochondral lesion. This pseudodefect should not be mistaken for an osteochondral lesion of the capitellum (Fig. 19.3). It is important for radiologists to be aware of the pseudodefect of the capitellum as it is a readily visible MR finding in approximately 85% of the general population.

Typical clinical scenario

A young teenage male presents with chronic elbow pain related to pitching. This clinical scenario can increase the possible likelihood of diagnosing a pseudodefect as an osteochondral lesion. If a lesion on MRI is suspected of being an osteochondral lesion, careful attention should be given to its location relative to the articular surface of the capitellum.

Differential diagnosis

The pseudodefect of the capitellum has a pathognomonic appearance and location on the distal humerus.

Teaching point

A pseudodefect of the capitellum should not be confused with an osteochondral injury of the capitellum. The pseudodefect occurs by the far posterolateral edge of the smooth articular surface of the capitellum. Osteochondral lesions occur classically at the central to anterolateral aspect of the capitellum rather than posterolaterally where the pseudodefect is found. Unstable osteochondral lesions will also have a rim of increased signal intensity or a fluid-filled cyst on the T2-weighted MR images while the pseudodefect will not.

READING LIST

Husarik DB, Saupe N, Pfirrmann CWA, *et al.* Ligaments and plicae of the elbow: normal MR imaging variability in 60 asymptomatic subjects. *Radiology* 2010; **257**:185–194.

Kijowski R, De Smet AA. MRI findings of osteochondritis dissecans of the capitellum with surgical correlation. *AJR Am J Roentgenol* 2005;**185**:1453–1459.

Rosenberg ZS, Beltran J, Cheung YY. Pseudodefect of the capitellum: potential MR imaging pitfall. *Radiology* 1994;**191**:821–823.

Pearls and Pitfalls in Musculoskeletal Imaging, ed. D. Lee Bennett and Georges Y. El-Khoury. Published by Cambridge University Press. © Cambridge University Press 2013.

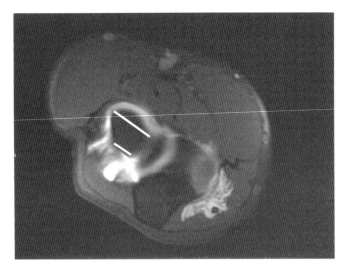

Figure 19.1 Elbow MR arthrogram. Transverse T1-weighted fat suppressed image demonstrates that the anterior aspect of the capitellum (long white line) is wider than the posterior aspect of the capitellum (short white line).

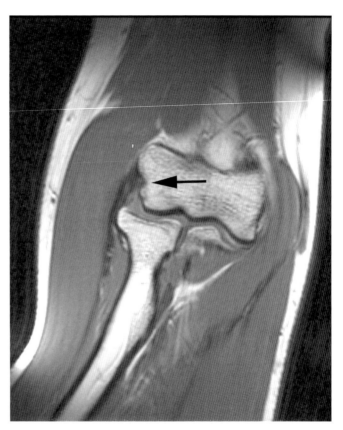

Figure 19.2 Elbow MRI image. Coronal T1-weighted image demonstrates the normal irregularity of the non-articular lateral aspect of the capitellum (arrow).

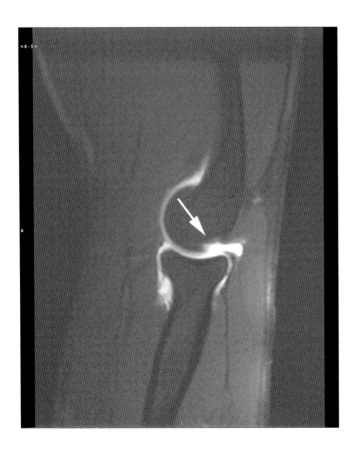

Figure 19.3 Elbow MR arthrogram. Sagittal T1-weighted fat-suppressed image demonstrates the normal pseudodefect of the capitellum (arrow) that can be confused with an osteochondral injury.

Imaging description

The trochlear groove is the large curved depression that articulates with the trochlea of the humerus. At the junction of the olecranon and coronoid process there is an osseous ridge without cartilage in this trochlear groove. There is also a waist or inward tapering of the trochlear groove at the level of the trochlear ridge that produces both medial and lateral cortical notches on the trochlear groove (Figure 20.1). These cortical notches are seen as pseudodefects (apparent small cortical interruptions) on sagittal MR and can be mistaken for an osteochondral fracture (Figure 20.2). In order for this cortical notch to be identified as an incidental pseudodefect there should be no abnormal MRI signal in the adjacent bone marrow of the olecranon.

Importance

This pseudodefect can be mistakenly diagnosed as an osteochondral fracture resulting in unnecessary treatment. It is important for radiologists to be aware of this pseudodefect as it is a common finding and present in nearly 100% of the population.

Typical clinical scenario

A patient presents for MR imaging with a history of subacute or chronic elbow pain of unknown etiology. This pseudodefect of the trochlear groove should not be misconstrued as pathology and should not be reported as a possible cause of the patient's elbow pain.

Differential diagnosis

There is no differential as the pseudodefect of the trochlear groove has a pathognomonic appearance and location in the olecranon.

Teaching point

A pseudodefect of the trochlear groove should not be confused with a fracture of the olecranon. The pseudodefect is present at the cortical notches on the trochlear groove that occurs at the junction of the olecranon and coronoid process. In addition, in order to identify the cortical notch as an incidental pseudodefect, the adjacent bone marrow signal on MR should be normal. A fracture would be expected to have abnormal MRI signal within the adjacent bone marrow.

READING LIST

Rosenberg ZS, Beltran J, Cheung Y, Broker M. MR imaging of the elbow: normal variant and potential diagnostic pitfalls of the trochlear groove and cubital tunnel. *AJR Am J Roentgenol* 1995; **164**:415–418.

Pearls and Pitfalls in Musculoskeletal Imaging, ed. D. Lee Bennett and Georges Y. El-Khoury. Published by Cambridge University Press. © Cambridge University Press 2013.

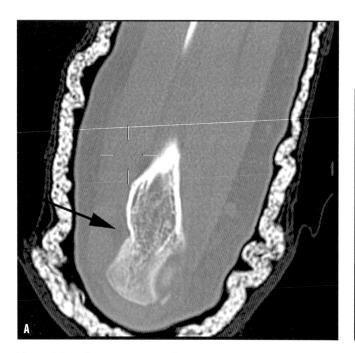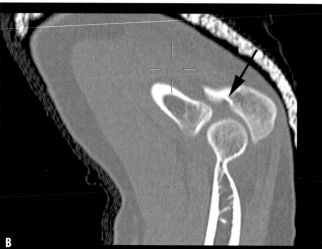

Figure 20.1 Elbow CT. A coronally oriented (**A**) CT image of the trochlear groove of the ulna demonstrates the normal waist or notch located on the medial aspect of the ulna in this patient (arrow). A sagittally oriented CT image (**B**) from the same patient demonstrates the cortical notch (arrow), which is a normal variant and should not be confused with a fracture or injury to the trochlear groove.

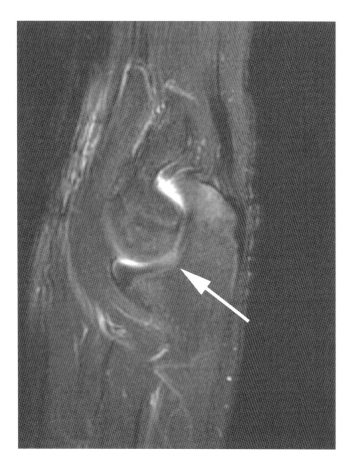

Figure 20.2 Elbow MRI. This *short tau inversion recovery* (STIR) image in the sagittal plane from an elbow MRI shows a normal cortical notch to the medial side of the trochlear groove (arrow). This should not be misdiagnosed as an injury or osteochondral defect.

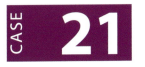

Transverse trochlear ridge versus osteophyte or post-traumatic deformity

Imaging description

The trochlear groove is the large curved depression that articulates with the trochlea of the humerus. At the junction of the olecranon and coronoid process there is an osseous ridge without cartilage in this trochlear groove called the trochlear ridge (Figure 21.1). This cartilage-free ridge can project above the articular surface of the trochlear groove by approximately 2–5 mm in 68% of the population. When a trochlear ridge is present, it does not cause impediment to smooth motion at the elbow and it does not decrease the range of motion at the elbow. However, when it approaches 3–5 mm in size it can be mistakenly confused for a central osteophyte (Figure 21.2). It has signal and morphologic characteristics of an osteophyte with projection from the articular surface with both cortical and medullary bone signal characteristics.

Importance

The trochlear ridge can be mistaken for a central osteophyte leading to an erroneous diagnosis of osteoarthritis if no other osteophytes are present and the joint space is still preserved. An erroneous diagnosis of osteoarthritis can lead to an incorrect assumption that the patient's elbow pain is from the incorrectly diagnosed osteoarthritis. Familiarity with the classic location of the trochlear ridge will help prevent this pitfall in interpretation.

Typical clinical scenario

A middle-aged patient presents for MR imaging with a history of chronic elbow pain of unknown etiology. The trochlear ridge should not be identified as a central osteophyte and thus lead to an erroneous diagnosis of osteoarthritis. This ridge of the trochlear groove should not be misconstrued as pathology and reported as a possible cause of the patient's elbow pain.

Differential diagnosis

The trochlear ridge is pathognomonic in appearance. It should not be confused with a central osteophyte of the trochlear groove.

Teaching point

Before the diagnosis of a central osteophyte of the trochlear groove is made, one should carefully make sure that the visualized osseous protrusion is not at the expected location of the trochlear ridge. This will help prevent an erroneous diagnosis of osteoarthritis.

READING LIST

Cotton A, Boutin RD, Resnick D. Normal anatomy of the elbow on conventional MR imaging and MR arthrography. *Semin Musculoskelet Radiol* 1998;**2**:133–140.

Rosenberg ZS, Beltran J, Cheung Y, Broker M. MR imaging of the elbow: normal variant and potential diagnostic pitfalls of the trochlear groove and cubital tunnel. *AJR Am J Roentgenol* 1995; **164**:415–418.

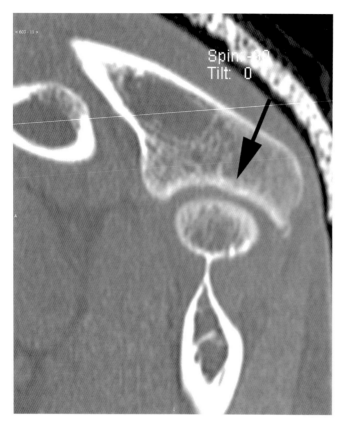

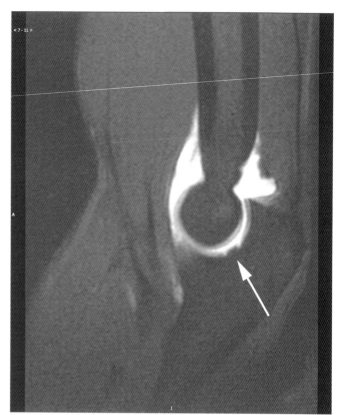

Figure 21.1 Elbow CT image reconstructed in the sagittal plane shows the subtle trochlear ridge seen as a small bump or raised area along the articular surface of the trochlear groove (arrow).

Figure 21.2 Elbow MR arthrogram. There is a normal transverse trochlear ridge located in the trochlear groove (arrow). It should not be confused with a central osteophyte on this T1-weighted fat-suppressed MR arthrographic image.

Imaging description

The flexed abducted supinated (FABS) positioning of the elbow for MRI is the optimal positioning for best visualization of the distal biceps. This positioning nicely demonstrates the full length of the distal biceps brachii from the musculotendinous junction to the radial tuberosity on only one slice/image in the majority of patients (Figure 22.1). The patient can be positioned for these images by first abducting the shoulder to 180° with the arm by the patient's head. Next, the elbow is flexed to 90° and the forearm is supinated to a thumb-up position with a coil placed around the elbow (Figure 22.2). In one study of 22 patients, this positioning demonstrated the full length of the distal biceps brachii on either one or two slices. This improves the visualization of both normal anatomy and pathology as this positioning moves the entire distal tendon and its attaching structures into a single plane instead of the tendon and its attaching structures being in multiple oblique planes.

Importance

Images obtained using the FABS positioning can aid the surgeon in their evaluation of the integrity (partial tear versus rupture) and the quality of the torn distal biceps tendon prior to surgical intervention (Figure 22.3).

Typical clinical scenario

The patient is usually a young to middle-aged adult male who sustained sudden, massive, eccentric contraction of the biceps (such as trying to catch a falling 250-pound rock) and felt sudden pain and a snap in the antecubital fossa region of the arm. MRI is typically ordered when the physical exam is equivocal for a complete rupture of the distal biceps or might be ordered for preoperative evaluation when the injury is subacute or chronic.

Teaching point

The FABS positioning is useful in demonstrating the full extent of the distal biceps brachii tendon from its musculotendinous junction to its insertion on only one or at most two sections. This improves the visualization of both normal anatomy and pathology.

READING LIST

Chew ML, Giuffrè BM. Disorders of the distal biceps brachii tendon. *Radiographics* 2005;**25**:1227–1237.

Giuffrè BM, Moss MJ. Optimal positioning for MRI of the distal biceps brachii tendon: flexed abducted supinated view. *AJR Am J Roentgenol* 2004;**182**:944–946.

Miyamoto RG, Elser F, Millett PJ. Distal biceps tendon injuries. *J Bone Joint Surg Am* 2010;**92**:2128–2138.

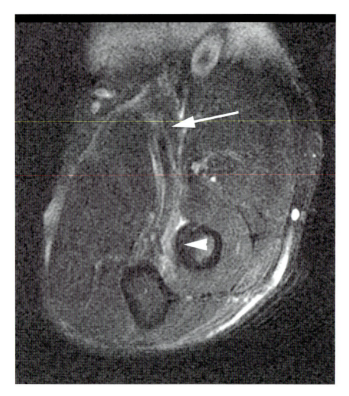

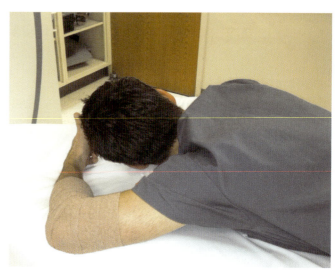

Figure 22.2 Patient in the flexed abducted supinated (FABS) position. The shoulder is abducted to 180°, the elbow is flexed to 90°, and the forearm is supinated with the hand in the thumb-up position.

Figure 22.1 Elbow MRI with arm in the flexed abducted supinated (FABS) position. One can easily see the full extent of the biceps tendon extending from its myotendinous junction (arrow) to near the level of the radial tuberosity (arrowhead) where it is ruptured.

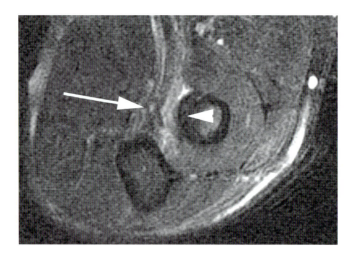

Figure 22.3 The distal biceps tendon can be readily evaluated in the flexed abducted supinated (FABS) position. This patient had rupture of the distal biceps tendon from the radial tuberosity (arrowhead) without significant retraction of the tendon (arrow).

23 Ulnar collateral ligament tear versus normal recess of the elbow

Imaging description

Medical imaging assessment of the integrity of the ulnar collateral ligament (UCL) is best performed using MR arthrography of the elbow. The ulnar collateral ligament consists of three bundles: anterior, transverse, and posterior. Clinically significant tears of the UCL involve the anterior bundle since the anterior bundle is the primary restraint to valgus force on the elbow from 20° to 120° of flexion. This bundle is best seen on coronally oriented MR images. When normal, it is seen as a uniformly low-signal intensity band extending from the base of the medial epicondyle to the medial aspect of the coronoid process (known as the sublime tubercle) (Figure 23.1). A normal subligamentous recess is seen between the medial surface of the trochlea and the undersurface of the anterior bundle of the UCL on elbow MR arthrography; however, the insertion of the anterior bundle on the sublime tubercle should be tight with no visible recess between the coronoid process and the UCL in young adults without ligamentous degeneration (Figure 23.2). A full thickness tear of the anterior bundle of the UCL is demonstrated by disruption of the fibers with abnormal insinuation of contrast into the tear (Figure 23.3). Full thickness tears most commonly occur in the midsubstance of the anterior bundle; however, avulsions at the epicondylar or tubercle attachments can occur.

Importance

Full thickness tears need to be identified by MR arthrography as the physical exam diagnosis of ruptures of the anterior bundle of the UCL can sometimes be difficult. If missed, this can cause an increase in patient morbidity due to a delay in diagnosis and definitive surgical treatment.

Typical clinical scenario

The patient is usually a young adult male that is an overhead throwing athlete (in the USA this is typically a baseball pitcher) who has slowly developed symptoms of medial elbow joint instability and/or medial opening that is worse during the acceleration phase of the throwing motion. Symptoms of ulnar neuropathy may also develop over time and may be present when the patient presents. Rarely, rupture of the anterior bundle of the UCL can also occur in severe acute trauma when elbow dislocation occurs and severe, acute, traumatic valgus stress is applied to the elbow.

Teaching point

The anterior bundle UCL subligamentous recess is normal and should not be confused with a tear. Diagnosis of a UCL tear by MR arthrography may be essential for diagnosis in cases where the physical exam is confusing or difficult. The exam can be difficult in that medial elbow pain can have multiple causes that can be difficult to distinguish from one another on physical exam such as valgus extension overload syndrome, ulnar neuropathy, and severe medial epicondylitis. MR can help in differentiating these entities.

READING LIST

Cain EL Jr, Dugas JR, Wolf RS, Andrews JR. Elbow injuries in throwing athletes: a current concepts review. *Am J Sports Med* 2003;**31**: 621–635.

Cotton A, Jacobson J, Brossmann J et al. MR arthrography of the elbow: normal anatomy and diagnostic pitfalls. *J Comput Assist Tomogr* 1997;**21**:516–522.

Kijowski R, Tuite M, Sanford M. Magnetic resonance imaging of the elbow. Part II: abnormalities of the ligaments, tendons, and nerves. *Skeletal Radiol* 2005;**34**:1–18.

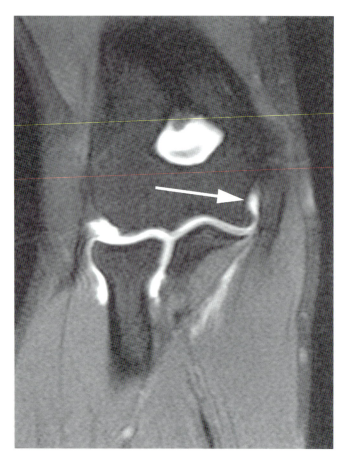 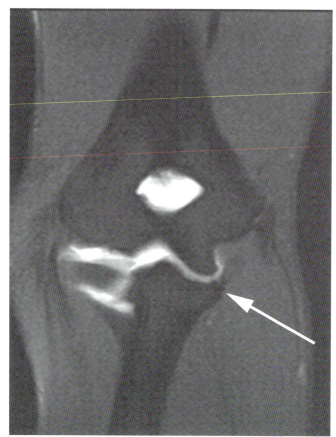

Figure 23.1 Elbow MR arthrogram. The white arrow points to the normal contrast filled subligamentous recess deep to the UCL and superficial to the medial edge of the trochlea on this T1-weighted fat-suppressed image.

Figure 23.2 Elbow MR arthrogram in a 21-year-old male. This coronal T1-weighted fat-suppressed image shows the tight insertion of the UCL on the sublime tubercle (arrow). In a young, healthy adult there should be no visible recess (or contrast) extending between the sublime tubercle and the distal aspect of the anterior band of the UCL.

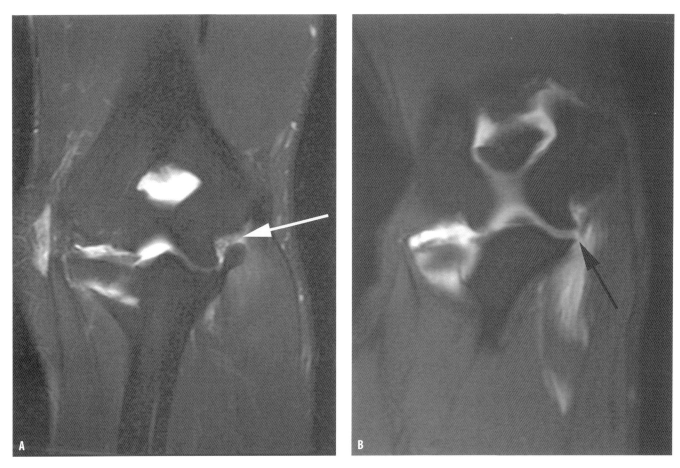

Figure 23.3 Elbow MR arthrogram. These are images demonstrating rupture (arrow) of the proximal aspect of the anterior band of the UCL (**A**) and, in a different patient, rupture (arrow) of the distal attachment of the anterior band of the UCL (**B**).

T-sign of undersurface partial tear of the ulnar collateral ligament

Imaging description

To reiterate, the anterior bundle of the ulnar collateral ligament (UCL) is best seen on coronally oriented MR arthrogram images. Based on prospective research, the insertion of the anterior bundle on the sublime tubercle should be tight with no visible recess between the coronoid process and the UCL in teenage and young adult baseball players. In young overhead-throwing athletes, an undersurface tear of the distal UCL is diagnosed if contrast is seen to extend between the sublime tubercle and the undersurface of the UCL. (Figure 24.1). This has been described as the T-sign. This finding or T-sign cannot be extrapolated as being abnormal in older adults as research has shown that this sign can be present in older adults in whom degenerative changes of the UCL may predominate.

Importance

Because of the difficulty in diagnosing partial tear of the anterior bundle of the UCL at physical examination and at arthroscopy, preoperative diagnosis with MR arthrography plays an important role in this injury. If this surgically treatable injury is missed, it causes an increase in patient morbidity and limitation in athletic performance due to a delay in the diagnosis.

Typical clinical scenario

The patient is usually a young adult male who is an overhead-throwing athlete (in the USA this is typically a baseball pitcher) and has slowly developed symptoms of medial elbow joint instability that are worse during the acceleration phase of the throwing motion.

Teaching point

Diagnosis of a partial thickness undersurface UCL tear at the sublime tubercle by MR arthrography is essential in diagnosis given the limitations of the physical exam and arthroscopy in diagnosing this injury. Caution should be exercised in extrapolating the T-sign as a definite partial tear of the UCL in older adults given the potential for this sign to be present when degenerative changes of the UCL have occurred. Finally, CT arthrography of the elbow can be used to diagnose partial thickness tears of the undersurface of the UCL in patients that have a contraindication to MRI.

READING LIST

Kijowski R, Tuite M, Sanford M. Magnetic resonance imaging of the elbow. Part II: abnormalities of the ligaments, tendons, and nerves. *Skeletal Radiol* 2005;**34**:1–18.

Munshi M, Pretterklieber ML, Chung CB *et al.* Anterior bundle of ulnar collateral ligament: evaluation of anatomic relationships by using MR imaging, MR arthrography, and gross anatomic and histologic analysis. *Radiology* 2004;**231**:797–803.

Timmerman LA, Schwartz ML, Andrews JR. Preoperative evaluation of the ulnar collateral ligament by magnetic resonance imaging and computed tomography arthrography. *Am J Sports Med* 1994;**22**:26–32.

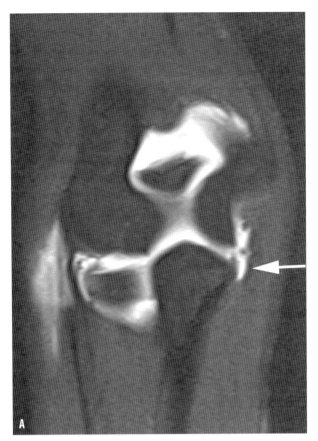

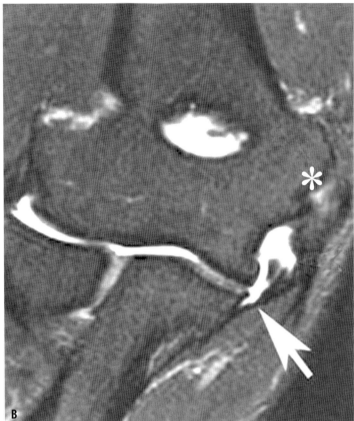

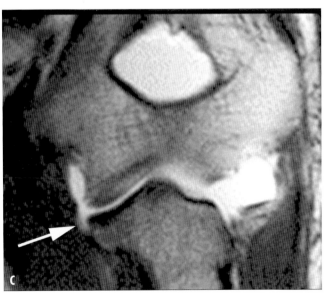

Figure 24.1 Images from three separate baseball pitchers who had received an MR arthrogram. The coronal T1-weighted fat-suppressed MR arthrogram image (**A**) demonstrates the T-sign of a partial tear of the UCL at its attachment to the sublime tubercle. There is abnormal contrast extension between the anterior band of the UCL and the subjacent sublime tubercle (arrow). In another baseball pitcher, a coronal T2-weighted fat-suppressed MR arthrogram image (**B**) not only demonstrates the partial tear of the UCL, but demonstrates increased signal within the common flexor wad origin (asterisk) consistent with tendinopathy. Lastly, a coronal T1-weighted MR arthrogram image (**C**) also demonstrates a partial tear of the UCL.

Lateral ulnar collateral ligament tears

Imaging description

On non-contrast MRI studies, tears of the lateral ulnar collateral ligament are best seen on coronal proton density fat-suppressed images that have a matrix equal to or greater than 256×512. If an MR arthrogram is performed, tears of this ligament are best seen on coronal T1-weighted fat-suppressed images. Normally, the lateral ulnar collateral ligament is seen as a uniformly low-signal intensity. It is attached proximally to the lateral epicondyle and extends distally to insert on the supinator crest of the ulna (Figure 25.1). Disruption or tearing of the lateral ulnar collateral ligament most commonly occurs at its proximal attachment to the lateral epicondyle. More recent research has shown that tearing of the lateral ligamentous complex attachment to the lateral epicondyle (be it the radial collateral ligament or the lateral ulnar collateral ligament) can result in posterolateral rotatory instability of the elbow. In addition, the lateral ulnar collateral ligament can be torn in its midportion, which is also associated with posterolateral rotatory instability of the elbow (Figure 25.2). Lastly, there are those that consider the lateral ligament complex to be a unified single structure (rather than separate radial collateral, lateral ulnar collateral, and annular ligaments) that extends from the lateral humeral epicondyle to attach to the supinator crest and the sigmoid notch. If this is true, then any disruption of this complex may lead to posterolateral rotatory instability at the elbow.

Importance

One of the major functions of the lateral ulnar collateral ligament is to provide stability to the elbow joint in extension and prevent posterolateral rotatory instability. In extension, the ulna will supinate into external rotation if the lateral ulnar collateral ligament is torn thus allowing the radial head to sublux or dislocate posteriorly relative to the capitellum; hence, allowing posterolateral rotatory instability (Figure 25.3).

Typical clinical scenario

The patient usually presents with painful clicking and snapping with extension of the elbow or the sensation that the elbow joint is unstable and giving way when extended. If the clinical physical exam for elbow instability is hampered by patient apprehension and guarding, MRI is useful in demonstrating rupture of the lateral ulnar collateral ligament and confirming a clinical history that is suspect for posterolateral rotatory instability of the elbow.

Teaching point

Diagnosis of a lateral ulnar collateral ligament tear can aid in the clinically suspected diagnosis of posterolateral rotatory instability of the elbow when the physical exam is hampered. MRI can also be useful in preoperative planning and evaluation for the patient with clinically confirmed elbow instability.

READING LIST

Bredella MA, Tirman PF, Fritz RC et al. MR imaging findings of lateral ulnar collateral ligament abnormalities in patients with lateral epicondylitis. AJR Am J Roentgenol 1999;**173**:1379–1382.

Carrino JA, Morrison WB, Zou HK et al. Lateral ulnar collateral ligament of the elbow: optimization of evaluation with two-dimensional MR imaging. Radiology 2001;**218**:118–125.

Charalambous CP, Stanley JK. Posterolateral rotatory instability of the elbow. J Bone Joint Surg Br 2008;**90**:272–279.

Kijowski R, Tuite M, Sanford M. Magnetic resonance imaging of the elbow. Part II: Abnormalities of the ligaments, tendons, and nerves. Skeletal Radiol 2005;**34**:1–18.

Potter HG, Weiland AJ, Schatz JA, Paletta GA, Hotchkiss RN. Posterolateral rotatory instability of the elbow: usefulness of MR imaging in diagnosis. Radiology 1997;**204**:185–198.

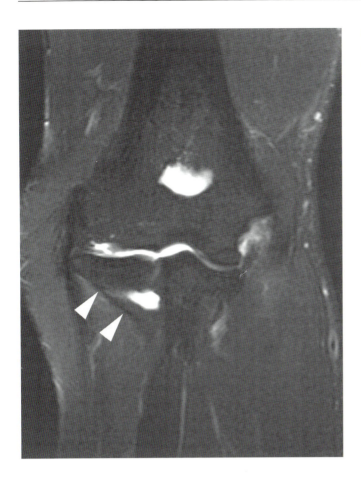

Figure 25.1 Elbow MRI. A coronal T2-weighted fat suppressed image demonstrating a normal lateral ulnar collateral band (arrowheads) extending distally to attach to the supinator crest.

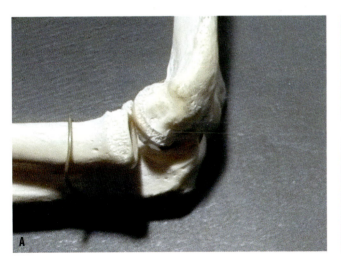
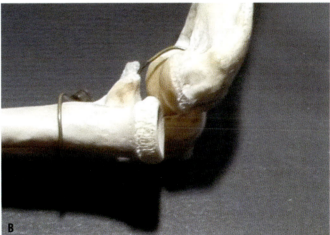

Figure 25.2 Demonstration of abnormal osseous motion when posterolateral rotatory instability of the elbow is present. Laterally oriented photograph of the elbow in pronation (**A**) with near anatomic alignment at the radiocapitellar articulation. When posterolateral rotatory instability is present, supination of the forearm results in posterior subluxation of the radius relative to the capitellum (**B**).

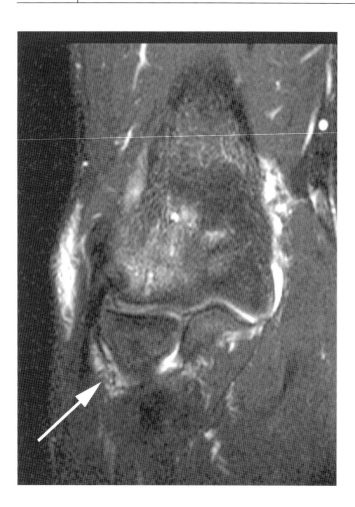

Figure 25.3 A 21-year-old male wrestler with clinical evidence of posterolateral rotatory instability of the elbow. The coronal MRI image demonstrates a ruptured lateral ulnar collateral ligament (arrow).

Locations and evaluation of loose bodies in the elbow joint

Imaging description

Loose bodies in the elbow are most commonly found in the anterior aspect of the joint within the coronoid fossa/recess (Figure 26.1). The second most common location is within the olecranon fossa/recess, posteriorly. On radiographs, ossified loose bodies can be seen as a typically round or ovoid osseous fragment (Figure 26.1). Non-ossified loose bodies (as well as ossified loose bodies) can be seen on CT arthrography or MRI. Ossified loose bodies on MRI can have fatty signal similar to fatty marrow. In general, loose bodies are seen as filling defects on CT arthrography. They can also be seen easily on MRI if there is fluid within the joint space of the elbow. In regard to imaging, CT arthrography has the best combined sensitivity (between 90–99%) and specificity (60–70%) for detecting elbow loose bodies. Radiographs have a similar specificity (but lower sensitivity) while MRI has a similar sensitivity (but lower specificity). Ultrasound (US) arthrography has also been reported to be more accurate than conventional US in the detection of loose bodies in the elbow.

Importance

Medical imaging plays an important role in the evaluation of the patient with limited range of motion of unknown etiology. One of the causes of this is the presence of an intra-articular loose body. Radiography is the initial imaging test of choice. If this is non-contributory and a loose body is clinically suspected, then CT arthrography would be the most helpful in accurately identifying a loose body. If the reason for the loss of range of motion is unknown, then MR would typically be the best imaging study (after radiography) given its overall utility in better identifying multiple different causes of elbow pathology (relative to US or CT arthrography).

Typical clinical scenario

The patient usually presents with elbow stiffness or loss of range of motion. The patient would typically have a history of significant arm use with their occupation, prior trauma, or a history of osteochondritis dissecans of the elbow.

Teaching point

If there is high clinical suspicion for a loose body in the elbow, then radiography is the initial imaging test of choice. This would be followed by CT arthrography if clinically warranted.

READING LIST

Bell MS. Loose bodies in the elbow. *Br J Surg* 1975;**62**:921–924.

Miller JH, Beggs I. Detection of intraarticular bodies of the elbow with saline arthrosonography. *Clin Radiol* 2001;**56**:231–234.

Quinn SF, Haberman JJ, Fitzgerald SW *et al*. Evaluation of loose bodies in the elbow with MR imaging. *J Magn Reson Imaging* 1994;**4**: 169–172.

Zubler V, Saupe N, Jost B *et al*. Elbow stiffness: effectiveness of conventional radiography and CT to explain osseous causes. *AJR Am J Roentgenol* 2010;**194**:W515–W520.

Pearls and Pitfalls in Musculoskeletal Imaging, ed. D. Lee Bennett and Georges Y. El-Khoury. Published by Cambridge University Press. © Cambridge University Press 2013.

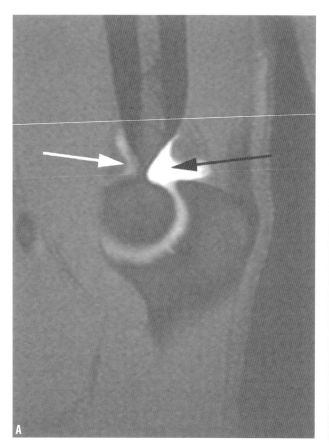

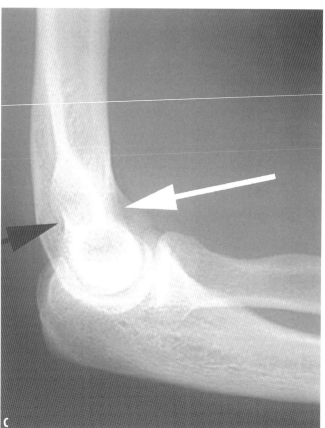

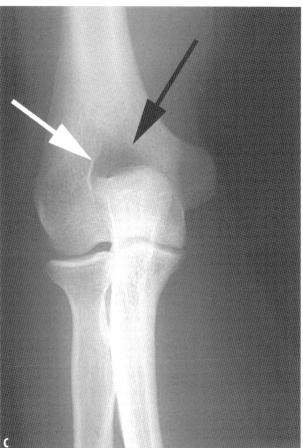

Figure 26.1 Elbow MR arthrogram. This sagittal view (**A**) with T1-weighting and fat suppression demonstrates the olecranon fossa (black arrow) and the coronoid fossa (white arrow). The olecranon (black arrow) and coronoid (white arrow) fossae are also pointed out on AP (**B**) and lateral (**C**) radiographs of the elbow.

Osteochondritis dissecans of the elbow: stable versus unstable

Imaging description

On radiography and CT, osteochondritis dissecans of the elbow is seen as a dome-shaped or somewhat circular-shaped lucency in the mid- or lateral aspect of the capitellum (Figure 27.1). However, in the advanced stage, it will be seen as a divot on the articular surface of the capitellum with a loose body/displaced fragment. The advanced stage of osteochondritis dissecans, will appear similarly on MRI. The earlier stages of osteochondritis dissecans without a loose body will appear as a dome-shaped, curvilinear lesion with a surrounding rim of low signal intensity on T1-weighted images with variable, heterogeneous signal intensity within the lesion. On T2-weighted images, lesions that are stable will also have a rim of low signal intensity and central heterogeneous, variable signal. However, when earlier lesions (those without fragment displacement) are unstable, they will have an intense rim of high signal on T2 or high signal cystic changes at the rim (Figure 27.2).

Importance

On MRI, it is important to identify stable lesions with an adjacent open distal humeral physis because these can be treated successfully with conservative therapy. The size of the lesion is also important as this can drive the type of surgical treatment (debridement with resection versus reconstruction of the injury – such as with osteochondral autograft transplantation surgery).

Typical clinical scenario

A 12-year-old male overhead-throwing athlete with elbow pain. The pain has been somewhat vague with insidious onset but progressive worsening. The pain is worse with the throwing activity. The patient has tenderness around the radiocapitellar articulation with some flexion contracture.

Teaching point

Radiographs will diagnose the majority of cases of osteochondritis dissecans of the elbow. However, in those cases where this disease is suspected and radiographs are normal, MRI is the next imaging study typically used to diagnose osteochondritis dissecans. MRI is also used to measure the size of the lesions and to determine whether it is stable or unstable since these findings will influence the treatment.

READING LIST

Chen NC. Osteochondritis dissecans of the elbow. *J Hand Surg Am* 2010;**35**:1188–1189.

Kijowski R, De Smet AA. MRI findings of osteochondritis dissecans of the capitellum with surgical correlation. *AJR Am J Roentgenol* 2005;**185**:1453–1459.

Ruchelsman DE, Hall MP, Youm T. Osteochondritis dissecans of the capitellum: current concepts. *J Am Acad Orthop Surg* 2010;**18**: 557–567.

Takahara M, Mura N, Sasaki J, Harada M, Oginio T. Classification, treatment, and outcome of osteochondritis dissecans of the humeral capitellum. *J Bone Joint Surg Am* 2007;**89**:1205–1214.

Pearls and Pitfalls in Musculoskeletal Imaging, ed. D. Lee Bennett and Georges Y. El-Khoury. Published by Cambridge University Press. © Cambridge University Press 2013.

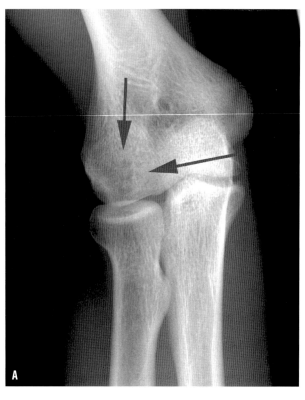

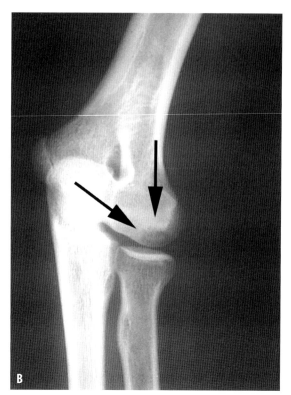

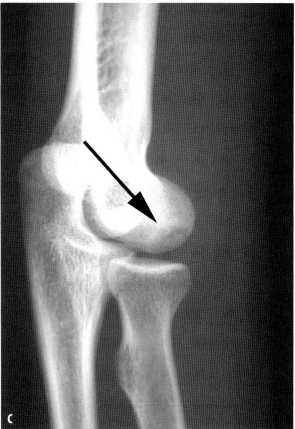

Figure 27.1 A 14-year-old male baseball pitcher with osteochondritis dissecans. Anteroposterior (**A**) and oblique (**B** and **C**) radiographs of the elbow reveal a somewhat circular-shaped lucency (arrows) in the mid- to lateral aspect of the capitellum. This lucency is the focus of osteochondritis dissecans.

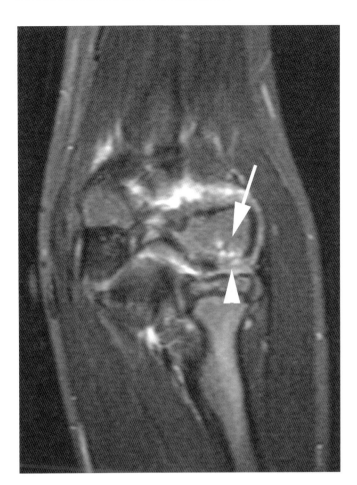

Figure 27.2 Elbow MRI coronally oriented STIR image. High signal cystic changes (arrow) are seen deep to the focus of osteochondritis dissecans (arrowhead) in this skeletally immature patient.

Imaging description

Little Leaguer's elbow was initially described to specifically indicate an injury to the medial epicondylar apophysis. More recently the term has been erroneously used to describe osteochondral injuries to the capitellum or tendinopathy of the common flexor tendon in the pediatric population. The radiographic appearance of Little Leaguer's elbow manifests in two ways. The first is separation of the medial epicondyle apophysis from the underlying humerus. The second appearance is fragmentation of this apophysis on the symptomatic side with the asymptomatic elbow not having any apophyseal fragmentation. Apophyseal separation is diagnosed when the subjacent physis is widened by more than 1 mm relative to the asymptomatic contralateral elbow (Figure 28.1). Additional associated abnormalities that can be seen on MRI include bone marrow-like edema in the apophysis/subjacent humerus, tendinopathy of the common flexor tendon, and a normal ulnar collateral ligament (UCL). Research suggests that injury to the UCL is not present in the pediatric patient with Little Leaguer's elbow.

Importance

It is important to know that this entity is usually diagnosed clinically. The imaging work-up, if indicated, consists of AP and lateral elbow radiographs. At present, research indicates that further evaluation with MRI is not warranted in patients with the classic clinical findings of Little Leaguer's elbow. This disease is usually treated conservatively, especially if the clinical findings are classic and the radiograph is normal or has minimal separation. MRI may be warranted if the patient does not respond to initial therapy and the radiographs are normal.

Typical clinical scenario

An 11-year-old male overhead-throwing athlete who has medial elbow pain. The patient is usually a baseball player and is either a pitcher or catcher. A pitcher is more likely to complain or present with the problem since pain with throwing has a greater effect on their effectiveness during a baseball game. The patient will have medial elbow tenderness with either direct palpation or valgus stress to the elbow. The average duration of pain before presentation is about one month. The patient may also have a mild flexion contracture (~5°) at the elbow.

Teaching point

Radiography is the medical imaging study of choice. MRI is rarely indicated in the setting of Little Leaguer's elbow. The term Little Leaguer's elbow should be reserved for injury to the medial epicondyle apophysis of the elbow.

READING LIST

Brogdon BG, Crow NE. Little Leaguer's elbow. *AJR Am J Roentgenol* 1960;**83**:671–675.

Hang DW, Chao CM, Hang YS. A clinical and roentgenographic study of Little League elbow. *Am J Sports Med* 2004;**32**:79–84.

Wei AS, Khana S, Limpisvasti O *et al*. Clinical and magnetic resonance imaging findings associated with Little League elbow. *J Pediatr Orthop* 2010;**30**:715–719.

Pearls and Pitfalls in Musculoskeletal Imaging, ed. D. Lee Bennett and Georges Y. El-Khoury. Published by Cambridge University Press. © Cambridge University Press 2013.

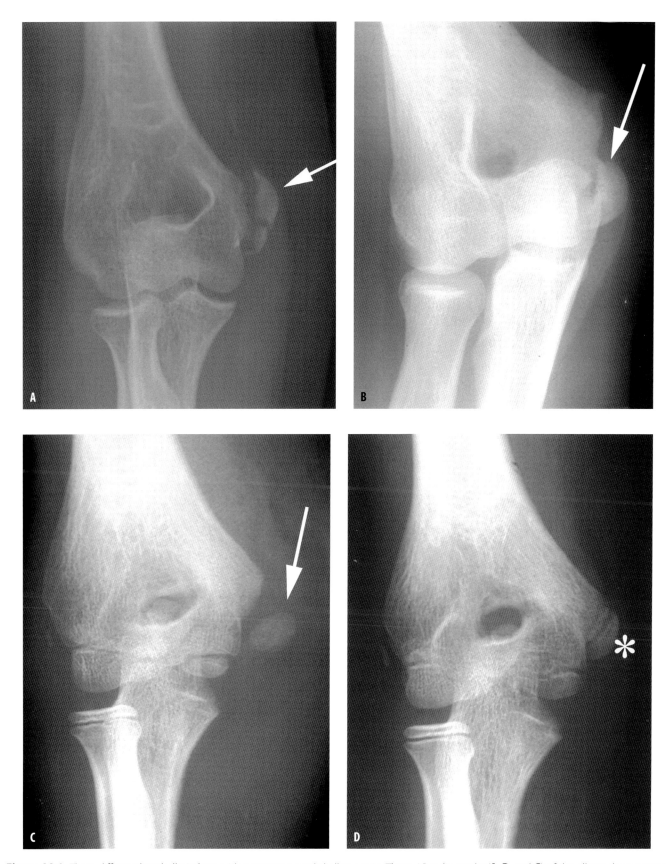

Figure 28.1 Three different baseball pitchers with worsening medial elbow pain. These AP radiographs (**A**, **B**, and **C**) of the elbow demonstrate avulsion fractures (arrows) of the medial epicondylar apophysis (or equivalent) in patients with varying degrees of skeletal maturity. Figure **D** demonstrates a normal elbow with a normally positioned medial epicondylar ossification center (asterisk).

Imaging description

Pseudocyst of the radial tuberosity is seen on radiographic or CT images of the forearm/elbow. A radial tuberosity pseudocyst is an apparent lytic lesion centered in the radial tuberosity. This apparent lytic lesion is caused by a focal area of increased stress on the trabecular bone relative to the surrounding trabeculae. Therefore, when this focal area of trabecular rarefaction (due to a focally different stress such as the attachment of a tendon) is visually compared with the surrounding bone without trabecular rarefaction, an apparent lytic lesion is seen (Figure 29.1). One of these areas of focal rarefaction of trabecular bone occurs in the radial tuberosity where the distal biceps tendon inserts. On MRI, this radial pseudocyst will have normal fatty marrow signal, since it is a normal variant (Figure 29.2).

Importance

It is important to know that this entity is a normal variant that can mimic an osseous lytic lesion. If there is still concern that a true lytic lesion is present in the radial tuberosity after careful evaluation of the radiographic images, an MRI can be performed. If the lesion seen on the radiographic images is a pseudocyst, it will have normal fatty marrow signal on the MRI images. On MRI, normal fatty marrow should demonstrate high signal intensity on T1-weighted images and low signal intensity on T2-weighted fat-suppressed or STIR images.

Typical clinical scenario

A 27-year-old male presents with elbow pain after trauma. An unexpected apparent lytic lesion is seen on the elbow radiographic study. This is most commonly a radial tuberosity pseudocyst, especially if the patient was asymptomatic prior to the trauma. Radial tuberosity pseudocysts should be painless; therefore, if there is bone pain associated with the lytic area, then one should be careful to not miss a true underlying lytic lesion.

Teaching point

An apparent lytic lesion at the radial tuberosity on radiography is typically a pseudocyst if the lytic lesion appears to be due to trabecular rarefaction in the underlying bone with no actual bone destruction. If there is concern that a true, neoplastic lytic lesion is present at the radial tuberosity, then an MRI can be performed to confirm the presence of tumor.

READING LIST

Bennett DL, El-Khoury GY. General approach to lytic bone lesions. *Appl Radiol* 2004;**33**:8–17.

De Wilde V, De Maeseneer M, Lenchik L *et al*. Normal osseous variants presenting as cystic or lucent areas on radiography and CT imaging: a pictorial overview. *Eur J Radiol* 2004;**51**:77–84.

Resnick D, Cone RO 3rd. The nature of humeral pseudocysts. *Radiology* 1984;**150**:27–28.

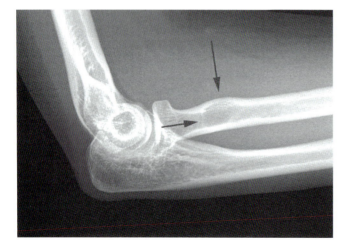

Figure 29.1 A lateral radiograph of the proximal forearm reveals a pseudocyst (arrows) at the radial tuberosity. There is no evidence of bone destruction on the radiograph.

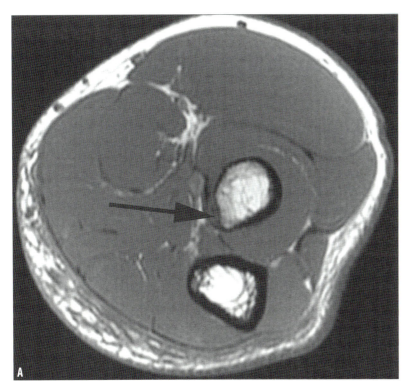

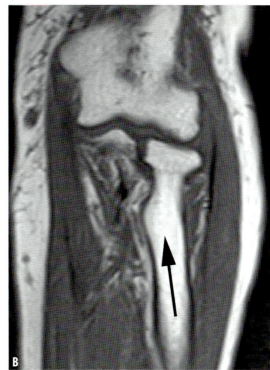

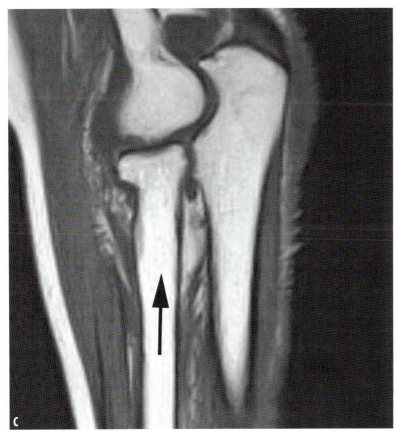

Figure 29.2 Transverse (A), coronal (B), and sagittal (C) T1-weighted MRI images at the level of the radial tuberosity demonstrates normal fatty marrow (arrow). A pseudocyst should have normal marrow signal characteristics on MRI.

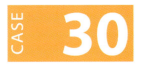
30 Unstable fracture/dislocations of the forearm

Imaging description

The more common unstable fracture/dislocations of the forearm are the Essex–Lopresti, Galeazzi, and Monteggia fracture/dislocations. The radiographic findings of an Essex–Lopresti fracture/dislocation are a comminuted radial head fracture coupled with dislocation of the distal radioulnar joint (DRUJ). The Galeazzi injury consists of a radial shaft fracture (usually mid to distal shaft) associated with a DRUJ dislocation. Finally, the Monteggia fracture/dislocation is a group of traumatic injuries having a dislocation of the elbow joint (usually radial head dislocation) associated with a fracture of the ulna at various levels (Figure 30.1).

Importance

These fracture/dislocation injuries are important because they are easily underdiagnosed (most likely due to the fact that they are not common) and need to be treated sooner rather than later with surgical intervention in order to obtain the best clinical outcome. The forearm functions biomechanically like a ring or unit structure, which means that an osseous injury to the radius or ulna that disrupts or alters its length will usually affect the DRUJ or elbow joint leading to an unstable injury. When the DRUJ is dislocated from these injuries it is due to disruption of the triangular fibrocartilage complex caused by sudden shortening of the radial length. When an elbow dislocation is a component of forearm fracture/dislocation injury, it dislocates due to rupture of the annular ligament about the proximal radius.

Typical clinical scenario

A 40-year-old male falls on an outstretched hand and suffers an elbow fracture. The radiograph demonstrates a comminuted radial head fracture. If the wrist is not carefully evaluated, a DRUJ dislocation may be missed leading to inappropriate treatment of the radial head fracture causing failure of treatment in several months due to forearm ring instability at the DRUJ.

Teaching point

With any comminuted radial head fracture or mid to distal radial shaft fracture, the wrist must be carefully evaluated so an unstable DRUJ dislocation is not missed. When an ulnar shaft fracture is present, the elbow should be carefully evaluated so that a radial head dislocation is not missed because an isolated ulnar shaft fracture (night stick fracture) is treated differently from a Monteggia fracture/dislocation. Always carefully check the adjacent joints when any of the above fractures are found to ensure a DRUJ or radial head dislocation is not missed.

READING LIST

Atesok KI, Jupiter JB, Weiss AP. Galeazzi fracture. *J Am Acad Orthop Surg* 2011;**19**:623–633.

Bock GW, Cohen MS, Resnick D. Fracture-dislocation of the elbow with inferior radioulnar dislocation: a variant of the Essex–Lopresti injury. *Skeletal Radiol* 1992;**21**:315–317.

Eathiraju S, Mudgal CS, Jupiter JB. Monteggia fracture-dislocations. *Hand Clin* 2007;**23**:165–177.

Pearls and Pitfalls in Musculoskeletal Imaging, ed. D. Lee Bennett and Georges Y. El-Khoury. Published by Cambridge University Press. © Cambridge University Press 2013.

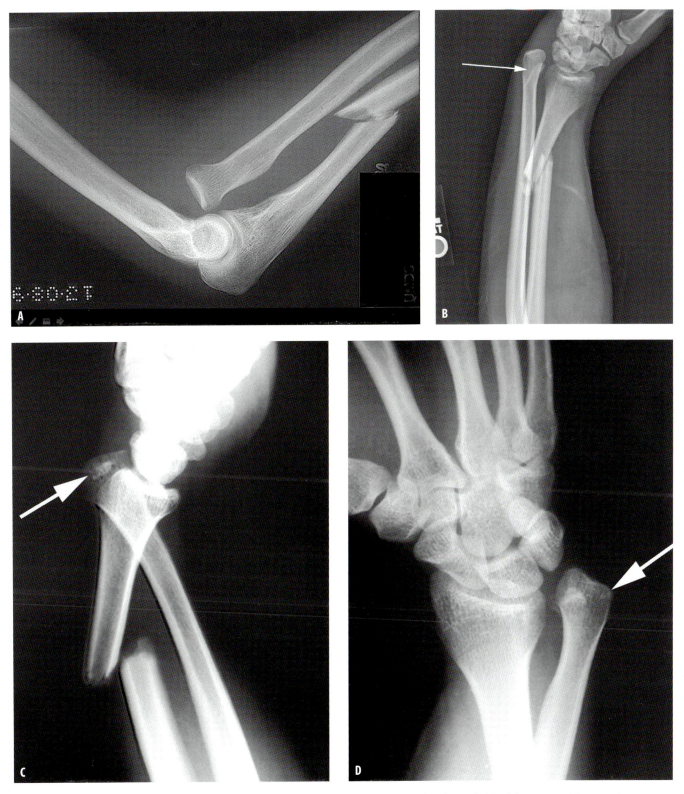

Figure 30.1 Radiographs of Monteggia and Galeazzi fracture/dislocation injuries. Lateral radiograph (**A**) of the proximal forearm shows an ulnar shaft fracture and a radial head dislocation of a Monteggia injury. Oblique radiographs (**B, C,** and **D**) of the distal forearm and wrist show a radial shaft fracture and distal ulnar dislocation of a Galeazzi injury. An ulnar styloid process fracture is also present (arrow).

Cat scratch disease: medial epitrochlear lymphadenopathy and pustules of the forearm

Imaging description

The majority of cases of medial epitrochlear lymphadenopathy are reactive or benign in origin. One of the more common benign causes is cat scratch disease. It can occasionally be seen with radiography as a soft tissue mass in the medial epitrochlear area. It is much more commonly seen on MRI as a soft tissue space-occupying lesion in the medial epitrochlear region. On MRI, the lesion is typically round or ovoid in shape, has slightly hyper-intense signal on T1-weighted images, has hyperintense signal on T2-weighted images, and shows homogeneous enhancement on postcontrast images (Figure 31.1). The lesion can contain areas of necrosis which are seen as areas of heterogeneous signal intensity and areas of no enhancement. The lesion in cat scratch disease is a reactive lymph node. The more common locations for reactive lymphadenopathy from cat scratch disease are the medial epitrochlear area, the axillary region, and the groin. Patients can have pustule formation in the wrist and distal forearm area as well. By US, the mass may have the appearance of a large reactive lymph node (Figure 31.2).

Importance

It is important to know that a medial epitrochlear mass is usually benign and most commonly is a manifestation of cat scratch disease so that unnecessary surgery does not occur. The lesion (reactive lymphadenopathy) does not need to be resected. Cat scratch disease is usually diagnosed clinically using the history, physical exam findings, and laboratory tests (serology for antibodies to *Bartonella henselae*). A history of a cat scratch or physical exam findings of a cat scratch involving the hand, wrist, or distal forearm helps confirm the diagnosis; however, it is not mandatory to make the diagnosis. In one larger study, the age range for this disease was 6–63 years old. It is important to suspect this disease when imaging a medial epitrochlear mass so that unnecessary work-up or surgery for malignancy is not performed.

Typical clinical scenario

A 12-year-old female presents with recent onset of a somewhat rapidly growing soft tissue mass in the medial epitrochlear area of the arm. Her family is worried about cancer. On physical exam, the mass may or may not be painful. The family does report that they own a cat; however, the patient denies any recent cat scratches. There are a few pustules present on the forearm near the wrist.

Teaching point

With any epitrochlear soft tissue mass, benign reactive lymphadenopathy should be included in a limited differential, the most common of which is cat scratch disease. This disease should be clinically excluded before any invasive work-up or surgery is performed. MRI coupled with clinical corroboration can help prevent unnecessary intervention, biopsy, or surgery.

READING LIST

Dong PR, Seeger LL, Yao L *et al.* Uncomplicated cat-scratch disease: findings at CT, MR imaging, and radiography. *Radiology* 1995;**195**: 837–839.

Garcia CJ, Varela C, Abarca K *et al.* Regional lymphadenopathy in cat-scratch disease: ultrasonographic findings. *Pediatr Radiol* 2000;**30**:640–643.

Gielen J, Wang XL, Vanhoenacker F *et al.* Lymphadenopathy at the medial epitrochlear region in cat-scratch disease. *Eur Radiol* 2003;**13**:1363–1369.

Holt PD, de Lang EE. Cat scratch disease: magnetic resonance imaging findings. *Skeletal Radiol* 1995;**24**:437–440.

Hopkins KL, Simoneaux SF, Patrick LE *et al.* Imaging manifestations of cat-scratch disease. *AJR Am J Roentgenol* 1996;**166**:435–438.

Pearls and Pitfalls in Musculoskeletal Imaging, ed. D. Lee Bennett and Georges Y. El-Khoury. Published by Cambridge University Press. © Cambridge University Press 2013.

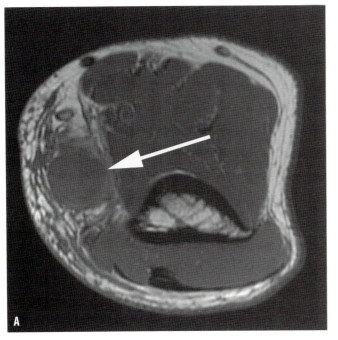

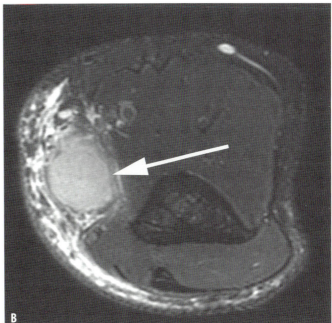

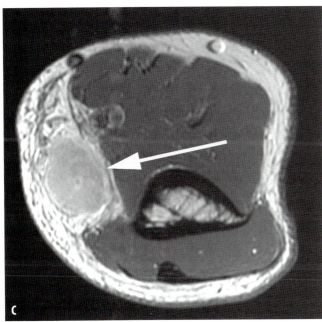

Figure 31.1 A 29-year-old male with cat scratch disease. Transverse MRI images in the epitrochlear region of the arm demonstrate an epitrochlear mass (arrows) that is hyperintense with T1-weighting (**A**), hyperintense with T2-weighting (**B**), and shows nearly uniform contrast enhancement (**C**) in this patient with cat scratch disease.

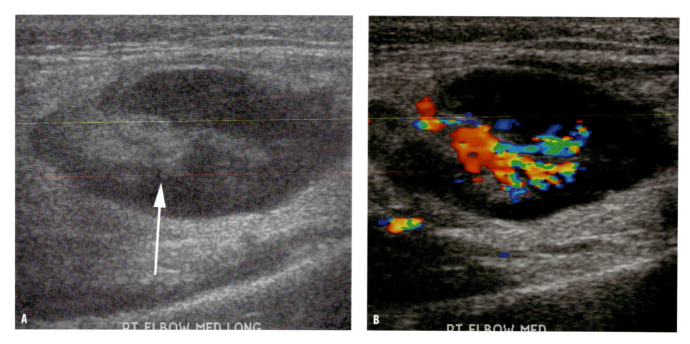

Figure 31.2 Ultrasound images of an epitrochlear mass in a patient with cat scratch disease. Image (**A**) demonstrates a large reactive lymph node with a fatty hilum that was hyperemic on color Doppler (**B**). The appearance is classic for a large reactive lymph node. This figure is presented in color in the color plate section.

Pseudotear of the triangular fibrocartilage (TFC): radial cartilage

Imaging description

Subjacent to the radial attachment of the triangular fibrocartilage (TFC) is the mildly increased signal of hyaline articular cartilage of the distal radius.

Importance

At radial attachment, the TFC inserts on hyaline cartilage and not on cortex; as a result, there is a focus of intermediate signal intensity that represents cartilage between the low-signal intensity radial cortex and low-signal intensity TFC (Figure 32.1).

Typical clinical scenario

A misdiagnosis of a TFC tear may be made if an intermediate to high signal intensity is noted at the radial attachment of the TFC.

Differential diagnosis

Radial hyaline cartilage should not be misinterpreted as a tear. The areas of increased signal intensity at the hyaline cartilage interface can be distinguished from tears by their lack of increased signal on MR images with T2-type contrast. A radial-sided TFC tear, which is usually slit-like, lies medial to the radial articular cartilage.

> ### Teaching point
>
> The MR imaging appearance of TFC is a hypointense disc in all sequences. However, the radial attachment of the TFC often shows an intermediate to high signal intensity which may be a potential imaging pitfall.

READING LIST

Pfirrmann CW, Zanetti M. Variants, pitfalls and asymptomatic findings in wrist and hand imaging. *Eur J Radiol* 2005;**56**:286–295.

Timins ME, O'Connell SE, Erickson SJ, Oneson SR. MR imaging of the wrist: normal findings that may simulate disease. *Radiographics* 1996;**16**:987–995.

Zlatkin MB, Rosner J. MR imaging of ligaments and triangular fibrocartilage complex of the wrist. *Radiol Clin North Am* 2006; **44**:595–623.

Pearls and Pitfalls in Musculoskeletal Imaging, ed. D. Lee Bennett and Georges Y. El-Khoury. Published by Cambridge University Press. © Cambridge University Press 2013.

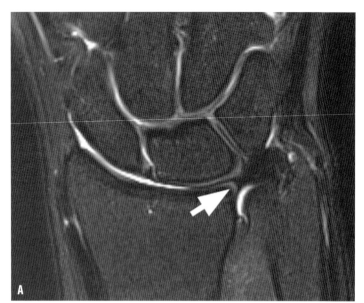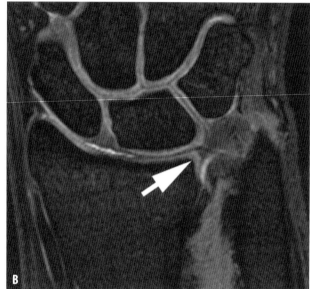

Figure 32.1 Pseudotear of the TFC: radial cartilage. Coronal fat-suppressed T2-weighted MR image (**A**) shows an area of increased signal intensity at the radial hyaline cartilage (arrow). Coronal gradient echo MR image (**B**), obtained in the same patient as in A, shows an area of increased signal intensity at the radial hyaline cartilage (arrow).

Imaging description

A triangular fibrocartilage (TFC) tear appears as a linear band of increased signal intensity (Figure 33.1). With complete tears the signal extends to the proximal and distal articular surfaces. MR imaging may demonstrate an asymptomatic defect of the TFC (Figure 33.2).

Importance

With increasing age, defects and central communication within the TFC increase in frequency. Non-communicating TFC defects are worthwhile to record specifically because they can be associated more reliably with symptomatic wrists than communicating TFC defects. Non-communicating and communicating defects of the TFC near the ulnar attachment have a more reliable association with symptomatic wrists than do radial communicating defects.

Typical clinical scenario

Patients with a TFC tear present with ulnar-sided pain. The radial-sided communicating TFC defects are commonly seen bilaterally and in asymptomatic wrists.

Differential diagnosis

Differential diagnosis includes TFC tear, asymptomatic defects, and pseudotear.

Teaching point

There are no specific differentiating features on MR imaging separating a traumatically induced tear of the TFC from one caused by degeneration. The appearance of these lesions may also be similar in symptomatic and asymptomatic individuals; therefore, determining the clinical relevance of these lesions and their correlation with patients' symptoms may be difficult.

READING LIST

Metz VM, Schratter M, Dock WI *et al.* Age-associated changes of the triangular fibrocartilage of the wrist: evaluation of the diagnostic performance of MR imaging. *Radiology* 1992;**184**:217–220.

Pfirrmann CW, Zanetti M. Variants, pitfalls and asymptomatic findings in wrist and hand imaging. *Eur J Radiol* 2005;**56**:286–295.

Zanetti M, Linkous MD, Gilula LA, Hodler J. Characteristics of triangular fibrocartilage defects in symptomatic and contralateral asymptomatic wrists. *Radiology* 2000;**216**:840– 845.

Zlatkin MB, Chao PC, Osterman AL *et al.* Chronic wrist pain: evaluation with high-resolution MR imaging. *Radiology* 1989;**173**:723–729.

Zlatkin MB, Rosner J. MR imaging of ligaments and triangular fibrocartilage complex of the wrist. *Radiol Clin North Am* 2006;**44**:595–623.

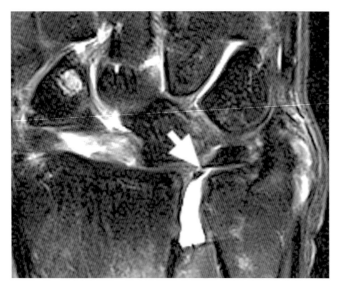

Figure 33.1 Triangular fibrocartilage (TFC) tear. Coronal fat-suppressed T2-weighted MR image demonstrates a linear increased signal intensity (arrow) extending to proximal and distal articular surfaces.

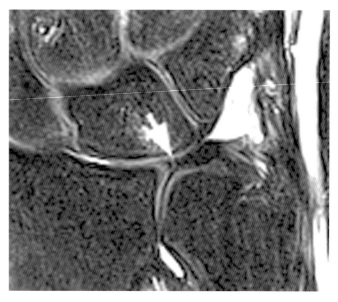

Figure 33.2 Asymptomatic radial-sided defect of triangular fibrocartilage (TFC). Coronal fat-suppressed T2-weighted MR image shows a radial-sided and slightly increased signal intensity (arrow).

Occult carpal fractures: imaging work-up

Imaging description

Plain radiography is the first step in the evaluation of carpal bone injuries such as a scaphoid fracture, and it is effective in diagnosing most but not all carpal fractures. If radiography is negative, and clinical suspicion persists, further investigation with special radiographic views, CT scan, or MR imaging is necessary. Criteria for an occult fracture on multi-detector CT are the presence of a sharp lucent line, a discontinuity in the trabecular meshwork, and a break or step-off in the cortex. MR imaging is exquisitely sensitive to bone marrow abnormalities and therefore renders even non-displaced fractures obvious (Figure 34.1). MR imaging helps in detecting non-displaced fractures by showing a hypointense fracture line on T1-weighted images and increased signal intensity in areas of trabecular injury on fluid-sensitive sequences.

Importance

Detection of the occult fracture can be crucial for treatment planning. In many clinical settings, the diagnosis of a scaphoid fracture on the basis of radiography is delayed up to 2 weeks or more after the injury. Follow-up radiography demonstrates the initially occult scaphoid fracture because hyperemia and bone resorption at the fracture site make the fracture line more visible.

Typical clinical scenario

Accurate diagnosis using CT or MR imaging initiates early treatment with immobilization for the wrist fractures.

Teaching point

Although conventional radiography remains the primary imaging modality for evaluation of suspected carpal fractures, they may be overlooked. Multi-detector CT may depict fractures that are occult at radiography. CT has a high sensitivity for occult wrist fractures, and MR imaging enables visualization of bone marrow abnormalities in non-displaced fractures.

READING LIST

Ahn JM, El-Khoury GY. Occult fractures of extremities. *Radiol Clin North Am* 2007;**45**:561–579.

Berger PE, Ofstein RA, Jackson DW *et al*. MRI demonstration of radiographically occult fractures: what have we been missing? *Radiographics* 1989;**9**:407–436.

Breitenseher MJ, Metz VM, Gilula LA *et al*. Radiographically occult scaphoid fractures: value of MR imaging in detection. *Radiology* 1997;**203**:245–250.

Eustace S. MR imaging of acute orthopedic trauma to the extremities. *Radiol Clin North Am* 1997;**35**:615–629.

Kaewlai R, Avery LL, Asrani AV *et al*. Multidetector CT of carpal injuries: anatomy, fractures, and fracture-dislocations. *Radiographics* 2008;**28**:1771–1784.

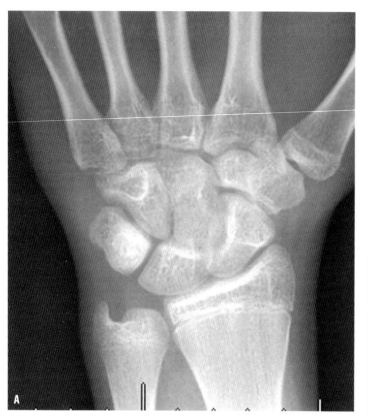

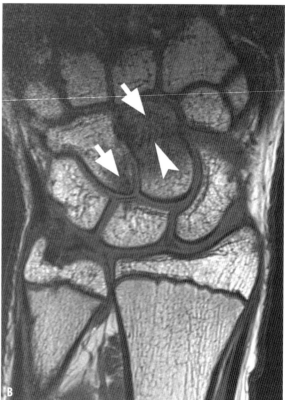

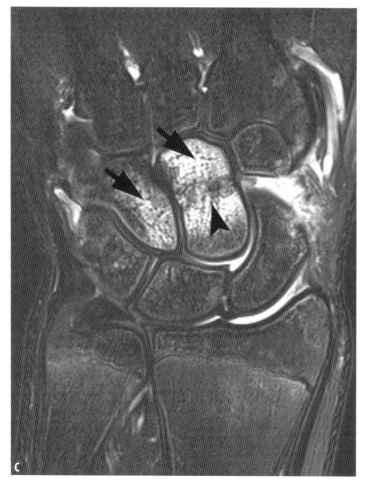

Figure 34.1 Occult fracture of the capitate. Posteroanterior projection (**A**) shows no fracture. Coronal T1-weighted MR image (**B**), obtained in the same patient as in A, demonstrates hypointense bone marrow edema in the capitate and hamate (arrows). A linear more hypointense band is noticed within the capitate (arrowhead), indicating a fracture. Coronal fat-suppressed T2-weighted MR image (**C**), obtained in the same patient as in A, demonstrates hyperintense bone marrow edema in the capitate and hamate (arrows). A linear hypointense band is noticed within the capitate (arrowhead), indicating a fracture.

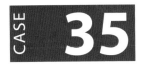

CASE 35

Carpal instability: are you looking at a true lateral view of the wrist?

Imaging description

On a lateral radiograph of the wrist, axes can be drawn and carpal relationships can be inferred based on the angle of these axes. A line parallel to the center of the radial shaft is its axis. The lunate axis is a line drawn perpendicular to the anterior and posterior distal lunate poles. To determine the scaphoid axis, a line is drawn connecting the proximal and distal ventral convexities of the scaphoid. This line is parallel to or is only a few degrees off the central axis of the scaphoid, and can easily be drawn on any adequate lateral wrist view. In the normal wrists, the longitudinal axes of the third metacarpal, capitate, lunate, and radius should all fall on the same plane.

The scapholunate angle normally ranges from 30 to 60°, average 47°. When the lunate is extended dorsally, it is called dorsal intercalated segmental instability (DISI) (Figure 35.1) and when it is tipped volarly, it is called volar intercalated segmental instability (VISI) (Figure 35.2). The scapholunate angle increases when the concave distal articular surface of the lunate faces or tilts dorsally, and the scaphoid stays in its normal position or tilts volarly. A scapholunate angle greater than 70° or 80° indicates DISI. VISI exists when the distal articular surface of the lunate faces volarly. In this situation, the lunate may tilt volarly more than the scaphoid, so that the scapholunate angle is less than 30°.

Importance

Carpal instability is often a confusing and challenging topic. Radiographic evaluation is an integral part of the diagnosis.

Typical clinical scenario

Patients may present with decreased wrist motion secondary to trauma or arthritis.

> ### Teaching point
>
> Recognition of carpal instability or malalignment requires locating the central axes of the radius, lunate, scaphoid, and capitate in the lateral view.

READING LIST

Carlsen BT, Shin AY. Wrist instability. *Scand J Surg* 2008;**97**: 324–332.

Gilula LA, Weeks PM. Post-traumatic ligamentous instabilities of the wrist. *Radiology* 1978;**129**:641–651.

Linscheid RL, Dobyns JH, Beabout JW, Bryan RS. Traumatic instability of the wrist. Diagnosis, classification, and pathomechanics. *J Bone Joint Surg Am* 1972;**54**:1612–1632.

Pearls and Pitfalls in Musculoskeletal Imaging, ed. D. Lee Bennett and Georges Y. El-Khoury. Published by Cambridge University Press. © Cambridge University Press 2013.

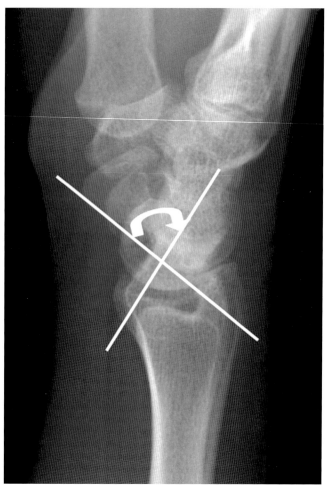

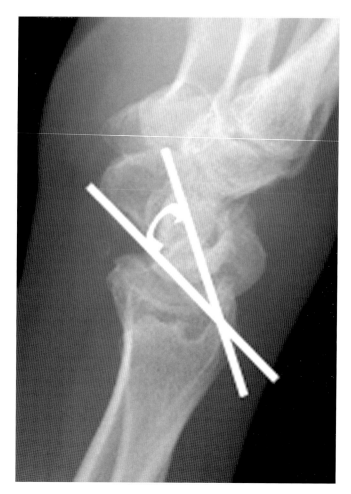

Figure 35.1 Dorsal intercalated segmental instability (DISI). When the lunate is extended dorsally, it is called dorsal intercalated segmental instability (DISI). The scapholunate angle (curved arrow) increases when the concave distal articular surface of the lunate faces or tilts dorsally.

Figure 35.2 Volar intercalated segmental instability (VISI). When the distal articular surface of the lunate faces volarly, the scapholunate angle decreases (curved arrow), suggestive of the volar intercalated segmental instability (VISI).

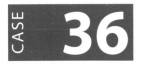

CASE 36

Extensor carpi radialis brevis and longus: synovial fluid versus tenosynovitis

Imaging description

Small amounts of fluid are commonly identified in the tendon sheaths of extensor tendons (Figure 36.1), particularly the extensor carpi radialis brevis and longus. The characteristic finding of the intersection syndrome on MR imaging is peritendinous edema around the first and second extensor compartment tendons, extending proximally from the crossover point.

Importance

Although the cause is unknown, fluid within the extensor tendon sheaths should not be mistaken for tenosynovitis unless the amount of fluid is excessive.

Typical clinical scenario

Tenosynovitis is an inflammatory condition that is diagnosed by noting hyperintense fluid that distends a tendon sheath and surrounds the indwelling tendon (Figure 36.2). Intersection syndrome is an inflammatory process of the second extensor compartment tendons of the forearm, characterized by pain and swelling 4–8 cm proximal to Lister's tubercle of the distal radius.

Differential diagnosis

The main differential diagnosis is de Quervain's tenosynovitis, which is characterized by tendinopathy and stenosing tenosynovitis affecting the abductor pollicis longus and the extensor pollicis brevis tendons and sheath.

Teaching point

Small quantities of fluid in the extensor tendon sheaths may be normal and not indicative of tenosynovitis. MR imaging can perform an important role in establishing the diagnosis of intersection syndrome of the forearm.

READING LIST

Bencardino JT. MR imaging of tendon lesions of the hand and wrist. *Magn Reson Imaging Clin N Am* 2004;**12**:333–347.

Costa CR, Morrison WB, Carrino JA. MRI features of intersection syndrome of the forearm. *AJR Am J Roentgenol* 2003;**181**:1245–1249.

Glajchen N, Schweitzer M. MRI features in de Quervain's tenosynovitis of the wrist. *Skeletal Radiol* 1996;**25**:63–65.

Timins ME, O'Connell SE, Erickson SJ, Oneson SR. MR imaging of the wrist: normal findings that may simulate disease. *Radiographics* 1996;**16**:987–995.

Pearls and Pitfalls in Musculoskeletal Imaging, ed. D. Lee Bennett and Georges Y. El-Khoury. Published by Cambridge University Press. © Cambridge University Press 2013.

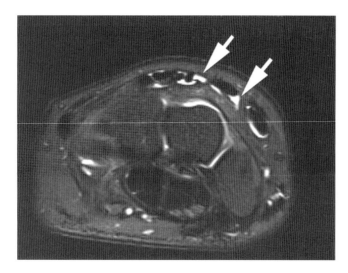

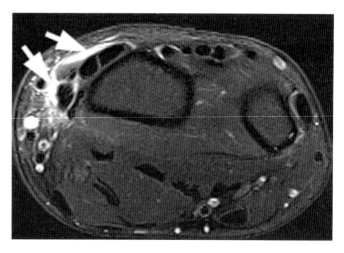

Figure 36.1 Normal synovial fluid. Small amounts of fluid (arrows) are commonly identified in the tendon sheaths of extensor tendons on fat-suppressed fluid-sensitive sequences.

Figure 36.2 Tenosynovitis. Tenosynovitis shows hyperintense fluid (arrows) on fat-suppressed fluid-sensitive sequences. The fluid distends a tendon sheath and surrounds the indwelling tendon.

37 Lunotriquetral carpal coalition: incidental finding

Imaging description

Radiographs may show lunotriquetral coalition with widened scapholunate joint space or a narrowed space between the lunate and triquetrum with cysts and sclerosis similar to pseudoarthrosis (Figure 37.1).

Importance

Lunotriquetral coalitions are frequently bilateral. The most common isolated carpal coalition is the lunotriquetral, followed by the capito-hamate.

Typical clinical scenario

Lunotriquetral coalitions are most commonly discovered as incidental findings during radiographic examinations. Patients with lunotriquetral coalition may poorly tolerate stress loading or trauma.

Differential diagnosis

Differential diagnosis includes lunotriquetral coalition, degenerative arthritis, and pseudoarthrosis.

Teaching point

Widening of the scapholunate joint space is a normal variant that is common in patients with lunotriquetral coalition.

READING LIST

Delaney TJ, Eswar S. Carpal coalitions. *J Hand Surg Am* 1992; **17**:28–31.

Metz VM, Schimmerl SM, Gilula LA, Viegas SF, Saffar P. Wide scapholunate joint space in lunotriquetral coalition: a normal variant? *Radiology* 1993;**188**:557–559.

Pfirrmann CW, Zanetti M. Variants, pitfalls and asymptomatic findings in wrist and hand imaging. *Eur J Radiol* 2005;**56**: 286–295.

Stäbler A, Glaser C, Reiser M, Resnick D. Symptomatic fibrous lunato-triquetral coalition. *Eur Radiol* 1999;**9**:1643–1646.

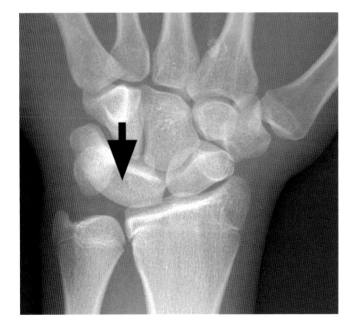

Figure 37.1 Lunotriquetral coalition. Posteroanterior projection shows osseous fusion of the lunate and triquetrum (arrow).

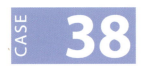

CASE 38 Skier's thumb and Stener lesion

Imaging description

Skier's thumb (also known as Gamekeeper's thumb) is a rupture of the ulnar collateral ligament (UCL) at the first metacarpophalangeal joint. The lesion is not readily visible on radiography unless there is an associated avulsion fracture at the ulnar-sided base of the first metacarpal (Figure 38.1). The soft tissue injury can be seen by MRI as a rupture of the UCL. The Stener lesion is when the ruptured UCL becomes displaced superficial to the adductor policis aponeurosis. On MRI a Stener lesion is seen when the ruptured UCL is seen superficial to the aponeurosis or when the yo-yo on a string sign is seen on MRI. The yo-yo on a string sign is caused by the ruptured distal end of the UCL being doubled back upon itself (Figure 38.2). In general, radiographic stress views of the first metacarpophalangeal joint are not currently recommended to aid in the diagnosis of a Stener lesion or skier's thumb.

Importance

Identification of a displaced avulsion fragment associated with a skier's thumb is important to identify. When this fragment is displaced, it usually will need to be treated surgically or with fixation to promote healing.

Typical clinical scenario

A 24-year-old male has sustained a "ski pole" injury to his right thumb. There is swelling and tenderness at the UCL of the first metacarpophalangeal joint. The physical exam is positive for rupture of the UCL. A radiograph is ordered usually to rule out an underlying avulsion fracture. If the physical exam is positive for a Stener lesion, an MRI may be ordered for preoperative planning based on the surgeon's preference.

Teaching point

In the clinical setting of a skier's thumb injury, a radiograph is usually ordered to rule out an associated fracture. Any significant displacement of the fracture fragment will usually result in fixation in addition to immobilization. Physical exam (sensitivity around 95%) has been reported to be as sensitive as or more sensitive than MRI or US in diagnosing a Stener lesion (sensitivity ranges from 75% to upper 90th percentile range). When an MRI is requested for preoperative planning, one should carefully look for superficial displacement of the torn UCL or the yo-yo on a string sign to confirm the physical exam diagnosis. One should also carefully evaluate for other unsuspected injuries that might be visualized by the MRI.

READING LIST

Haramati N, Hiller N, Dowdie J *et al.* MRI of the Stener lesion. *Skeletal Radiol* 1995;**24**:515–518.

Lohman M, Vasenius J, Kivisaari A, Kivisaari L. MR imaging in chronic rupture of the ulnar collateral ligament of the thumb. *Acta Radiol* 2001;**42**:10–14.

Papendrea RF, Fowler T. Injury at the thumb UCL: is there a Stener lesion? *J Hand Surg Am* 2008;**33**:1882–1884.

Pearls and Pitfalls in Musculoskeletal Imaging, ed. D. Lee Bennett and Georges Y. El-Khoury. Published by Cambridge University Press. © Cambridge University Press 2013.

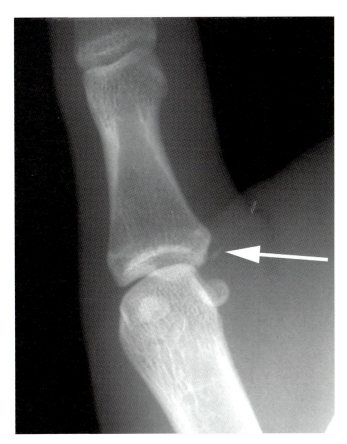

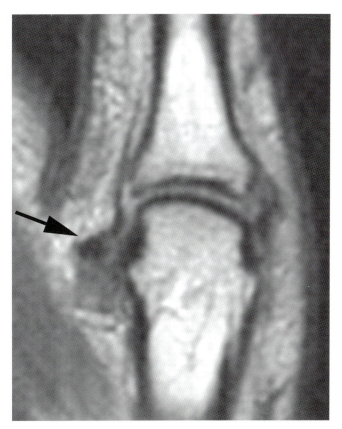

Figure 38.1 Skier's thumb fracture. The AP radiograph of the thumb demonstrates a small avulsion fracture fragment (arrow) from the ulnar-sided base of the proximal phalanx. The fragment has been avulsed by the ulnar collateral ligament of the first metacarpophalangeal joint due to an injury causing valgus angulation at this joint.

Figure 38.2 Stener lesion. T1-weighted MR image shows the yo-yo on a string sign (arrow) which is the "balled-up" or yo-yo appearance of the proximally displaced ulnar collateral ligament. The more distal "string" represents the aponeurosis that is preventing the "balled-up" ulnar collateral ligament from reaching the ulnar base of the proximal phalanx of the thumb.

Bennett versus Rolando fracture

Imaging description

A Bennett fracture is an intra-articular, simple, oblique fracture at the base of the first metacarpal (Figure 39.1). A Rolando fracture is an intra-articular, comminuted fracture at the base of the first metacarpal (Figure 39.2).

Importance

It is important to identify a Bennett fracture due to its instability coupled with the need for early treatment with near anatomic reduction and fixation. If a Bennett fracture heals with greater than 1 mm of step-off at the metacarpal base articular surface, the patient is at increased risk for symptomatic first carpometacarpal joint osteoarthritis in 5–7 years. Unfortunately, the Bennett fracture tends not to hold its reduced, anatomic position with just closed reduction and Spica casting. In a Bennett fracture, the main substance of the metacarpal head and shaft are left intact, but they are avulsed off of a large portion of the volar-ulnar aspect of the metacarpal base. The base is held in place by a strong intermetacarpal ligament while the main portion of the metacarpal (small part of the radial base, the shaft, and the head) is displaced radially and dorsally primarily by the abductor pollicis longus tendon. This displacement leads to an incongruous first carpometacarpal joint followed by early, symptomatic osteoarthritis. A Rolando fracture that is only minimally comminuted and has large fragments is usually treated similar to a Bennett fracture (if near anatomic reduction can be achieved). Unfortunately, a severely comminuted Rolando fracture cannot be anatomically reduced and the usual outcome is post-traumatic osteoarthritis.

Typical clinical scenario

A 30-year-old female with a jamming injury, i.e. an axial loading injury, to the thumb presents with severe pain and deformity at the base of the thumb. Radiographs are performed to see if the injury is a Bennett fracture or a minimally comminuted Rolando fracture so that early reduction and fixation can be accomplished to prevent symptomatic post-traumatic osteoarthritis. If a severely comminuted Rolando fracture is present and cannot be anatomically reduced, then simpler immobilization is provided.

Teaching point

It is important to identify a Bennett fracture in the setting of thumb trauma since this injury requires good reduction and fixation to prevent osteoarthritis. The same also holds true for a minimally comminuted Rolando fracture. If a Bennett fracture is missed, then the patient has the likelihood of developing symptomatic osteoarthritis in just a few years.

READING LIST

Bennett EH. The classic. On fracture of the metacarpal bone of the thumb. By Edward H. Bennett, 1886. *Clin Orthop Relat Res* 1987; **220**:3–6.

Huang JI, Fernandez DL. Fractures of the base of the thumb metacarpal. *Instr Course Lect* 2010;**59**:343–356.

Soyer AD. Fractures of the base of the first metacarpal: current treatment options. *J Am Acad Orthop Surg* 1999;7:403–412.

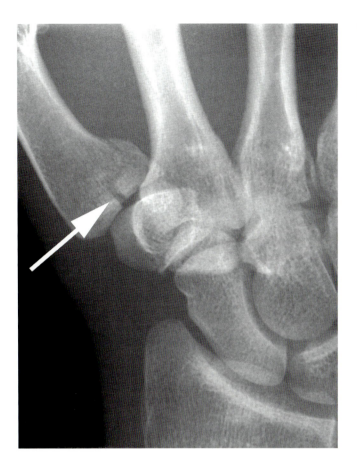

Figure 39.1 Bennett fracture. This image is a coned down AP view of the wrist. The arrow points to a simple intra-articular fracture at the base of the first metacarpal. If reduction cannot be maintained with casting/splinting, then the fracture will have to be treated with percutaneous pinning until osseous healing starts.

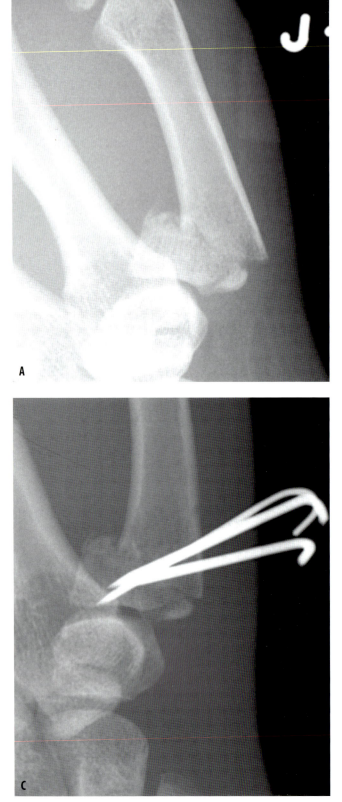

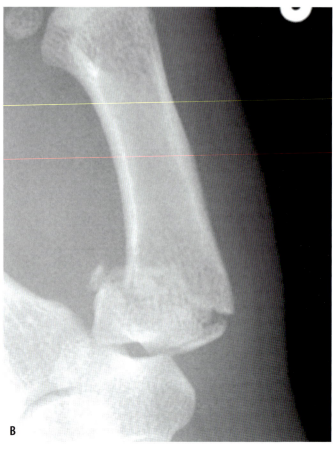

Figure 39.2 An intra-articular, comminuted fracture (Rolando fracture) can be seen at the base of the first metacarpal on images (A) and (B). Since this particular patient's fracture was only mildly comminuted, reduction and percutaneous pinning was attempted as seen in image (C).

Imaging description

Mallet (or baseball) finger is used to describe traumatic avulsion of the extensor tendon from the dorsal base of the distal phalanx or a traumatic avulsion fracture of bone from the dorsal base of the distal phalanx. This traumatic avulsion is caused by sudden flexion at the distal interphalangeal (DIP) joint while the finger is extended. If the injury is confined to the soft tissues, then radiographic images will demonstrate soft tissue swelling and fullness centered about the DIP joint of the involved digit. If the mallet finger involves an avulsion fracture, then this is best seen on the lateral radiographic view of the digit. The avulsion fragment is seen to arise from the dorsal base of the distal phalanx (Figure 40.1). Advanced imaging is usually not indicated.

Importance

A mallet finger injury must be identified, as it needs to be treated early to prevent proximal migration and retraction of the extensor mechanism of the digit. After retraction of the tendon occurs, it becomes more difficult to treat mallet finger and requires surgical intervention. Untreated mallet finger will lead to increasing imbalanced extensor tone at the proximal interphalangeal joint relative to the DIP joint. This imbalance will cause development of a biomechanically debilitating swan neck deformity of the involved digit. Both the mallet finger injury confined to the soft tissues and the mallet finger injury with a non-displaced small avulsion fracture fragment (<50% of the articular surface) are treated with a simple splint for several weeks. A displaced fracture or a large fracture requires reduction and fixation by a surgeon.

Typical clinical scenario

A 21-year-old male presents with a left long finger that was jammed while trying to catch a softball line drive with the bare hands. There is focal soft tissue swelling centered about the DIP joint of this long finger. Given this clinical scenario and physical exam findings, a mallet finger is diagnosed. A radiograph is obtained to determine if the injury involves a displaced avulsion fracture fragment or a large fracture fragment. The treatment (splinting versus reduction and fixation) is based on the radiographic findings.

Teaching point

When the history of a jammed finger is known, a mallet finger can be diagnosed if there is focal soft tissue swelling about the DIP joint or if there is an avulsion fracture from the dorsal aspect of the base of the distal phalanx. This fracture is treated conservatively with splinting unless there is a displaced fracture (>2 mm) or a large fracture fragment (>50% of the articular surface involved). Even though this fracture is commonly treated conservatively, it must be treated diligently with a splint for several weeks to prevent a debilitating swan neck deformity of the finger. Strict splinting is usually done for at least 8 weeks to ensure the injury is well on its way to healing before any significant motion is allowed at the DIP joint.

READING LIST

Bendre AA, Hartigan BJ, Kalainov DM. Mallet finger. *J Am Acad Orthop Surg* 2005;**13**:336–344.

Leinberry C. Mallet finger injuries. *J Hand Surg Am* 2009;**34**: 1715–1717.

Okafor B, Mbubaegbu C, Munshi I, Williams DJ. Mallet deformity of the finger. Five-year follow-up of conservative treatment. *J Bone Joint Surg Br* 1997;**79**:544–547.

Schaffer TC. Common hand fractures in family practice. *Arch Fam Med* 1994;**3**:982–987.

Pearls and Pitfalls in Musculoskeletal Imaging, ed. D. Lee Bennett and Georges Y. El-Khoury. Published by Cambridge University Press. © Cambridge University Press 2013.

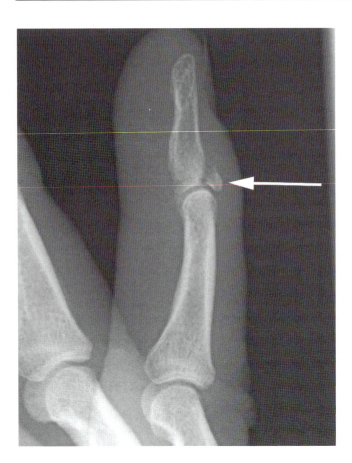

Figure 40.1 A dorsal avulsion fracture fragment is seen at the base of the distal phalanx of this finger (arrow). Since this fracture involved less than 50% of the articular surface, it was treated with closed reduction and splinting.

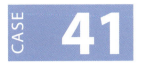

CASE 41

Volar plate injuries of the finger

Imaging description

A volar plate fracture of the finger is used to describe a traumatic avulsion fracture of bone from the volar lip of the base of the middle phalanx. The fracture fragment is best seen on the lateral radiographic view of the finger and is seen to arise from the volar lip of the middle phalangeal base (Figure 41.1). This avulsion fracture is caused by sudden traumatic hyperextension at the proximal interphalangeal (PIP) joint while the finger is mildly flexed. Because the connective tissue of the volar plate is thick, an isolated rupture of the volar plate without an avulsion fracture is rare. Advanced imaging is usually not indicated.

Importance

A volar plate fracture of the middle phalanx must be identified, as it needs to be treated early to prevent chronic pain, stiffness, and swelling. Untreated volar plate fractures will lead to increasing pain, instability, and stiffness. A non-displaced, small (<30% of the articular surface) volar plate fracture can be treated conservatively with a splint for a few weeks. If the fragment is displaced or larger, the injury should be evaluated by and potentially treated by a surgeon.

Typical clinical scenario

A 22-year-old male presents with a right ring finger injury that was caused by forced hyperextension of the finger while playing football the night before. There is significant focal pain and swelling about the PIP of the ring finger. The treating physician closely examines the digit to ensure there is no appreciable instability at the joint. A radiograph of the ring finger is obtained to determine if there is a displaced or large fracture fragment, as this will require evaluation by a surgeon with potential surgical treatment. The radiograph is also obtained to ensure there is no significant subluxation at the PIP joint of the right ring finger as this may also require evaluation by a surgeon.

Teaching point

A volar plate fracture of the middle phalanx can be diagnosed if there is an avulsion fracture from the volar aspect of the base of the middle phalanx. This fracture is treated conservatively with short-term splinting unless there is persistent dorsal subluxation of the PIP joint associated with the fracture or a large fracture fragment (>30% of the articular surface involved) is present. Even though this fracture is commonly treated conservatively, it must be treated surgically if there is any evidence of instability in order to prevent chronic pain and stiffness of the PIP joint.

READING LIST

Bendre AA, Hartigan BJ, Kalainov DM. Mallet finger. *J Am Acad Orthop Surg* 2005; **13**:336–344.

Calfee RP, Sommerkamp TG. Fracture-dislocation about the finger joints. *J Hand Surg Am* 2009;**34**:1140–1147.

Schaffer TC. Common hand fractures in family practice. *Arch Fam Med* 1994;**3**:982–987.

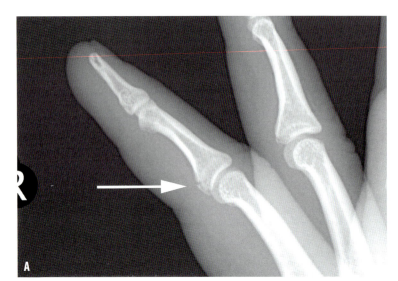
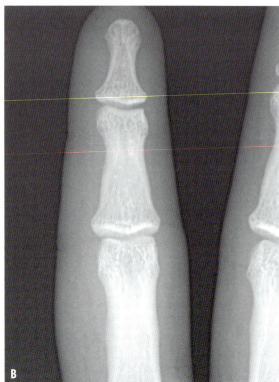

Figure 41.1 A subtle volar rim fracture (white arrow) at the base of the middle phalanx of the right index finger is present on this lateral radiograph (**A**). The PA radiograph of the index finger (**B**) demonstrates soft tissue swelling at and proximal to the proximal interphalangeal joint of this digit.

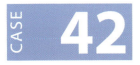

CASE 42

Subungual glomus tumor of the distal phalanges

Imaging description

A subungual glomus tumor is usually not visible on radiographs unless it is causing erosion of the dorsal surface of the distal phalanx (Figure 42.1). This is readily differentiated from exostosis, which is seen as an osseous protuberance rather than an erosion (Figure 42.2). MRI has visualized subungual glomus tumors as small as 2mm in size. The classic MRI appearance is iso- or hypointense on T1-weighted images, hyperintense on T2-weighted images, and strong enhancement with IV contrast.

Importance

Subungual glomus tumors need to be preoperatively identified. Subungual glomus tumors can be suspected by their characteristic clinical manifestation. However, because glomus tumors cannot be detected by visual inspection or palpation, they are sometimes diagnosed wrongly. Even if the clinical diagnosis is correct, surgery without knowing the exact size and location of the glomus tumor may result in incomplete excision, and thus recurrence. It is possible that no tumor is found by surgery leading to unnecessary deformity of the nail bed and finger. The combination of the correct clinical manifestation and MRI appearance is helpful in preventing unwarranted or unsuccessful surgeries.

Typical clinical scenario

A 50-year-old female presents with tenderness and pain in the nail bed of the right thumb. The pain has been present for a few years with severe attacks of pain when the digit is exposed to cold. The nail bed is painful with palpation; however, no definite mass is palpable. A radiograph was normal; however, an MRI showed a T1 isointense, T2 hyperintense, and intensely enhancing mass in the subungual area of the thumb. This was diagnosed as a subungual glomus tumor.

Teaching point

With the correct clinical history, the radiographic finding of a dorsal erosion on the dorsal aspect of the distal phalanx is diagnostic for a subungual glomus tumor of the digit. MRI is also useful in appropriate preoperative planning as well as the diagnosis (when radiographs are non-contributory) of a glomus tumor.

READING LIST

Baek HJ, Lee SJ, Cho KH et al. Subungual tumors: clinicopathologic correlation with US and MR imaging findings. *Radiographics* 2010;**30**:1621–1636.

Drapé JL, Idy-Peretti I, Goettmann S et al. Subungual glomus tumors: evaluation with MR imaging. *Radiology* 1995;**195**:507–515.

Koc O, Kivrak AS, Paksoy Y. Subungual glomus tumour: magnetic resonance imaging findings. *Australas Radiol* 2007;**51**: B107–B109.

Opdenakker G, Gelin G, Palmers Y. MR imaging of a subungual glomus tumor. *AJR Am J Roentgenol* 1999;**172**:250–251.

Takemura N, Fujii N, Tanaka T. Subungual glomus tumor diagnosis based on imaging. *J Dermatol* 2006; **33**:389–393.

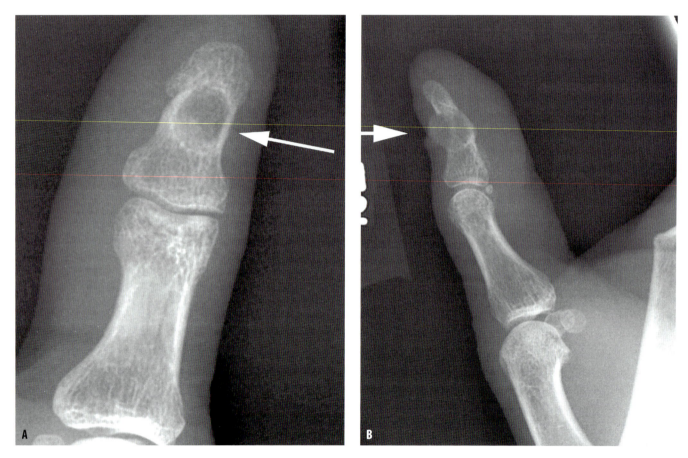

Figure 42.1 A 50-year-old female with a glomus tumor of the right thumb. The AP radiograph (**A**) demonstrates an apparent intraosseous lytic lesion in the distal phalanx; however, the lateral radiograph (**B**) shows that this lesion is an erosion along the dorsal aspect of this phalanx cause by a subungual glomus tumor (arrow).

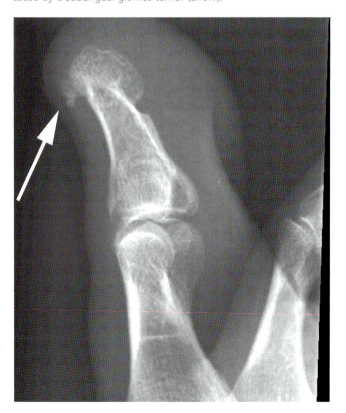

Figure 42.2 Lateral radiograph of the great toe showing a subungual exostosis (arrow) arising from the dorsal surface of the distal phalanx.

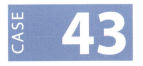
Imaging description

Two normal muscle variants that are commonly described in the literature are the accessory abductor digiti minimi muscle and the extensor digitorum brevis manus muscle (Figure 43.1). On MRI, normal variant muscle tissue signal characteristics will follow that of normal muscle. The accessory abductor digiti minimi can originate at the palmar carpal ligament, the tendon of the palmaris longus muscle, or the antebrachial fascia of the forearm. It inserts at the volar, ulnar aspect of the base of the proximal phalanx of the small finger. On transverse MR images, it is a fusiform mass with the signal characteristics of muscle located volar, lateral to the pisiform bone. The extensor digitorum brevis manus originates from the distal radius and dorsal radiocarpal ligament with an insertion on the index or long finger. On MRI, it is identified as an accessory muscle just ulnar to the extensor tendon of the index or long finger at or distal to the wrist.

Importance

These muscles can be misdiagnosed clinically as a mass or inflammatory process. This usually occurs when these variant muscles are prominent or hypertrophied. The accessory abductor digiti minimi muscle is somewhat common, occurring in as many as 25% of the population. In addition, when an accessory abductor digiti minimi muscle is prominent it can cause a compressive neuropathy of the ulnar nerve.

Typical clinical scenario

A 35-year-old male presents with a somewhat soft palpable mass along the volar, ulnar aspect of the fifth metacarpal. The mass is slightly difficult to palpate on physical exam, but it appears to be somewhat soft. An MRI is ordered to confirm the clinical suspicion of a ganglion cyst. The MRI does not reveal a ganglion cyst; however, it demonstrates an accessory abductor digiti minimi muscle at the location of the suspected mass.

Teaching point

MRI easily identifies the above normal variant muscles since their signal characteristics are identical to normal muscle. These normal muscle variants can be clinically confused with a neoplastic mass, ganglion cyst, or inflammatory mass. The accessory abductor digiti minimi can also be a cause of compressive ulnar neuropathy when it is hypertrophic or prominent.

READING LIST

De Smet L. Median and ulnar nerve compression at the wrist caused by anomalous muscles. *Acta Orthop Belg* 2002;**68**:431–438.

Harvie P, Patel N, Ostlere SJ. Prevalence and epidemiological variation of anomalous muscles at Guyon's canal. *J Hand Surg Br* 2004;**29**:26–29.

Stein JM, Cook TS, Simonson S, Kim W. Normal and variant anatomy of the wrist and hand on MR imaging. *Magn Reson Imaging Clin N Am* 2011;**19**:595–608.

Timins ME. Muscular anatomic variants of the wrist and hand: findings on MR imaging. *AJR Am J Roentgenol* 1999;**172**:1397–1401.

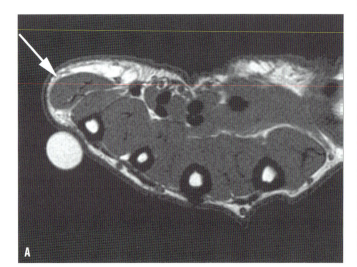
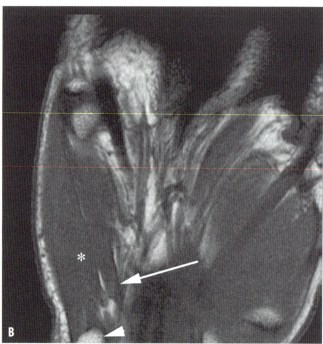

Figure 43.1 A 35-year-old male with a palpable mass just lateral to the neck of the fifth metacarpal. An MRI was performed to rule out a soft tissue mass. On T1-weighted transverse images, there is prominent musculature just medial to the fifth metacarpal neck (arrow) corresponding to the palpable abnormality (**A**). Coronal T1-weighted MR images (**B**) demonstrated an accessory muscle (arrow) located lateral to the pisiform (arrowhead) and the normal abductor digiti minimi (asterisk). It was felt the accessory muscle was either an accessory abductor digit minimi or an accessory abductor digiti minimi longus. The palpable abnormality had signal characteristics of muscle on all MRI sequences. It was felt that the accessory muscle contributed to the palpable prominence of the abductor digiti minimi in this patient.

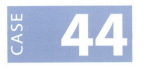

Painful intraosseous hand enchondroma: pathologic fracture

Imaging description

Radiographically, an enchondroma in the hand is seen as a geographic lytic lesion. Approximately 50% of the time it will contain calcifications characteristic of a chondroid matrix, with popcorn-like dots, arcs, and whirls (Figure 44.1). Enchondromas can cause visible endosteal scalloping or thinning of the cortex; however, an isolated enchondroma should not have an aggressive appearance. MRI is not indicated usually for enchondromas involving the hand. Pathologic fractures can be a frank, easily seen displaced fracture; however, they may also demonstrate only subtle discontinuity of the cortex on radiographs (Figure 44.2).

Importance

An enchondroma involving the hand should not be painful. If pain is present, then one must carefully look for a subtle fracture (Figure 44.2). If a fracture is not present, then the lesion is not likely to be an enchondroma and further evaluation would be warranted. Pathologic fractures of an enchondroma may not have an antecedent history of trauma, especially if the overlying cortex is fairly thin. Pathologic fractures of enchondromas account for approximately 80% of pathologic fractures in the hand. Most of the fractures occur in the proximal phalanx (approximately 51% of hand pathologic fractures) and in the small finger (approximately 45%).

Typical clinical scenario

A 25-year-old female presents with a two-week history of pain over the proximal phalanx of the right index finger. The pain started while she was washing dishes. She has no known trauma. A radiograph was taken that demonstrated an enchondroma with a subtle pathologic fracture (Figure 44.2). This fracture was treated and the pain resolved.

Teaching point

Benign enchondromas of the hand should not be associated with pain. If the radiograph demonstrates an apparent enchondroma, then one should carefully examine the image for a subtle pathologic fracture. Approximately 50% of enchondromas will contain calcifications indicating the presence of a chondroid matrix.

READING LIST

Eisenberg RL. Bubbly lesions of bone. *AJR Am J Roentgenol* 2009;**193**: W79–W94.

Shenoy R, Pillai A, Reid R. Tumours of the hand presenting as pathological fractures. *Acta Orthop Belg* 2007;**73**:192–195.

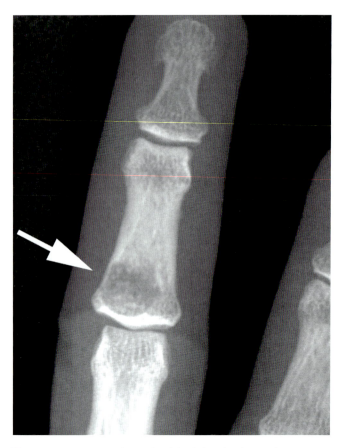

Figure 44.1 An AP radiograph of the left index finger shows popcorn-like dots (arrow) within the enchondroma of the middle phalanx.

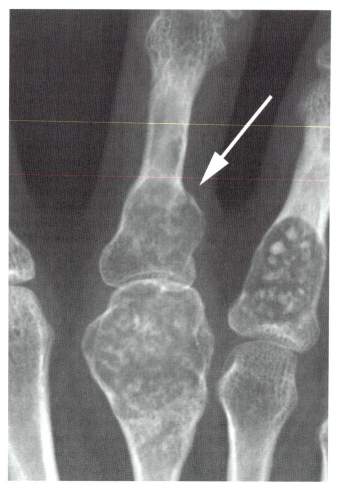

Figure 44.2 A 25-year-old female with Ollier's disease and new onset of pain in the proximal phalanx of the long finger. This AP radiograph of the left long finger reveals a subtle, lucent disruption of the cortex (arrow) near the base of the proximal phalanx. This was a non-displaced pathologic fracture of the enchondroma at this location, and it was responsible for the new onset of the patient's pain.

Femoroacetabular impingement: cam- versus pincer-type

Imaging description

Femoroacetabular impingement (FAI) is a common cause of hip pain and eventual osteoarthritis of the hip. It is screened for using an AP radiograph of the pelvis. The radiograph must be aligned as perfectly as possible with the coccyx centered at the symphysis pubis so that no rotation of the pelvis is present. Femoroacetabular impingement is broken down into three major categories: cam-type, pincer-type, and mixed type. Patients with the mixed type of FAI have coexistence of both the cam- and pincer-type. The cam-type can be thought of as abnormal formation/development of the femoral head/neck junction. This can be seen as an osseous bump or as a pistol grip deformity (loss of normal concavity) at the femoral head/ neck junction (Figure 45.1). The pincer-type of FAI is abnormal coverage or positioning of the acetabulum. The pincer-type can be diagnosed on radiographs by the presence of coxa profunda, acetabular protrusion, or acetabular retroversion. Coxa profunda and acetabular protrusion are diagnosed radiographically by abnormal positioning of the femoral head and acetabulum relative to the ilioischial line (Figure 45.2). Acetabular retroversion can be diagnosed by presence of the cross-over sign, posterior acetabular wall sign, or the prominent ischial spine sign (Figure 45.3).

Importance

Femoroacetabular impingement is important to recognize in patients with hip pain as treatment of this disease has the best outcome if it is recognized early so that osteoarthritis has not yet developed. Development of osteoarthritis is felt to be the eventual outcome in symptomatic FAI patients if the disease goes untreated. The basic pathology is abnormal abutment of the femoral head/neck junction on the acetabular rim during flexion. This abutment causes labral and cartilage damage at the hip leading to incongruity of the hip joint. Continued usage of an incongruous joint leads to the development of osteoarthritis.

Symptomatic cam-type FAI is most common in young athletic males while symptomatic pincer-type FAI is most common in athletic middle-aged women. It is important to know that at present, radiographic findings of FAI are not treated if the patient is asymptomatic; that is, if the findings are incidental. At present, the eventual outcome of patients with so-called asymptomatic FAI is not known.

Typical clinical scenario

A 20-year-old male football player presents with groin pain especially with deep flexion. The pain has become progressively worse. It is exacerbated by prolonged walking, athletic activities, and prolonged sitting. Radiographic screening studies of the pelvis demonstrated cam-type FAI. A MR arthrogram of the hip demonstrated a labral tear. The patient was treated successfully with surgery.

Teaching point

Femoroacetabular impingement is a cause of hip pain. Treatment of FAI is more successful if diagnosed prior to the development of osteoarthritis. Asymptomatic radiographic findings indicating FAI are not treated at present.

READING LIST

Anderson SE, Siebenrock KA, Tannaast M. Femoroacetabular impingement. *Eur J Radiol* 2012;**81**:3740–3744.

Imam S, Khanduja V. Current concepts in the diagnosis and management of femoroacetabular impingement. *Int Orthop* 2011;**35**:1427–1435.

Laborie LB, Lehmann TG, Engesæter IØ et al. Prevalence of radiographic findings thought to be associated with femoroacetabular impingement in a population-based cohort of 2081 healthy young adults. *Radiology* 2011;**260**:494–502.

Werner CM, Copeland CE, Ruckstuhl T et al. Radiographic markers of acetabular retroversion: correlation of the cross-over sign, ischial spine sign and posterior wall sign. *Acta Orthop Belg* 2010;**76**:166–173.

Pearls and Pitfalls in Musculoskeletal Imaging, ed. D. Lee Bennett and Georges Y. El-Khoury. Published by Cambridge University Press. © Cambridge University Press 2013.

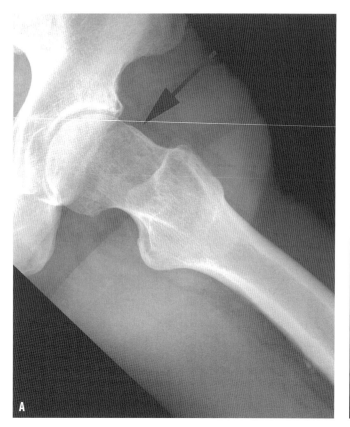

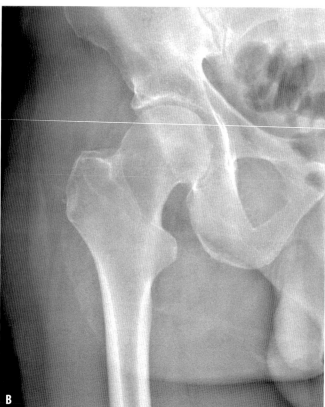

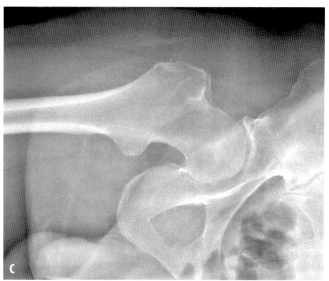

Figure 45.1 A frog-leg lateral view of the left hip (**A**) demonstrates an abnormal osseous bump (arrow) at the junction of the femoral head and neck. This osseous abnormality can be associated with cam-type femoroacetabular impingement. The AP views of a right hip (**B** and **C**) demonstrate the pistol grip deformity. This is easier to conceptualize on the rotated AP view (**C**) where one can see how the proximal femur and femoral head have the appearance of an old-fashioned pistol grip.

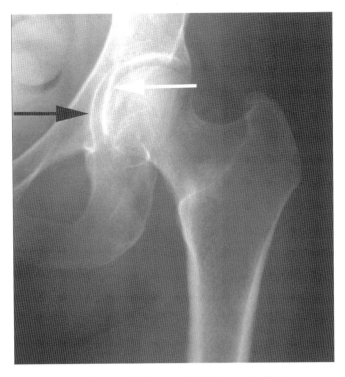

Figure 45.2 A 32-year-old female with left hip pain. This is a cropped image from an AP pelvis radiograph isolated to the left hip. One can see that coxa profunda is present in that the acetabulum (black arrow) projects medial to the ilioischial line (white arrow). Coxa profunda can be associated with symptomatic pincer-type femoroacetabular impingement.

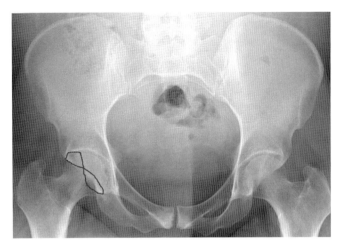

Figure 45.3 A 25-year-old female with bilateral hip pain. This AP radiograph of the pelvis demonstrates a cross-over sign at both hips, which is a sign of acetabular retroversion. Acetabular retroversion can be a cause of hip pain from femoroacetabular impingement. On this image, the cross-over sign is traced on the right acetabulum for demonstration purposes.

Imaging description

Snapping hip can be classified as either the external type or the internal type. The external type is readily diagnosed by clinical evaluation so medical imaging is seldom performed. The external type is usually caused by a thickened or tight iliotibial band or by thickening of the anterior edge of the gluteus maximus. This thickened edge can be associated with atrophy of the bulk of the gluteus maximus muscle.

The internal type of snapping hip is related to intra-articular pathology or to snapping of the iliopsoas tendon over the iliopectineal eminence (Figure 46.1). Ultrasound is the medical imaging test of choice if a radiograph does not demonstrate any evidence of intra-articular pathology or osteoarthritis. Dynamic US will show an abnormal, sudden jerky motion of the iliopsoas tendon when the patient repeats the hip motion that causes the snapping. If the patient is unable to voluntarily repeat the motion that causes the painful snapping, then the patient is placed in a supine position and instructed to move the hip and leg from a position of flexion, external rotation, and abduction (the so-called frog-leg position) into a position of full extension, adduction, and internal rotation. This may cause a reproduction of the painful snapping.

Static US imaging in the transverse and sagittal planes is done of the iliopsoas tendon along the course of the tendon to its attachment to the lesser trochanter. The tendon is easily seen as a hyperechoic structure surrounded by the more hypoechoic muscle tissue about the tendon (Figure 46.2).

Importance

When external types of hip snapping have been ruled out, medical imaging plays an important role in diagnosing the cause of the internal hip snapping. The most common approach is radiography of the pelvis and affected hip. If this is negative and snapping of the iliopsoas is a possibility, a static and dynamic US of the hip is performed. The combination of radiography and US evaluation has been shown to diagnose the cause of the internal type of hip snapping in approximately 80% of the patients. MR evaluation is reserved if the painful hip snapping persists and the combined radiographic and US evaluation was non-diagnostic.

Typical clinical scenario

A 20-year-old male football player presents with hip snapping and groin pain especially with flexion. The pain has become progressively worse. It is exacerbated by prolonged walking, athletic activities, and prolonged sitting. Radiographic screening studies of the pelvis were normal. Dynamic US demonstrated a snapping iliopsoas tendon. Another advantage of US is that if snapping of the iliopsoas is demonstrated then contemporaneous conservative treatment with corticosteroid injection can be performed.

Teaching point

Radiography and US evaluation are the mainstay medical imaging paradigm when evaluating for internal types of painful hip snapping. MRI is a useful adjunct when radiography and US fail. MR can demonstrate labral pathology, osteonecrosis, loose bodies, and other pathology that may have been missed by radiography or US. MR arthrography is the preferred medical imaging test if labral pathology is suspected.

READING LIST

Blankenbaker DG, De Smet AA, Keene JS. Sonography of the iliopsoas tendon and injection of the iliopsoas bursa for diagnosis and management of the painful snapping hip. *Skeletal Radiol* 2006;**35**:565–571.

Krishnamurthy G, Connolly BL, Naravanan U, Babyn PS. Imaging findings in external snapping hip syndrome. *Pediatr Radiol* 2007;**37**:1272–1274.

Tatu L, Parratte B, Vuillier F, Diop M, Monnier G. Descriptive anatomy of the femoral portion of the iliopsoas muscle. Anatomical basis of anterior snapping of the hip. *Surg Radiol Anat* 2001;**23**:371–374.

Wunderbaldinger P, Bremer C, Matuszewski L *et al.* Efficient radiological assessment of the internal snapping hip syndrome. *Eur Radiol* 2001;**11**:1743–1747.

Pearls and Pitfalls in Musculoskeletal Imaging, ed. D. Lee Bennett and Georges Y. El-Khoury. Published by Cambridge University Press. © Cambridge University Press 2013.

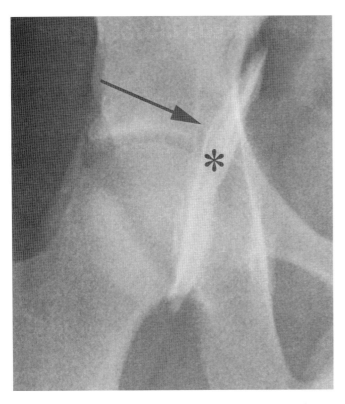

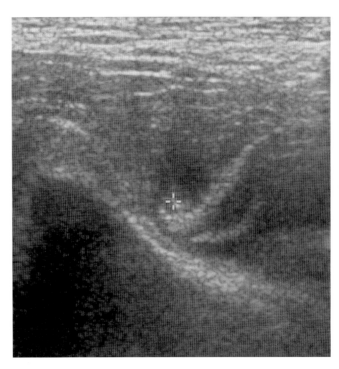

Figure 46.1 This is a spot image from a fluoroscopic study of the iliopsoas tendon sheath, which is outlined with contrast (*). This tendon extends by the iliopectineal eminence (arrow).

Figure 46.2 Transverse US image of the iliopsoas tendon as it extends by the iliopectineal eminence. The hyperechoic tendon (+) is seen surrounded by the more hypoechoic muscle tissue.

Labral tear versus cleft versus labral recess

Imaging description

With medical imaging, labral tears of the hip are best diagnosed using MR arthrography. Tears are diagnosed usually when there is intralabral or sublabral interposition of contrast (Figure 47.1). Regardless of the contour or shape of sublabral contrast interposition, any contrast material interposition occurring in the upper one-half of the anterior labrum should be considered a tear. However, sublabral contrast material interposition that occurs in the anteroinferior aspect of the labrum (typically the 8 o'clock position), has a linear shape, is partial thickness, and is not associated with perilabral pathology/cysts should be considered a normal recess (Figure 47.2).

Importance

Initial reports of the sensitivity of MR arthrography for labral tears were around 92%. However, a few more recent studies have reported sensitivity as low as approximately 66%. One of the potential reasons for this discrepancy is misdiagnosing a labral tear as a sublabral recess. It is important for radiologists to be aware of morphologic variants located in the anterior labrum because most labral tears occur in this area as well. It is important to recognize that sublabral contrast material interposition that is partial-thickness, linear, has no associated perilabral pathology, and is located near the 8 o'clock position should be considered a normal variant (sublabral recess). Incorrectly diagnosing a sublabral recess as a labral tear may lead to unnecessary surgery and its associated morbidity.

Typical clinical scenario

A 35-year-old male with chronic left hip pain presents for evaluation. His pain is worse with activity, especially ascending and descending stairs. The pain is exacerbated by prolonged sitting and becomes sharp when he rises from a sitting position. On examination, he has left groin pain, reproduction of his symptoms with forced flexion with internal rotation of the hip. He also exhibits log rolling of the left lower extremity. There is clinical concern for intra-articular pathology of the left hip; however, the initial pelvis and hip radiographs are negative. A hip MR arthrogram was ordered to rule out a labral tear or other intra-articular pathology.

Differential diagnosis

If sublabral contrast material interposition is seen on the study at the anteroinferior aspect of the labrum the differential would be a labral tear versus a sublabral recess. Partial-thickness interposition of contrast, a smooth linear line of contrast, and absence of a perilabral cyst would favor a recess. Full-thickness interposition, rough and irregular contour, and the presence of a perilabral cyst would favor a labral tear.

Teaching point

Sublabral recesses occur as normal variants in the anteroinferior labrum (at approximately the 8 o'clock position). A linear shape and only partial interposition of contrast under the labrum coupled with the 8 o'clock position are characteristic findings of a normal sublabral recess.

READING LIST

Czerny C, Hofmann S, Urban M et al. MR arthrography of the adult acetabular capsular-labral complex: correlation with surgery and anatomy. AJR Am J Roentgenol 1999;**173**:345–349.

Ghebontni L, Roger B, El-khoury J, Brasseur JL, Grenier PA. MR arthrography of the hip: normal intra-articular structures and common disorders. Eur Radiol 2000;**10**:83–88.

Studler U, Kalberer F, Leunig M et al. MR arthrography of the hip: differentiation between an anterior sublabral recess as a normal variant and a labral tear. Radiology 2008;**249**:947–954.

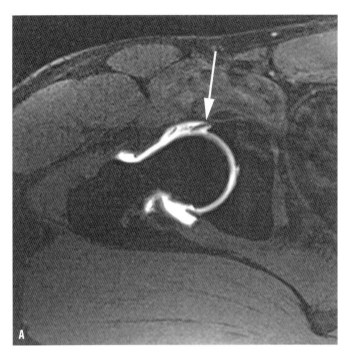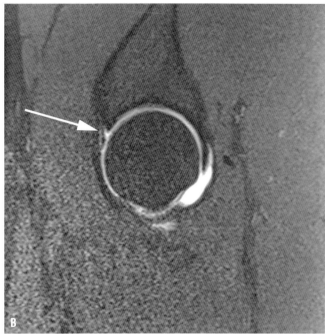

Figure 47.1 Right hip MR arthrogram in a 28-year-old male with right hip pain. The oblique axial image (**A**) and the parasagittal image (**B**) demonstrate intralabral and sublabral interposition of contrast (white arrow) at the anterosuperior aspect of the labrum (approximately the 10:30 o'clock position).

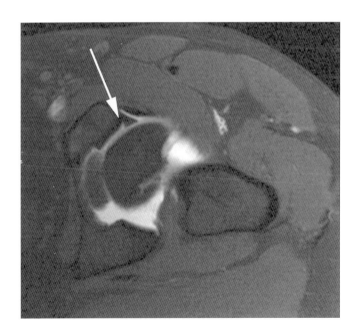

Figure 47.2 Left hip MR arthrogram in a 35-year-old male with a normal labral recess. This oblique axial MR image demonstrates a normal sublabral recess (white arrow) at the 8:00 o'clock position. Note its smooth contour and its only partial labral thickness extension.

Imaging description

When visible on radiographs, transient osteoporosis and osteonecrosis are quite distinct. Transient osteoporosis of the hip demonstrates radiographically marked osteoporosis. The osteoporosis can be so profound that the subchondral cortex of the head becomes nearly invisible. In contradistinction, when osteonecrosis is visible radiographically, it will have patchy areas of sclerosis or increased density (Figure 48.1). As the osteonecrosis progresses, areas of subchondral collapse and eventual osteoarthritis will develop.

In the earlier course of both of these diseases, the radiographs can be negative. However, MRI will be abnormal. Transient osteoporosis (or transient bone marrow edema of the hip, if osteoporosis never develops) demonstrates diffuse hypointense signal on T1-weighted images and diffuse high signal intensity on water-sensitive sequences (Figure 48.2). MRI of osteonecrosis of the hip may also demonstrate diffusely abnormal bone marrow signal that appears edematous; however, there should be a superimposed focus of infarct. This area of infarct will be seen as a large area of high T1-weighted signal surrounded by a serpentine border of low signal intensity (Figure 48.3). This border may also exhibit the double-line sign of adjacent marked high and low signal on T2-weighted images.

One should also remember that both transient osteoporosis and osteonecrosis are susceptible to superimposed insufficiency fractures. This will have the classic appearance of a fracture line and will parallel the subchondral bone of the femoral head (Figure 48.4).

Importance

The distinction between transient osteoporosis (transient bone marrow edema) and osteonecrosis is important because of their different outcomes. Transient osteoporosis is a self-limited disease that usually spontaneously resolves in 6–12 months. Treatment is palliative pain control until the disease resolves. Osteonecrosis is generally a progressive disease that eventually develops subchondral bone collapse causing loss of congruency of the hip joint. This loss of congruency leads to the development of severe secondary osteoarthritis over time. Most commonly this disease is eventually treated with a hip prosthesis when the symptoms become intolerable for the patient.

Typical clinical scenario

Transient osteoporosis is most commonly observed in middle-aged men. It has also been described in pregnancy during the third trimester. The clinical course of this disease has three phases. The initial phase is typically heralded by rapid onset of hip pain. The pain worsens until the plateau phase is reached. During the plateau phase the pain can persist for several months with no change. Eventually, the disease enters the final phase of pain resolution where the pain slowly subsides with the eventually disappearance of all symptoms by 6–12 months.

Osteonecrosis of the hip presents as the gradual onset of groin pain that can radiate to the knee. The pain is exacerbated by movement of the hip, especially internal rotation.

Differential diagnosis

Somewhat diffuse bone marrow edema of the hip can be seen with transient osteoporosis, osteonecrosis, and subchondral insufficiency fracture.

Teaching point

Transient osteoporosis and osteonecrosis of the hip should be distinguished from one another based on their MRI appearance. Osteonecrosis should have a focal necrotic area in the subchondral bone. Bone marrow edema of the femoral head can also be caused by a subchondral insufficiency fracture, which has a characteristic fracture line located just below the subchondral bone of the hip and paralleling the subchondral bone. Subchondral fractures can occur as a complication of both transient osteoporosis and osteonecrosis of the hip.

READING LIST

Vande Berg BC, Lecouvet FE, Koutaissoff S, Simoni P, Malghem J. Bone marrow edema of the femoral head and transient osteoporosis of the hip. *Eur J Radiol* 2008;**67**:68–77.

Watson RM, Roach NA, Dalinka MK. Avascular necrosis and bone marrow edema syndrome. *Radiol Clin North Am* 2004;**42**:207–219.

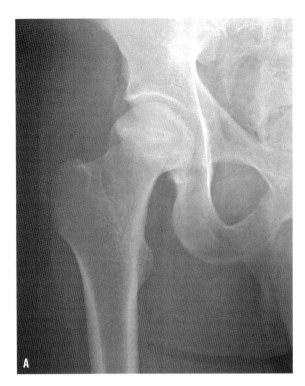
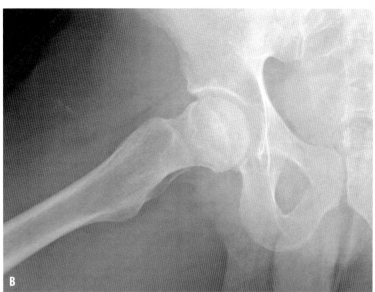

Figure 48.1 A 41-year-old male with osteonecrosis of the right hip. Anteroposterior (**A**) and lateral (**B**) views of the right hip demonstrate areas of patchy sclerosis and patchy lucency in the femoral head, which is a radiographic sign of osteonecrosis that can precede subchondral collapse.

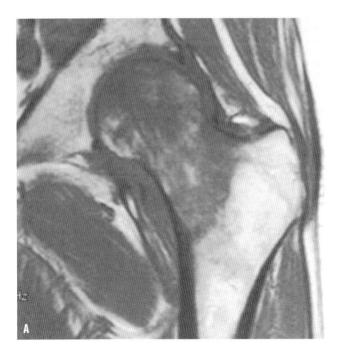
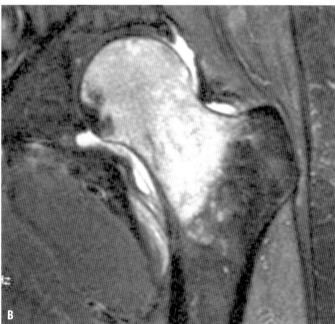

Figure 48.2 A 40-year-old male with a diagnosis of transient osteoporosis of the left hip. MR images with both T1-weighted (**A**) and STIR (**B**) sequences show the classic appearance of diffuse hypointense signal (**A**) and hyperintense signal (**B**) on T1-weighted and STIR sequences, respectively. A joint effusion is also present, which can be seen with transient osteoporosis of the hip.

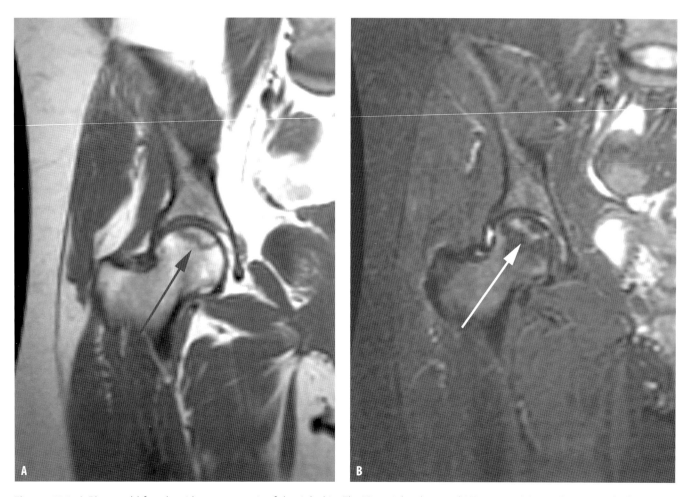

Figure 48.3 A 53-year-old female with osteonecrosis of the right hip. The T1-weighted coronal MR images (**A**) reveal an area of infarct that has hyperintense signal surrounded by a serpentine low signal border (arrow). The STIR sequence (**B**) also shows the area of infarct (arrow).

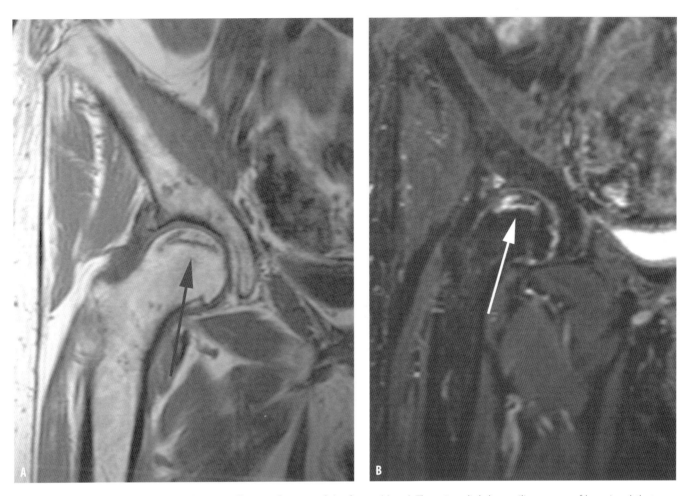

Figure 48.4 A 60-year-old female with an insufficiency fracture of the femoral head. There is a slightly curvilinear area of low signal that parallels the convex surface of the femoral head (arrow) on the coronal T1-weighted MR image (**A**). This fracture line can be seen as a corresponding area of hyperintense signal on the STIR sequence (arrow) (**B**).

Hip fractures in the elderly

Imaging description

The MRI appearance of a fracture is that of a linear or curvilinear focus of hypointensity on T1-weighted images that is either hyper- or hypointense on T2-weighted or STIR images (Figure 49.1). A limited MRI study with only coronal images is highly effective in ruling out a radiographically occult hip fracture in the elderly. Depending on the study, anywhere from 10–67% of hip fractures in the elderly seen on MRI are not visible on radiographs.

Importance

Between 10–67% of hip fractures in the elderly seen on MRI are not visible on radiographs. Early detection of occult hip fractures in the elderly has been shown to lower the risk of complications such as osteonecrosis, reduce the length of the hospital stay, and to reduce the overall cost for the patient. MRI can also demonstrate other causes of post-traumatic hip pain such as muscle strains, muscle ruptures, or pubic rami fractures (Figure 49.2).

Typical clinical scenario

An 80-year-old female presents to the emergency treatment center from an assisted living institution. Her caregiver reports that she is no longer ambulating. The patient does not remember any trauma or a fall. She describes some vague pain over the right hip. A radiograph was negative; however, an MRI demonstrated a basicervical hip fracture.

Teaching point

In an elderly patient with post-traumatic hip pain or in a patient that is a poor historian, MRI is used to rule out radiographically occult hip fractures to prevent unnecessary complications and potentially lower the overall morbidity.

READING LIST

Hossain M, Barwick C, Sinha AK, Andrew JG. Is magnetic resonance imaging (MRI) necessary to exclude occult hip fracture? *Injury* 2007;**38**:1204–1208.

Nachtrab O, Cassar-Pullicino VN, Lalam R *et al*. Role of MRI in hip fractures, including stress fractures, occult fractures, avulsion fractures. *Eur J Radiol* 2011, in press [Epub ahead of print].

Pandey R, McNally E, Ali A, Bulstrode C. The role of MRI in the diagnosis of occult hip fractures. *Injury* 1998;**29**:61–63.

Pearls and Pitfalls in Musculoskeletal Imaging, ed. D. Lee Bennett and Georges Y. El-Khoury. Published by Cambridge University Press. © Cambridge University Press 2013.

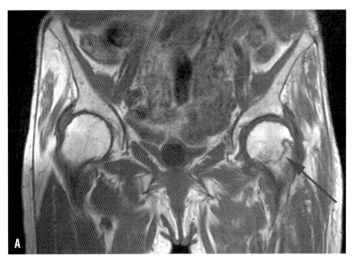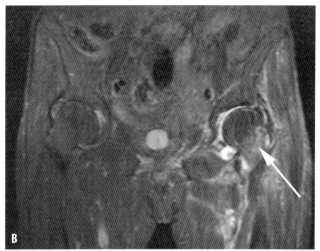

Figure 49.1 An 80-year-old female with a non-displaced left hip fracture that was radiographically occult. Coronal MR images demonstrate a hypointense fracture line (arrow) through the femoral neck on T1-weighted imaging (**A**). The fracture line is also hypointense on the STIR image (**B**) (arrow) with some surrounding bone marrow-like edema within the femoral neck.

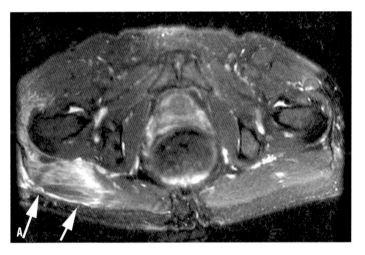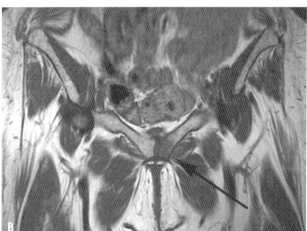

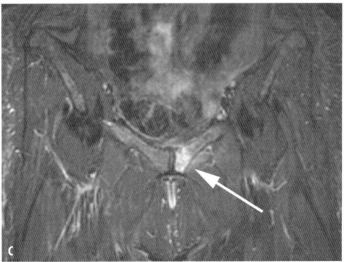

Figure 49.2 Magnetic resonance images in elderly patients demonstrating a traumatic muscle strain (arrows) of the gluteus maximus on an axial fat-suppressed T2-weighted image (**A**). A non-displaced pubic bone fracture can be seen on coronal T1-weighted (**B**) and STIR (**C**) images as shown by the arrows.

Insufficiency fractures of the pelvis

Imaging description

Radiographic studies of the pelvis may demonstrate insufficiency fractures of the pelvis. Pelvic insufficiency fractures most commonly occur in the sacrum, inferior pubic ramus, superior pubic ramus, ilium, and acetabulum. When insufficiency fractures of the pelvis are radiographically occult, they can be demonstrated by MRI. The MRI appearance of a fracture is that of a linear or curvilinear focus of hypointensity on T1-weighted images that is either hyper- or hypointense on T2-weighted or STIR images (Figure 50.1).

Importance

Pelvic insufficiency fractures can be a source of groin or pelvic pain in elderly women with underlying osteoporosis. In elderly women with a history of cancer, development of groin or pelvic pain can obviously raise concerns for recurrent or metastatic disease. Pelvic insufficiency fractures are frequently unrecognized on radiographs due to their subtle or occult appearance. When the radiograph is negative in this type of clinical scenario, MRI is helpful in differentiating tumor from an insufficiency fracture as the cause of the new pain. Finally, pelvic insufficiency fractures can also be seen in any patient that has an underlying condition that has caused secondary osteoporosis or altered normal bone metabolism.

Typical clinical scenario

An 80-year-old female with a history of breast cancer presents to the family care clinic with new onset of right groin pain. One of the concerns of her physician is that she might have recurrent breast cancer in the form of metastatic disease to the osseous pelvis. A pelvic radiograph was performed and demonstrated an osteopenic appearance to the bones, but it was negative for any focal bone lesions. An MRI was then performed to rule out radiographically occult metastatic disease to the osseous pelvis. The MRI demonstrated insufficiency fractures involving the right pubic rami.

Teaching point

In a patient with osteoporosis or altered bone metabolism, new onset of groin pain or lower back (sacral) pain can be the result of a pelvic insufficiency fracture. If the radiographic exam fails to elucidate a cause of the pain, MRI is useful in demonstrating radiographically occult pelvic insufficiency fractures as well as other non-osseous causes of the pain. Finally, fatigue stress fractures in the pelvis can occur at the same location as insufficiency fractures in patients suffering from stress-related hip, buttock, or groin pain (Figure 50.1).

READING LIST

Grangier C, Garcia J, Howarth NR, May M, Rossier P. Role of MRI in the diagnosis of insufficiency fractures of the sacrum and acetabular roof. *Skeletal Radiol* 1997;**26**:517–524.

Kiuru MJ, Pihlajamaki HK, Ahovuo JA. Fatigue stress injuries of the pelvic bones and proximal femur: evaluation with MRI imaging. *Eur Radiol* 2003;**13**:605–611.

Otte MT, Helms CA, Fritz RC. MR imaging of supra-acetabular insufficiency fractures. *Skeletal Radiol* 1997;**26**:279–283.

Pearls and Pitfalls in Musculoskeletal Imaging, ed. D. Lee Bennett and Georges Y. El-Khoury. Published by Cambridge University Press. © Cambridge University Press 2013.

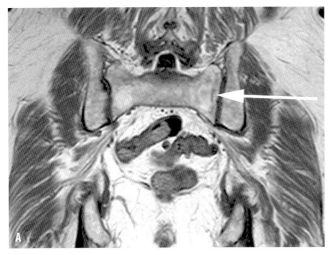

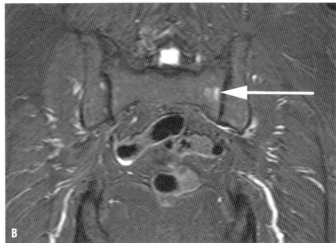

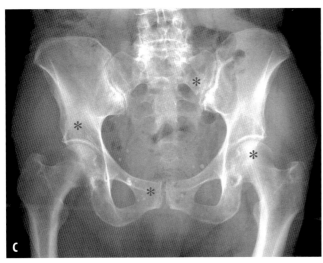

Figure 50.1 Coronal T1-weighted (**A**) and STIR (**B**) MR images demonstrate a vertically oriented insufficiency fracture (arrows) in the left sacral ala of this patient with a clinical diagnosis of osteoporosis. An AP radiograph of the pelvis (**C**) is shown with common locations for insufficiency fractures marked with asterisks. These common locations include the sacral ala, acetabular roof, femoral head/neck, and pubic rami.

Mild-to-moderate acetabular maldevelopment in the adult hip

Imaging description

Medical imaging evaluation of hip dysplasia or acetabular maldevelopment is primarily done by radiography. Strict attention to detailed technique is essential for accurately measuring the degree or severity of hip dysplasia. The most commonly used view is the AP radiograph of the pelvis. It should be done in the standing position with approximately 20° of internal rotation of the lower limbs. The focus film distance should be 100 cm. The imaging criteria for acceptance of a radiograph to evaluate for hip dysplasia are symmetric appearance of the obturator foramina, symmetric appearance of the iliac crests, and near superimposition of the coccyx with the symphysis pubis. Common measurements obtained on the pelvic AP radiograph are the center-edge angle, the horizontal toit externe angle, and the percentage of femoral head coverage. Some of these measurements require identification of the most medial point of the weight bearing acetabulum. The weightbearing portion of the acetabulum is identified by its sclerotic, arched appearance known as the sourcil (eyebrow) (Figure 51.1).

The second most commonly used radiographic view for measuring the degree of acetabular dysplasia is the false profile view. This view is obtained with the patient in the standing position with the pelvis rotated 65° relative to the film or detector. The imaging appearance criteria for acceptance of a false profile image as adequate for measuring acetabular dysplasia is if the distance between the two femoral heads is approximately the size of one femoral head. The vertical-center-anterior edge angle is measured on the false profile view (Figure 51.2). This view may also show early signs of osteoarthritis (small osteophytes and/or mild joint space narrowing) that is not yet seen on the AP view of the pelvis.

Computed tomography can also be used to evaluate for the severity of hip dysplasia in the adult population. A standardized CT technique is used for these acetabular measurements. First, a frontal scout view is obtained. Using the scout view for alignment, next a CT slice is obtained in the transverse plane. The plane should pass through the center of both femoral heads. From this transaxial CT image, the anterior acetabular sector angle, the posterior acetabular sector angle, and the horizontal acetabular sector angle can be measured (Figure 51.3).

Importance

Hip dysplasia can cause significant hip pain in the young adult, which may have been undiagnosed and asymptomatic throughout childhood. Symptomatic hip dysplasia that is left untreated can lead to early development of hip osteoarthritis in the young adult. Surgical outcomes for treating hip dysplasia discovered in adulthood are better if there is not significant osteoarthritis present at the time of surgery. There are currently available surgical treatments that can alleviate the hip pain and help prevent early onset of hip osteoarthritis. The measurements described above are most useful to the radiologist in diagnosing adult hip dysplasia when the dysplasia is not grossly severe on the radiograph.

Typical clinical scenario

A 25-year-old female presents with a two-week history of pain in both hips and the groin. The pain has been progressively getting worse over the past few years. Radiographs were obtained, and they revealed bilateral hip dysplasia. The hip dysplasia was treated with periacetabular osteotomies, and the patient is now asymptomatic.

Teaching point

In a young adult with hip pain, one should carefully scrutinize the pelvic radiographic study to rule out adult hip dysplasia as a potential cause. Measurements described above are useful if there is concern that dysplasia might be present. It is important to make this diagnosis so that surgical intervention can be provided to alleviate the patient's hip pain and to prevent potential hip osteoarthritis.

READING LIST

Delaunay S, Dussault RG, Kaplan PA, Alford BA. Radiographic measurements of dysplastic adult hips. *Skeletal Radiol* 1997;**26**:75–81.

Garbuz DS, Masri BA, Haddad F, Duncan CP. Clinical and radiographic assessment of the young adult with symptomatic hip dysplasia. *Clin Orthop Relat Res* 2004;**418**:18–22.

Jacobsen S. Adult hip dysplasia and osteoarthritis. Studies in radiology and clinical epidemiology. *Acta Orthop Suppl* 2006;**77**:1–37.

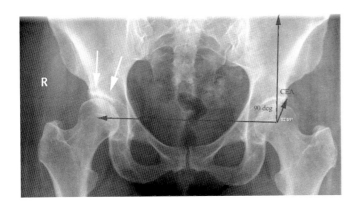

Figure 51.1 A 27-year-old female with bilateral hip dysplasia. An AP radiograph of the pelvis demonstrates (black arrows) how to measure the center-edge angle (CEA). The horizontal arrow connects the center point of both femoral heads. The vertical arrow is drawn perpendicular to the horizontal arrow with its base in the center of the femoral head. The oblique arrow extends from the center of the femoral head to the lateral lip of the acetabulum. The CEA is formed by the vertical and oblique arrows. The sourcil is present (white arrows); if it is absent, it usually indicates severe dysplasia of the hip.

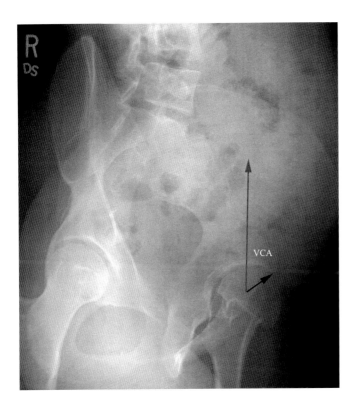

Figure 51.2 A 27-year-old female with hip dysplasia. This profile radiographic view shows (black arrows) how to measure the vertical-center-anterior edge angle (VCA). A vertical arrow is drawn with its base in the center of the femoral head. The oblique arrow connects the center of the femoral head with the anterior lip of the acetabulum.

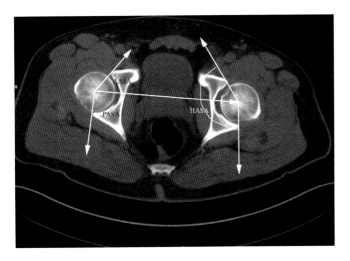

Figure 51.3 A 27-year-old female with hip dysplasia. This CT image demonstrates (white arrows) how to measure the anterior acetabular sector angle (AASA), the posterior acetabular sector angle (PASA), and the horizontal acetabular sector angle (HASA). The measurements are to be done on the transaxial slice through the center of both femoral heads.

Calcific tendinitis of the hip

Imaging description

Calcific tendinitis (also known as hydroxyapatite deposition disease) is best recognized on radiographic images. It appears as an area of amorphous calcification in the gluteal tendons near the greater trochanter, the iliopsoas tendon near the lesser trochanter, or the gluteus maximus tendon near the gluteal tuberosity of the femur (Figure 52.1). On MRI, the surrounding soft tissues will be edematous as evidenced by hyperintense signal on T2-weighted or STIR sequences.

Importance

Calcific tendinitis about the shoulder is well described and documented in the literature. Therefore, it is a well-known clinical entity. It is important to remember that calcific tendinitis is not confined to the shoulder but can occur within tendons at many different locations throughout the body. The hip is one of the more common locations for calcific tendinitis. When evaluating radiographic studies that include images of the hip, it is important to exclude amorphous calcifications near tendinous insertions as calcific tendinitis is a source of hip pain that can be readily treated with injection and aspiration.

Typical clinical scenario

A 44-year-old female presents with a 24-hour history of severe, debilitating left hip pain. The pain is non-radiating and is exacerbated significantly by any motion of the hip. There is significant pain with palpation over the greater trochanter. A radiograph demonstrated amorphous calcifications within the gluteus medius tendon near the greater trochanter. The calcification was aspirated under fluoroscopic guidance and then a corticosteroid/local anesthetic injection was performed. The patient exhibited immediate decrease in pain after the procedure.

Teaching point

As in the shoulder, amorphous calcifications about the hip at tendinous insertion sites are a sign of calcific tendinitis. This can be treated with imaging-guided aspiration and injection.

READING LIST

Bancroft LW, Blankenbaker DG. Imaging of the tendons about the pelvis. *AJR Am J Roentgenol* 2010;**195**:605–617.

Chow HY, Recht MP, Schils J, Calabrese LH. Acute calcific tendinitis of the hip: case report with magnetic resonance imaging findings. *Arthritis Rheum* 1997;**40**:974–977.

Kuroda H, Wada Y, Nishiguchi K *et al.* A case of probable hydroxyapatite deposition disease (HADD) of the hip. *Magn Reson Med Sci* 2004;**3**:141–144.

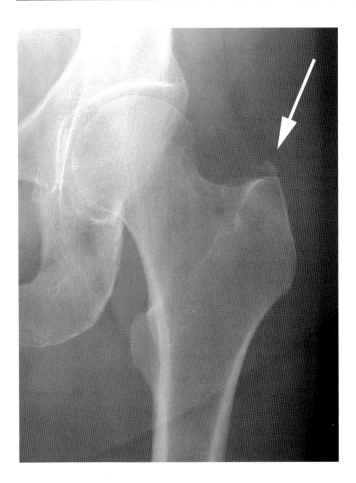

Figure 52.1 A 49-year-old male with left hip pain. An AP radiograph of the left hip demonstrates an amorphous calcification (arrow) immediately superior to the greater trochanter. This is calcific tendinitis involving the gluteus medius near its insertion.

Imaging description

Periprosthetic fractures involving the femur in the setting of hip arthroplasty are not rare. Periprosthetic acetabular fractures in the setting of arthroplasty are rare. Periprosthetic femur fractures are classified using the Vancouver classification system since it is reproducible and helps determine the type of treatment to be used. Fractures can occur at or about the femoral component or distal to the femoral component (Figure 53.1). They are readily detected on radiographs. A faint longitudinal linear lucency seen about the femoral stem tip in the immediate post-operative period may represent an artifact or longitudinal fracture; however, it can be treated conservatively (Figure 53.2).

Importance

Lesser trochanter and greater trochanter periprosthetic fractures are usually treated conservatively while femoral shaft perihardware fractures are treated with reduction and internal fixation (as long as the prosthesis is not loose). If there is hardware loosening present in addition to the fracture, then a revision arthoplasty with or without a graft is performed. A faint longitudinal linear lucency seen about the femoral stem tip in the immediate post-operative period may represent an artifact; however, it can be treated conservatively as well.

Typical clinical scenario

A 70-year-old female with a history of a right total hip arthroplasty 4 months ago presents with sudden onset of hip and right leg pain after a fall. She is unable to bear weight on the right leg. Radiographs demonstrate a femoral shaft fracture about the femoral stem of the right hip prosthesis. There is no evidence of perihardware loosening, and she has no clinical evidence of infection. The fracture was treated with reduction and interval fixation.

Teaching point

Trochanteric periprosthetic fractures are usually treated conservatively. Femoral shaft periprosthetic fractures in well-fixed prostheses usually require reduction and internal fixation with or without a graft. Loosened prostheses with a femoral shaft fracture generally require a revision arthroplasty. A faint longitudinal linear lucency seen about the femoral stem tip in the immediate postoperative period may represent an artifact; however, it can be treated conservatively.

READING LIST

Gaski GE, Scully SP. In brief: classifications in brief: Vancouver classification of postoperative periprosthetic femur fractures. *Clin Orthop Relat Res* 2011;**469**:1507–1510.

Masri BA, Meek RM, Duncan CP. Periprosthetic fractures evaluation and treatment. *Clin Orthop Relat Res* 2004;**420**:80–95.

Pearls and Pitfalls in Musculoskeletal Imaging, ed. D. Lee Bennett and Georges Y. El-Khoury. Published by Cambridge University Press. © Cambridge University Press 2013.

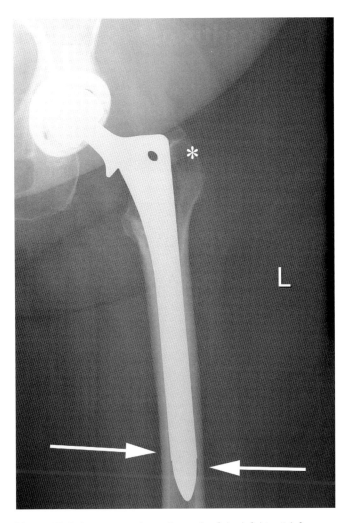

Figure 53.1 Anteroposterior radiograph of the left hip. A left total hip arthroplasy is present. The more common locations for periprosthetic fractures are near the distal portion of the femoral component (arrows) and at the area of the greater trochanter (asterisk).

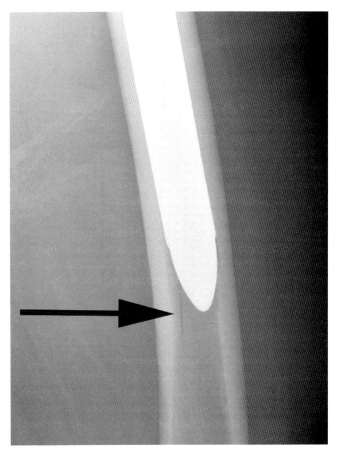

Figure 53.2 A 50-year-old male with an AP radiograph of the left hip demonstrating a non-displaced longitudinal fracture at the tip of the femoral prosthesis (arrow). This was treated conservatively and healed without the need for further surgical intervention.

54 Linea aspera versus periostitis of the femur

Imaging description

The linea aspera is an elevated crest or longitudinal ridge along the posterior aspect of slightly more than the middle third of the femur. Technically, the linea aspera refers only to the attachment sight of several musculotendinous structures while the term pilaster refers to the elevated crest and longitudinal ridge. Some of the musculotendinous attachments to the femur along the linea aspera are the adductor magnus, adductor longus, and short head of the biceps femoris. In the skeletally mature adult, the linea aspera is seen on a lateral radiographic view of the femur as an area of increased posterior cortical thickness with a rough or scalloped surface (Figure 54.1). This appearance can be mistaken for periostitis.

Importance

If one is not aware of the typical appearance of the linea aspera in the adult, it can be mistaken for periostitis along the posterior aspect of the femur. This can result in unnecessary work-up for an infectious or neoplastic process. In the literature, it has also been confused with or erroneously reported as Paget's disease.

Typical clinical scenario

Usually a femur radiograph is performed for trauma, pain, or other coincidental history, and the irregular thickening of the linea aspera is seen along the posterior aspect of the femur. It should not be confused with periostitis or Paget's disease since this can lead to unnecessary work-up of an incidental finding.

Teaching point

In the skeletally mature adult, the linea aspera has been reported to be confused with periostitis or Paget's disease. One should be aware of the linea aspera's normal appearance in the skeletally mature patient so that periostitis or Paget's disease is not erroneously diagnosed.

READING LIST

Gheorghia D, Leinenkugel A. The linea aspera-pilaster complex as a possible cause of confusion with the 'flame sign': a case report. *Acta Orthop Traumatol Turc* 2010;**44**:254–256.

Hoeffel C, Munier G, Hoeffel JC. The femoral linea aspera: radiological pattern. *Eur Radiol* 1993;**3**:357–358.

Pitt MJ. Radiology of the femoral linea aspera-pilaster complex: the track sign. *Radiology* 1982;**142**:66.

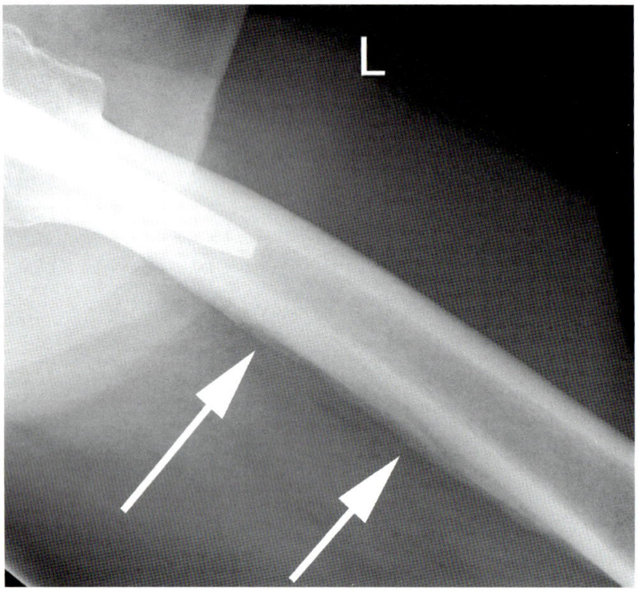

Figure 54.1 A frog-leg lateral view of the femur in a 59-year-old male. This image demonstrates the normal rough, scalloped appearance (arrows) that can be seen on the surface of the linea aspera. This should *not* be confused with periostitis.

Pearls and Pitfalls in Musculoskeletal Imaging, ed. D. Lee Bennett and Georges Y. El-Khoury. Published by Cambridge University Press. © Cambridge University Press 2013.

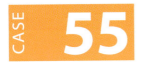

Imaging description

Morel–Lavallée lesions of the thigh and hip region are most commonly diagnosed by MR imaging. Their shape and location are helpful in their diagnosis. A Morel–Lavallée lesion should be located in the deep subcutaneous and perifascial space superficial to the tensor fascia lata (Figure 55.1). They should have well-defined margins and have an oval or fusiform shape. Their signal intensity is non-specific on T1-weighted images since they can be hypo-, iso-, or hyperintense on this sequence. However, they should be hyperintense on T2-weighted images. Their signal intensity can be hetero- or homogeneous. These lesions can demonstrate patchy internal enhancement with contrast and rim enhancement. Ultrasound can demonstrate a fluid collection in the typical locations that may contain hyperechoic nodules, which represent remnants of fat within the lesion.

Importance

Morel–Lavallée lesions can be pathognomonically diagnosed on MRI; therefore, one should be knowledgeable of their appearance so that unnecessary work-up for a neoplasm doesn't occur. They may also require treatment with sclerosing agents or with surgical resection as they can repeatedly accumulate after aspiration alone. The Morel–Lavallée lesion is an internal degloving injury from trauma caused by separation of the hypodermis from the underlying deep fascia. This results in disruption of the rich vascular and lymphatic plexus that pierces the tensor fascia lata. This disruption of capillaries and lymphatics may lead to continuous fluid and lymphatic drainage into this perifascial virtual cavity filling it with blood, lymph, and debris.

Typical clinical scenario

A 12-year-old male presented to the clinic three weeks after an all-terrain vehicle accident. He was seen the day of the accident in the emergency treatment center; however, no traumatic injury was found. He has now developed progressive upper left thigh swelling and pain for the past two weeks. An MRI demonstrated a Morel–Lavallée lesion. The lesion was resected surgically; however, he returned to the clinic eight weeks later with recurrence of the lesion. At this time it was treated with a US-guided sclerotherapy injection, and it has not recurred.

Teaching point

One should be aware of the classic appearance and location of a Morel–Lavallée lesion to prevent unnecessary work-up for a neoplasm. Imaging-guided aspiration, surgical aspiration, or surgical resection may be used to initially treat Morel–Lavallée lesions. These lesions may need to be treated with sclerotherapy injection using imaging guidance if they recur after aspiration.

READING LIST

Choudhary AK, Methratta S. Morel–Lavallée lesion of the thigh: characteristic findings on US. *Pediatr Radiol* 2010;**40 Suppl 1**:S49.

Mellado JM, Pérez del Palomar L, Diaz L, Ramos A, Sauri A. Long-standing Morel–Lavallée lesions of the trochanteric region and proximal thigh: MRI features in five patients. *AJR Am J Roentgenol* 2004;**182**:1289–1294.

Parra JA, Fernandez MA, Encinas B, Rico M. Morel–Lavallée effusions in the thigh. *Skeletal Radiol* 1997;**26**:239–241.

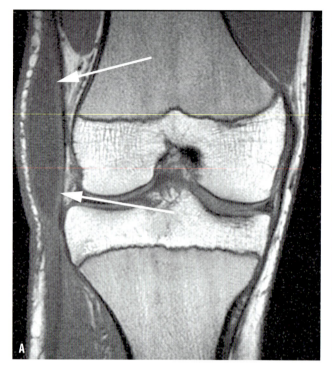

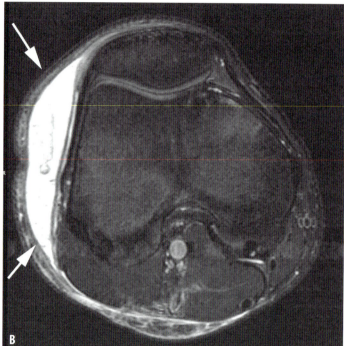

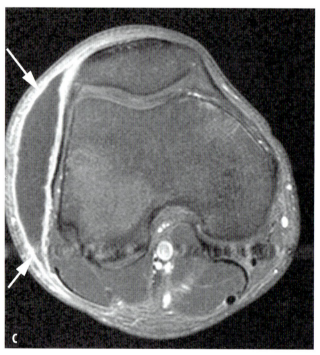

Figure 55.1 A 34-year-old male with a past history of a motorcycle collision with a history of a soft tissue injury to the right knee. A Morel–Lavallée lesion can be seen just superficial to the iliotibial band (arrows). This lesion is hypointense on T1-weighted imaging (**A**), hyperintense on T2-weighted imaging with fat suppression (**B**), and has no internal enhancement on the T1-weighted, fat-suppressed, post-contrast imaging (**C**).

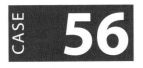

CASE 56

Intraneural ganglion cyst of the peroneal nerve

Imaging description

Imaging features of intraneural ganglion cyst of the peroneal nerve are the same as those of ganglion cyst of other locations. Intraneural ganglion occurs within a variety of nerves, but the most frequent location is the common peroneal nerve at the fibular neck. MRI may reveal an elongated, lobulated mass posterolateral to the fibular neck (Figure 56.1). The mass shows homogeneous low signal intensity on T1-weighted images, high signal intensity on T2-weighted images, and no to minimal peripheral enhancement after IV contrast. The lesions are often closely related to the proximal tibiofibular joint. Ultrasound shows a hypoechoic lesion along the common peroneal nerve.

Importance

Intraneural ganglions are typically contained in the epineurium of the peripheral nerve, frequently associated with nerve palsy due to compression. Early diagnosis and surgical removal is important to prevent permanent axonal injuries. Previous report on patients with intraneural ganglion of the peroneal nerve noted that the patients with good results either had no preoperative paralysis or had footdrop for four months or less before surgical decompression.

Typical clinical scenario

Male patients are more commonly affected (about 80%) than female with a peak incidence in the fourth decade of life. The patient presents with a palpable mass on the lateral aspect of the fibular head with a varying degree of symptoms from compression of the common peroneal nerve. The symptoms include pain in the anterolateral aspect of the leg and dorsum of foot, muscle weakness of the anterior compartment of the leg, and complete peroneal nerve palsy. Sensory loss is usually less obvious than motor deficit.

Pathogenesis

The exact pathogenesis of intraneural ganglion cyst of the peroneal nerve is unknown. The articular theory is based on the existence of a genuine ganglion owing to synovial fluid migration from an adjacent joint via an articular branch of the nerve. The connection has been reported in 40% of the cases. The degeneration theory proposes that degeneration of the connective tissue of the epineurium or perineurium proceeds in accordance with myxoid degeneration. The neoplastic theory proposes that the cyst originates from degeneration of a peripheral nerve sheath tumor as a result of intralesional necrosis.

Differential diagnosis

Magnetic resonance imaging of an elongated, cystic mass posterolateral to the fibular neck along the course of the common peroneal nerve is highly diagnostic for this entity, which reportedly includes peripheral nerve sheath tumor with extensive cystic changes. Simple ganglion cysts may potentially cause similar symptoms due to intraneural ganglion cysts.

Teaching point

An elongated, cystic mass lesion posterolateral to the fibular neck on MRI is characteristic for the diagnosis of intraneural ganglion cyst of the peroneal nerve. Early diagnosis is important to facilitate microscopic dissection of the ganglion and to prevent permanent common peroneal nerve injuries.

READING LIST

Kili S, Perkins RD. Common peroneal nerve ganglion following trauma. *Injury* 2004;**35**:938–939.

Lowenstein J, Towers J, Tomaino MM. Intraneural ganglion of the peroneal nerve: importance of timely diagnosis. *Am J Orthop (Belle Mead NJ)* 2001;**30**:816–819 .

Pedrazzini M, Pogliacomi F, Cusmano F *et al*. Bilateral ganglion cyst of the common peroneal nerve. *Eur Radiol* 2002;**12**:2803–2806 .

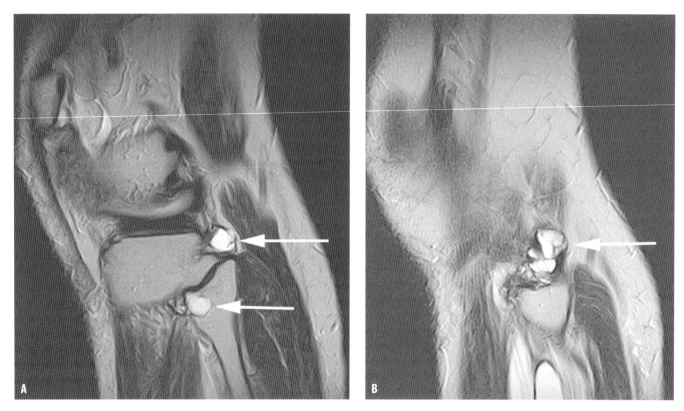

Figure 56.1 Sagittal PD-weighted (**A**) and T2-weighted (**B**) MR images of the right knee of a 50-year-old male with a palpable mass on the lateral aspect of the right knee reveal an elongated area of high signal posterolateral to the proximal fibula (arrows).

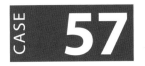

CASE 57

Tibial bowing: intrauterine deformation versus neurofibromatosis

Imaging description

Tibial bowing is a collective term to describe congenital abnormalities associated with tibial bowing deformity. Straight AP and lateral radiographs are diagnostic to document direction of the bowing (apex side) and associated findings such as a skin dimple and foot deformity.

Importance

Identifying the direction of the apex side of the bowing is important to suggest the underlying conditions and, therefore, to predict the prognosis. For most of the cases, the bowing is the result of intrauterine positioning (deformation), in which postero-medial (or postero-lateral) bowing of the tibia and fibula occurs (Figure 57.1). Thickening of the bone on the concave side and thinning and dimpling of the skin on the convex side may be seen. This is considered to be a benign, self-resolving condition. Anterolateral bowing of the tibia is rare and may lead to pseudoarthrosis. Anterolateral bowing is commonly associated with neurofibromatosis type I (NF1) (Figure 57.2). Anteromedial bowing is also a rare condition, which may be associated with fibular hemimelia (postaxial hypoplasia of the lower extremity).

Typical clinical scenario

In congenital postero-medial bowing of the tibia and fibula, the bowing is seen at birth with a calcaneovalgus deformity. It corrects spontaneously for most of the cases. Rapid resolution of angulation occurs in the first year of life. However, persistent residual deformity may require surgical intervention. Anterolateral bowing of the tibia and fibula is most likely a presentation of tibial dysplasia in infancy or early childhood in patients with NF1. This form is considered as part of infantile pseudarthrosis since fracture and non-union commonly follow.

Differential diagnosis

The radiographic findings are helpful for the differential diagnosis and following the condition. Anterolateral tibial bowing in NF1 tends to have a fracture and incomplete fusion when associated with extensive cortical thickening, medullary canal narrowing, cystic change, and decreased tibial diameter at the point of maximum angulation. Congenital anterolateral tibial bowing and polydactyly has been reported to be a distinct entity with a favorable prognosis. Degree of fibular hypoplasia in fibular hemimelia can be assessed radiographically. Other associated conditions of tibial bowing include fibrous dysplasia, osteogenesis imperfecta, rickets, and campomelic syndrome.

> ### Teaching point
>
> Direction of the tibial bowing is important to suggest the underlying etiologies and prognosis. Postero-medial (posterolateral) bowing is common and self-resolving for most of the cases. Anterolateral bowing is likely associated with NF1 and may develop a fracture and non-union.

READING LIST

Johari AN, Dhawale AA, Salaskar A, Aroojis AJ. Congenital postero-medial bowing of the tibia and fibula: is early surgery worthwhile? *J Pediatr Orthop B* 2010;**19**:479–486.

Lemire EG. Congenital anterolateral tibial bowing and polydactyly: a case report. *J Med Case Reports* 2007;**1**:54 .

Stevenson DA, Carey JC, Viskochil DH *et al.* Analysis of radiographic characteristics of anterolateral bowing of the leg before fracture in neurofibromatosis type 1. *J Pediatr Orthop* 2009;**29**: 385–392.

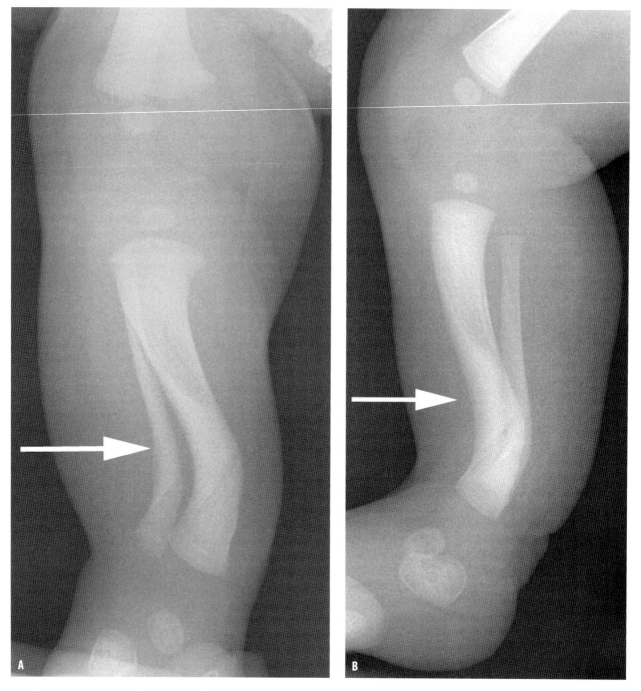

Figure 57.1 Anteroposterior (**A**) and lateral (**B**) radiographs of a 16-day-old male with the right leg deformity show postero-medial bowing of the tibia and fibula. Cortical thickening is seen on the concave sides (arrows). Spontaneous resolution was seen on the six-month follow-up study.

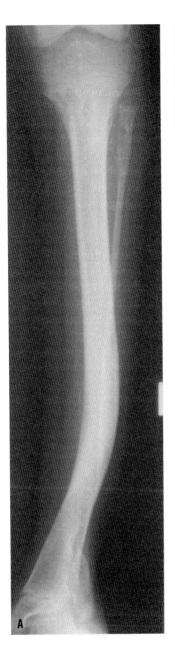 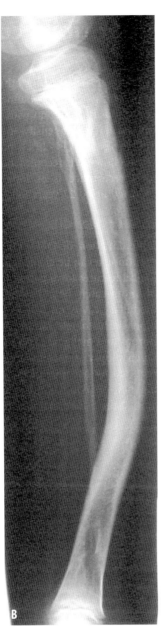

Figure 57.2 Anteroposterior (**A**) and lateral (**B**) radiographs of the tibia and fibula show anterolateral bowing of the tibia and fibula of a patient with neurofibromatosis type I. Multiple osteolytic lesions are seen in the tibia and fibula.

Osteofibrous dysplasia and other cystic lesions of the anterior tibial cortex

Imaging description

Osteofibrous dysplasia (OFD) almost exclusively occurs in the diaphysis of the tibia. Multiple cystic lesions are seen in the anterior cortex of the middle to proximal diaphysis of the tibia (Figure 58.1). There may be mild expansion with increased sclerosis in the surrounding cortex. Ipsilateral fibula may be involved. Similarly, adamantinoma most often occurs in the tibia, and typically involves the middle diaphysis. Adamantinoma is often purely lytic, eccentric, and expansile involving the anterior cortex (Figure 58.2). Ipsilateral fibula is occasionally involved.

Importance

Osteofibrous dysplasia is a benign fibroosseous lesion, named by Campanacci in 1976 in reference to histologic resemblance to fibrous dysplasia. Osteofibrous dysplasia most frequently occurs in the first two decades of life. Adamantinoma is a low-grade malignant bone tumor that typically affects patients older than 20 years. There is an intermediate entity called OFD-like adamantinoma or differentiated adamantinoma supporting the concept that these lesions are related. Immunohistochemical staining for cytokeratin confirms the epithelial nature of these lesions. There are well-documented cases, in which patients initially diagnosed as OFD or OFD-like adamantinoma have developed classic adamantinoma. Whether one lesion can progress or regress to another remains controversial. Surgical management is necessary for adamantinoma. The treatment of OFD-like adamantinoma is not well established. Because of the benign nature of OFD the treatment is based on the symptoms. Some recommend observation without surgical intervention for OFD as it ceases to progress towards skeletal maturity.

Typical clinical scenario

Osteofibrous dysplasia occurs most frequently in children under the age of 10 years. Lower leg swelling with or without pain or anterior bowing is a common clinical presentation. Osteofibrous dysplasia can be incidentally found on the radiographs obtained for other reasons. Adamantinoma tends to present in a similar manner to the patients with OFD. Both conditions may present with a pathological fracture. Adamantinoma has a propensity to both local recurrence (19–32%) and metastasis (15–29%), predominantly to the lung. Long-term follow-up is recommended because the mean duration to local recurrence is as long as 7 years and the metastasis reported up to 27 years following the diagnosis.

Differential diagnosis

Differentiation of OFD, OFD-like adamantinoma, and adamantinoma can be challenging as their radiological and histological features form part of a spectrum. Radiographic features of moth-eaten lytic lesions with complete involvement of medullary cavity on MRI suggest classic adamantinoma. The biphasic histologic nature of classic adamantinoma (benign fibrous and malignant epithelial) can lead to a sampling error. Open biopsy is recommended as ample diagnostic tissue is required for accurate diagnosis. Other cortical lesions including non-ossifying fibroma and chondromyxoid fibroma are among the differential diagnoses.

Teaching point

Close follow-up is recommended even if the lesion is radiographically typical for OFD. Biopsy is generally considered to confirm the diagnosis.

READING LIST

Kahn LB. Adamantinoma, osteofibrous dysplasia and differentiated adamantinoma. *Skeletal Radiol* 2003;**32**:245–258.

Khanna M, Delaney D, Tirabosco R, Saifuddin A. Osteofibrous dysplasia, osteofibrous dysplasia-like adamantinoma and adamantinoma: correlation of radiological imaging features with surgical histology and assessment of the use of radiology in contributing to needle biopsy diagnosis. *Skeletal Radiol* 2008;**37**:1077–1084.

Most MJ, Sim FH, Inwards CY. Osteofibrous dysplasia and adamantinoma. *J Am Acad Orthop Surg* 2010;**18**:358–366.

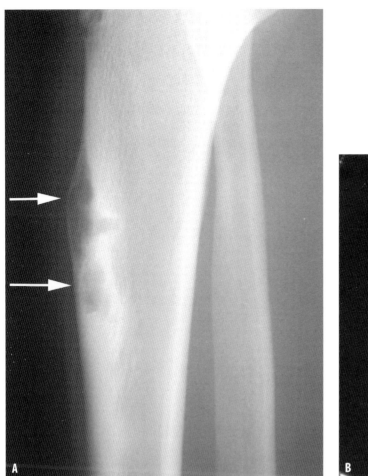
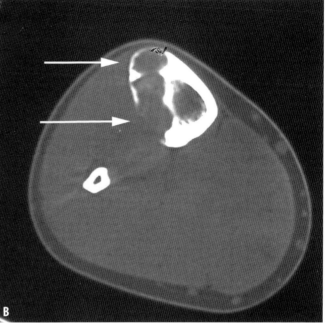

Figure 58.1 Lateral radiograph (**A**) of the tibia/fibula of a 16-year-old male with osteofibrous dysplasia shows a cortical-based, multi-cystic lesion in the anterior cortex of the proximal to middle tibia (arrows). The lesion is mildly expansile and has surrounding sclerosis. Computed tomography of the tibia/fibula of the same patient (**B**) clearly demonstrates an anterolateral cortical location of the lesion (arrows).

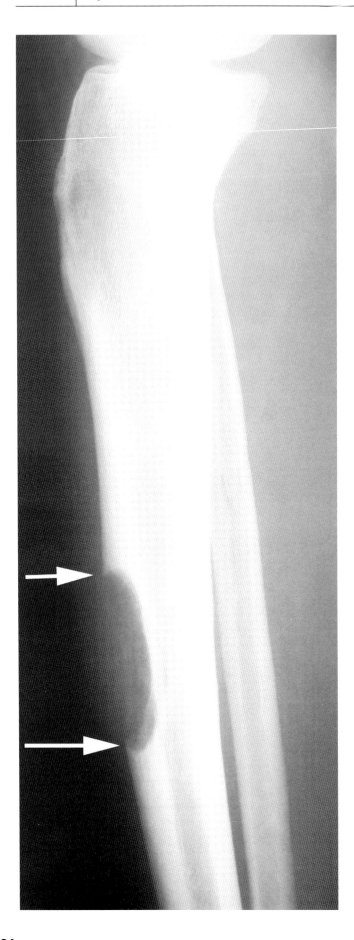

Figure 58.2 Lateral radiograph of the tibia/fibula of a 39-year-old female shows a slightly expansile, lytic lesion in the anterior cortex of the middle tibia (arrows) consistent with adamantinoma.

Less common stress fractures of the tibia and fibula

Imaging description

Stress fractures affect most frequently tibia and rarely fibula. When the fibula is involved, stress fractures affect the distal 1/3 and very rarely proximal 1/3. Radiographic findings of the stress fractures of the fibula may be identical to the stress fractures occurring to other common locations, which include a focal periosteal reaction (Figure 59.1), a focal cortical thickening, and a band of sclerosis. Focal cortical thickening may be associated with a lucent line (black line) perpendicular to the cortex. Longitudinal stress fractures are uncommon, usually occurring in the tibia. Radiography may show irregular cortical thickening and medullary sclerosis in a longitudinal fashion (Figure 59.2A). Axial images of CT (Figure 59.2B) demonstrate a cortical disruption (fracture) at multiple slices. Coronal images of CT and MRI (Figure 59.2C) or planer images of bone scan may better delineate its longitudinal extension.

Importance

Sensitivity of radiography for stress fractures is suboptimal. The diagnosis of stress fracture can be made clinically with pertinent clinical history even with negative radiographs. The diagnosis may be challenging with atypical clinical presentations, uncommon locations, and atypical imaging findings. Imaging findings may be misinterpreted as more aggressive lesions, particularly infection or tumor. Familiarity of these uncommon presentations of stress fractures is important to avoid unnecessary biopsy and to reach a correct diagnosis.

Typical clinical scenario

Stress fractures occur to a healthy bone with repetitive physical activities (fatigue fracture) and to a pathologically weak bone with usual daily activities (insufficiency fracture). The diagnosis of stress fracture is typically made from pertinent clinical history and characteristic radiographic findings. As mentioned above, negative radiography should not exclude the diagnosis of stress fracture. For patients with atypical clinical history or unusual radiographic findings, CT, MRI, or bone scan may be helpful. The symptoms subside with rest. Delayed healing or progression to a complete fracture, however, could occur in patients with poor compliance.

Differential diagnosis

Radiographic differential diagnoses for a focal cortical thickening include osteoid osteoma and infection. Nidus of osteoid osteoma or cortical microabscess may not be seen on the radiographs. Focal cortical thickening may be due to hyperostosis associated with an adjacent, benign, soft tissue lesion such as hemangioma. Bilateral stress fracture of the tibia has been reported as a presenting pathology in a patient with oncogenic osteomalacia (paraneoplastic syndrome).

Teaching point

Unusually presentations of common pathologies pose diagnostic challenges. Radiologists need to be aware of possible involvement of the fibula and an atypical, longitudinal orientation in stress fractures. Cross-sectional imaging, most importantly axial images of CT, may confirm the diagnosis of longitudinal stress fracture.

READING LIST

Craig JG, Widman D, van Holsbeeck M. Longitudinal stress fracture: patterns of edema and the importance of the nutrient foramen. *Skeletal Radiol* 2003;**32**:22–27.

Hong SH, Chu IT. Stress fracture of the proximal fibula in military recruits. *Clin Orthop Surg* 2009;**1**:161–164.

Kozlowski K, Azouz M, Hoff D. Stress fracture of the fibula in the first decade of life. Report of eight cases. *Pediatr Radiol* 1991;**21**:381–383.

Ohashi K, Ohnishi T, Ishikawa T *et al.* Oncogenic osteomalacia presenting as bilateral stress fractures of the tibia. *Skeletal Radiol* 1999;**28**:46–48.

Pearls and Pitfalls in Musculoskeletal Imaging, ed. D. Lee Bennett and Georges Y. El-Khoury. Published by Cambridge University Press. © Cambridge University Press 2013.

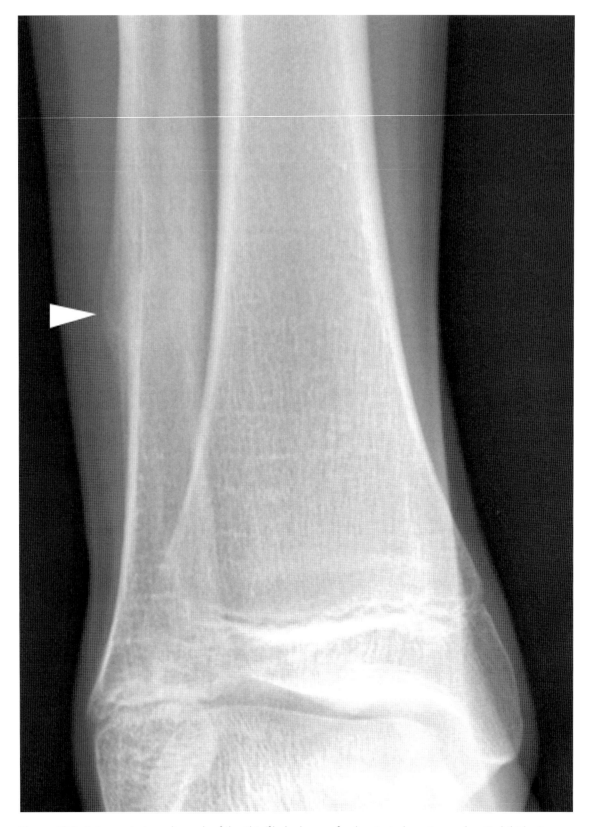

Figure 59.1 Anteroposterior radiograph of the tibia/fibula shows a focal periosteal reaction and cortical thickening (arrowhead) at the distal fibula of a 13-year-old male, a long-distance runner, consistent with a stress fracture.

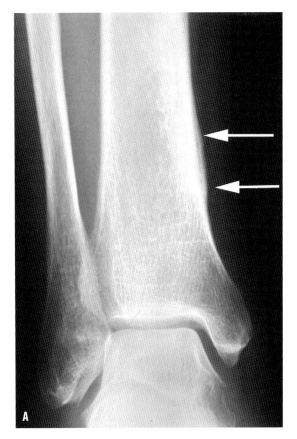

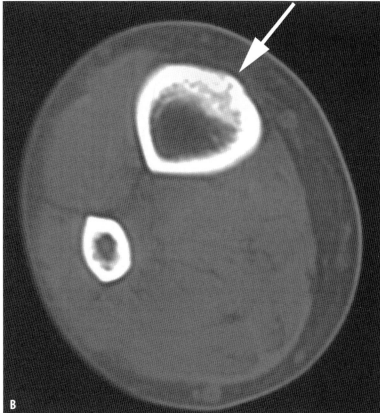

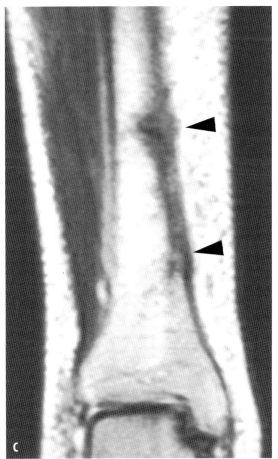

Figure 59.2 Mortise radiographic view (**A**) of the ankle shows a focal periosteal reaction and increased medullary sclerosis (arrows) along the medial cortex of the distal tibia of a 62-year-old physically active female. Axial CT image (**B**) through the distal tibia/fibula shows cortical disruption (arrow) in the anteromedial cortex of the tibia associated with medullary sclerosis. These findings were seen on multiple continuous images and consistent with a longitudinal stress fracture. A coronal T2-weighted MR image of the distal tibia (**C**) reveals longitudinal dark signal (arrowheads) along the medial cortex, which is associated with diffuse bone marrow edema.

Imaging description

Posterior impingement occurs between the distal tibia and calcaneus posteriorly. A lateral ankle radiograph may or may not show os trigonum, a triangular-shaped ossicle, posterior to the talus (Figure 60.1). Although this entity is often called "os trigonum syndrome," impingement associated with os trigonum is considered as a subset of posterior impingement. Sources of impingement can be other bony structures or soft tissues such as flexor hallucis longus (FHL) and posterior intermalleolar ligament. Prominent lateral tubercle, a lateral border of the groove for FHL, is called Stieda's process (Figure 60.2). Other bony variations associated with posterior impingement include a prominent superior calcaneal tuberosity and downward sloping posterior tibial plafond. MRI may show localized bone marrow edema (Figure 60.3) and evidence of inflammation in surrounding soft tissues including FHL, posterior talofibular ligament, and intermalleolar ligament.

Importance

Os trigonum is a common accessory bone seen in 13–25% of adults. When present, it is bilateral in 50% of patients. Posterior impingement is often associated with os trigonum. However, most individuals including athletes with os trigonum are asymptomatic. Other common etiologies causing posterior ankle pain (see below) should be excluded. Diagnostic injection of local anesthetic under fluoroscopy or ultrasound may be helpful for elusive cases.

Typical clinical scenario

Patients with posterior impingement syndrome may manifest posterior ankle pain with forceful plantar flexion. This syndrome often affects ballet dancers and soccer players, who are involved in plantar hyperflexion of the ankle. Os trigonum and posterior process are the most common causes of posterior ankle impingement. On physical examination, tenderness is noted behind the peroneal tendons in the back of the lateral malleolus. Reproducible pain by forced passive plantar flexion of the ankle is called the plantar flexion sign. The patients initially receive conservative treatments including modification of activities, anti-inflammatory drugs, and physical therapy. Excisional surgery may be indicated when conservative therapy has failed.

Differential diagnosis

Radiographic differentials for an ossicle posterior to the talus include os trigonum (with and without tear of synchondrosis) and fracture of the prominent posterior tubercle (Stieda's process). The differential diagnosis of posterior ankle pain includes posterior tubercle fracture, talocalcaneal coalition, ganglion, and tendon pathologies of FHL, peroneal, and Achilles tendons.

Teaching point

Precise knowledge of anatomy and normal variations of the talus is important to understand the mechanisms of posterior impingement syndrome. Given the fact that this condition is often overdiagnosed by paramedical practitioners, MR imaging may be considered for patients with suspected posterior ankle impingement.

READING LIST

Hamilton WG. Posterior ankle pain in dancers. *Clin Sports Med* 2008;**27**:263–267.

Rathur S, Clifford PD, Chapman CB. Posterior ankle impingement: os trigonum syndrome. *Am J Orthop* (*Belle Mead NJ*) 2009;**38**: 252–253.

Russell JA, Kruse DW, Koutedakis Y, McEwan IM, Wyon MA. Pathoanatomy of posterior ankle impingement in ballet dancers. *Clin Anat* 2010;**23**:613–621.

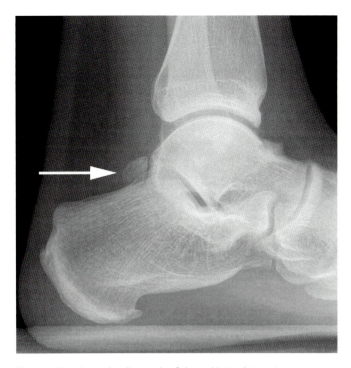

Figure 60.1 Lateral radiograph of the ankle in this patient demonstrates an os trigonum (arrow). It is a triangular-shaped ossicle, posterior to the talus, that can be associated with posterior impingement at the ankle.

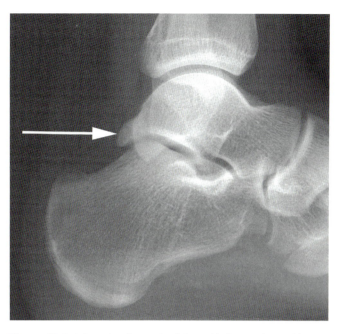

Figure 60.2 A lateral radiograph of the ankle in a patient with a prominent Stieda's process (arrow). This prominent osseous process can be associated with posterior impingement at the ankle.

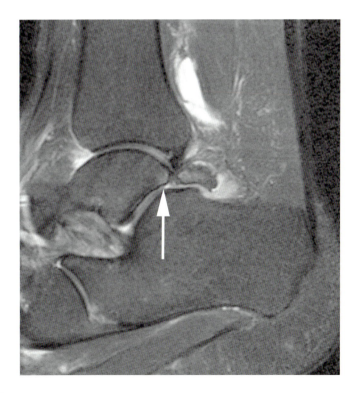

Figure 60.3 This patient had posterior ankle pain with plantar flexion. The sagittal STIR MR image demonstrates the MRI findings of posterior impingement associated with an os trigonum or an old Stieda's process fracture. The findings of posterior impingement are bone marrow edema in the talus and osseous process (arrow) with surrounding soft tissue edema.

Haglund's syndrome

Imaging description

Haglund's triad consists of insertional Achilles tendinosis, retrocalcaneal bursitis, and Haglund's deformity. Haglund's deformity refers to hypertropic bony projection of the bursal projection (Figure 61.1). Haglund's syndrome is a common cause of posterior heel pain characterized by a painful soft tissue swelling (pump-bump) at the Achilles tendon insertion. Dr. Haglund coined this entity in 1928 based on the symptom (heel pain) and physical findings typically for those who wore stiff low-back shoes while playing golf or hockey. MRI may show distension of the retrocalcaneal and possibly retro Achilles bursa with fluid signals and thickening of the Achilles tendon with or without signal changes (Figure 61.2).

Importance

Lateral radiograph may detect Haglund's deformity, distension of retrocalcaneal bursa, thickening of Achilles tendon (>9 mm, 2 cm above the bursal projection), and soft tissue swelling posterior to the Achilles tendon insertion (retro Achilles bursitis). These findings need to be correlated with the symptoms and physical findings for the diagnosis of Haglund's syndrome. Inflammatory arthropathy such as reactive arthritis may present with similar findings. Parallel pitch lines (PPL) (Figure 61.3) can be used to determine the prominence of the bursal projection (Haglund's deformity). However, this can be positive in about one third of asymptomatic individuals. MRI clearly visualizes the components of Haglund's syndrome.

Typical clinical scenario

Patients present with heel pain that is aggravated by rigid low-back shoes. A palpable posterolateral prominence at the posterior superior border of the calcaneus may be associated with erythema. Lateral radiograph and MRI confirm the Haglund's deformity, Achilles tendinosis and associated bursitis. Most of the patients are successfully treated by conservative treatments; the success of which depends on the duration of symptom before initiation of the treatment. Approximately 25% of patients with Haglund's triad fail non-operative treatment.

Differential diagnosis

Bony proliferative changes at the bursal projection of the calcaneus can be seen in seronegative arthropathy such as reactive arthritis and psoriasis. Bursitis around the Achilles tendon can be seen in patients with systemic inflammatory conditions such as rheumatoid arthritis and gout. Swelling of the Achilles tendon can be caused by trauma (tendon tear) or systemic conditions such as hyperlipidemia (xanthoma) and gout (tophus).

Teaching point

Haglund's syndrome is a clinical entity, in which not all three components of the Haglund's triad may present. Lateral radiographs of the calcaneus are helpful to support the diagnosis. MRI can visualize precise pathology and help guide the treatment for patients with Haglund's syndrome.

READING LIST

Alfredson H, Lorentzon R. Chronic Achilles tendinosis: recommendations for treatment and prevention. *Sports Med* 2000;**29**:135–146 .

DeVries JG, Summerhays B, Guehlstorf DW. Surgical correction of Haglund's triad using complete detachment and reattachment of the Achilles tendon. *J Foot Ankle Surg* 2009;**48**:447–451.

Pavlov H, Heneghan MA, Hersh A, Goldman AB, Vigorita V. The Haglund syndrome: initial and differential diagnosis. *Radiology* 1982;**144**:83–88.

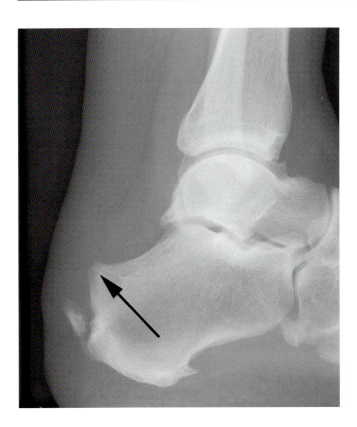

Figure 61.1 Lateral radiograph of the ankle of a 57-year-old male shows spurring of the bursal projection (arrow) consistent with Haglund's deformity. Marked thickening of the Achilles tendon is seen with ossification. Increased soft tissue opacity in the pre-Achilles fat pad suggests distension of retrocalcaneal bursa. Overall findings suggest Haglund's syndrome.

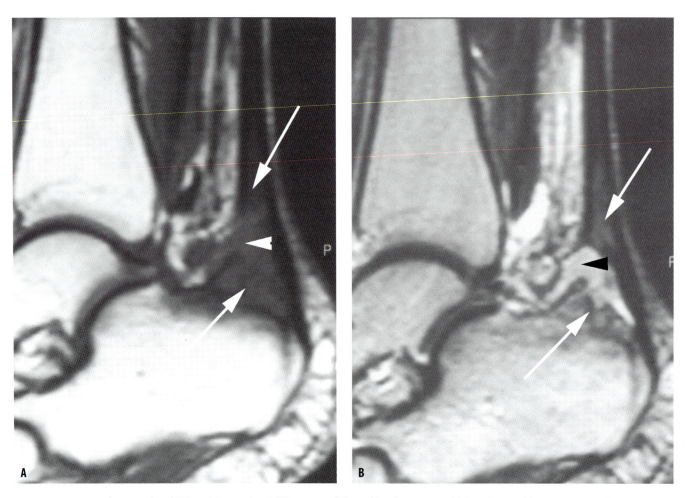

Figure 61.2 Sagittal T1-weighted (**A**) and T2-weighted (**B**) images of the ankle of a 59-year-old female reveal bone marrow edema (arrows at calcaneus) at the bursal projection, fluid in the retrocalcaneal bursa (arrowheads), and thickening and increased signals of the Achilles tendon (arrows at the Achilles tendon).

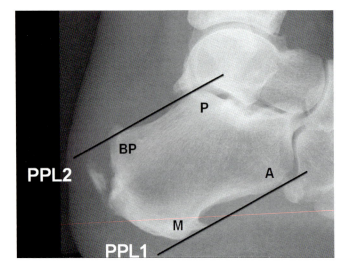

Figure 61.3 The parallel pitch lines (PPL) are used to determine the prominence of the bursal projection (BP). The lower PPL (PPL1) is the baseline tangent to the anterior tubercle (A) and the medial tuberosity (M). The upper PPL (PPL2) is drawn parallel to the baseline through the posterior edge of the posterior talar facet (P). The bursal projection (BP) is above the upper PPL (same patient as in Figure 61.1). A BP touching or below the upper PPL is normal, not prominent.

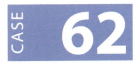

CASE 62

Accessory anterolateral facet of the talus

Imaging description

Accessory anterolateral facet of the talus is a normal variation involving the anterolateral aspect of the lateral process of the talus, which articulates with an extended facet of the anterior process of the calcaneus (Figure 62.1). Combined with the extended facet of the calcaneus, this opposing structure looks like an anterior extension of the posterior subtalar joint. Detection on the lateral radiographs may be difficult particularly in the presence of a valgus hindfoot deformity. Cross-sectional studies especially MRI can detect articular cartilage in the interface (Figure 62.2). This variation was seen in 34% of the 79 pediatric cadaveric specimens.

Importance

Painful talocalcaneal impingement associated with this variation has been reported in a small number of pediatric patients with rigid flatfoot. Although tarsal coalitions are the most common etiology of the rigid flatfoot in adolescents and young adults, lateral talocalcaneal impingement associated with accessory anterolateral facet of the talus can be a cause of painful rigid foot. Interestingly the accessory anterolateral facet is commonly associated with dorsal talar beaking (29%).

Typical clinical scenario

Pediatric to young adult patients may present with painful rigid flatfoot deformity. Subtalar motion is restricted with the pain localized to the sinus tarsi. Lateral radiographs may show flatfoot deformity with dorsal talar beaking. CT or MRI may be requested for possible tarsal coalition. Accessory anterolateral facet can be detected on these cross-sectional studies.

MRI demonstrates bone marrow edema on both talar and calcaneal sides along the accessory articulation. Surgical resection of accessory anterolateral facet provides improvement in symptoms.

Differential diagnosis

Tarsal coalitions are the most common etiology of the rigid flatfoot deformities for pediatric population. Talocalcaneal and calcaneonavicular coalitions are the two most common types. Adult patients with acquired flatfoot deformity may develop extra-articular lateral hindfoot (talocalcaneal) impingement with hindfoot valgus deformity.

> ## Teaching point
>
> Accessory anterolateral facet of the talus is a normal variation that can be associated with painful rigid flatfoot deformity. Lateral foot radiographs may show dorsal talar beaking with no evidence of tarsal coalition. Radiologists should look for the findings of talocalcaneal impingement on the MRI when tarsal coalition is suspected.

READING LIST

Malicky ES, Crary JL, Houghton MJ et al. Talocalcaneal and subfibular impingement in symptomatic flatfoot in adults. J Bone Joint Surg Am 2002;84-A:2005–2009.

Martus JE, Femino JE, Caird MS et al. Accessory anterolateral talar facet as an etiology of painful talocalcaneal impingement in the rigid flatfoot: a new diagnosis. Iowa Orthop J 2008;28:1–8.

Martus JE, Femino JE, Caird MS et al. Accessory anterolateral facet of the pediatric talus. An anatomic study. J Bone Joint Surg Am 2008;90:2452–2459.

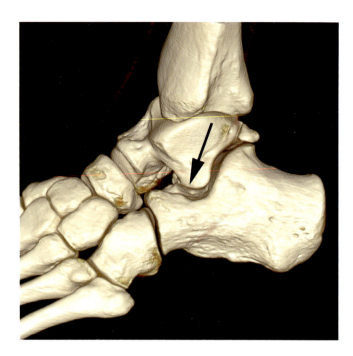

Figure 62.1 Three-dimensional volume-rendered image of the left foot shows an accessory anterolateral facet of the talus (arrow). CT was performed for a 21-year-old male with anterolateral foot pain to rule out coalition. This figure is presented in color in the color plate section.

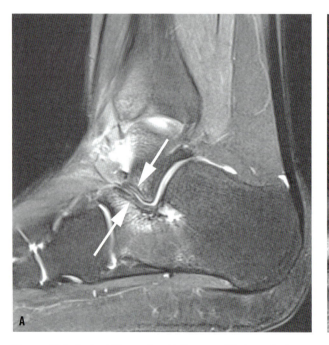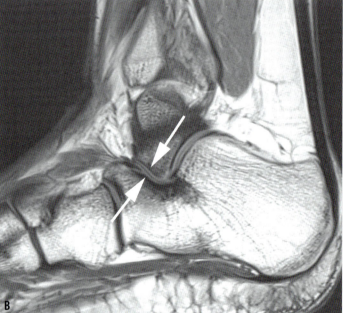

Figure 62.2 Sagittal T2-weighted MR image (**A**) through the accessory anterolateral facet of the talus shows articular cartilage (arrows) associated with bone marrow edema. MR imaging was performed for a 14-year-old female who previously had resection of calcaneonavicular coalition. Sagittal T1-weighted MR image (**B**) through the accessory anterolateral facet of the talus shows articular cartilage (arrows) associated with bone marrow edema.

Imaging description

Maisonneuve fracture has been described for the ankle injury characterized by a high fibular fracture with disruption of the tibiofibular syndesmosis. The diagnosis of a Maisonneuve fracture should be considered in each of the following situations: (1) widening of the medial or lateral clear space without evident fracture (Figure 63.1); (2) an apparent isolated displaced fracture of the medial malleolus; and (3) an apparent isolated fracture of the posterior malleolus (Figure 63.2). On such occasions, full-length views of the tibia and fibula should be obtained to identify the high fibular fracture. Stress radiography of the ankle may help for subtle cases of medial clear space widening. Lack of overlap of the distal fibula with the tibial tuberosity is a helpful sign for syndesmotic injury.

Importance

Maisonneuve fracture is considered as a severe ankle injury with syndesmotic disruption. The diagnosis is often delayed or missed because the patients rarely report pain in the proximal fibula most likely due to the presence of a more painful ankle injury. Early operative treatment is recommended for the majority of patients with Maisonneuve fracture. Therefore, recognizing the injury pattern of Maisonneuve fracture from ankle radiographs is important for a correct diagnosis. Radiologists should recommend radiographic evaluation of the entire tibia and fibula to confirm the proximal extent of the injury.

Typical clinical scenario

Maisonneuve fracture occurs in adult patients with a wide age range (17–73 years), more commonly in males. The injury pattern is most commonly classified as a pronation external rotation injury. The patients rarely complain of pain in the proximal fibula because of severe and painful soft tissue injuries in the ankle. Therefore, proximal fibular fracture and syndesmotic injury may be missed on the initial examination. Most patients with Maisonneuve fracture are managed operatively. A review of the literature revealed excellent to good functional outcome based on 61 patients with Maisonneuve fracture.

Differential diagnosis

Widening of the medial clear space indicates a deltoid ligament tear, which necessitates violent force. Isolated deltoid ligament tears without a fracture are rare. Isolated fractures of the posterior malleolus can be seen in extreme plantar flexion injuries of the foot. However, the fractures at this location are more commonly associated with rotation injuries and therefore, a high fibular fracture should be sought before the diagnosis of an isolated posterior malleolar fracture.

Teaching point

Maisonneuve fracture is typically associated with severe soft tissue injuries of the ankle. On the lateral side, interosseous membrane tear extends proximally to the level of the high fibular fracture, which is not seen on the ankle radiographs. Certain radiographic patterns of the ankle suggest Maisonneuve fracture (see above).

READING LIST

Kalyani BS, Roberts CS, Giannoudis PV. The Maisonneuve injury: a comprehensive review. *Orthopedics* 2010;**33**:196–197 .

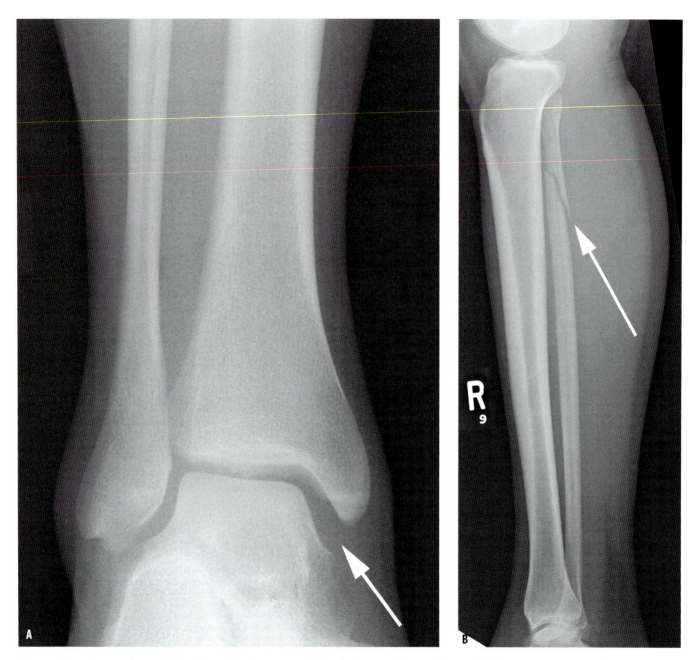

Figure 63.1 Mortise radiograph (A) of the ankle of a 28-year-old female shows widening of the medial clear space (arrow). No fracture is seen in the distal tibia or fibula. Lateral view of the tibia/fibula (B) reveals a high fibular fracture (arrow).

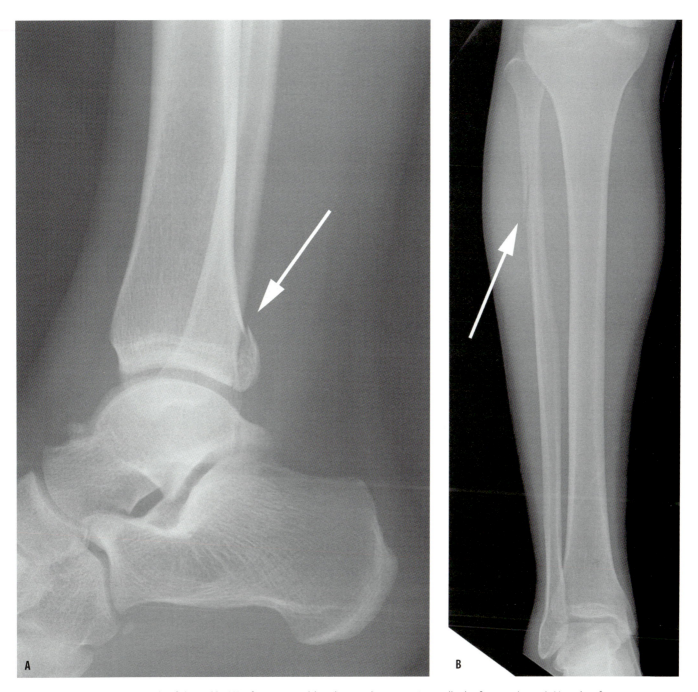

Figure 63.2 Lateral radiograph of the ankle (**A**) of a 21-year-old male reveals a posterior malleolar fracture (arrow). No other fracture was seen on the AP and mortise views. AP radiograph of the tibia/fibula (**B**) shows a high fibular fracture (arrow).

Imaging description

Triplane fracture occurs in the distal tibia before complete closure of the physis. As the name implies there are three fracture planes. Coronal oblique fracture is seen in the posterior metaphysis on the lateral radiograph (Figure 64.1). Sagittal epiphyseal fracture is seen on the AP or mortise view (Figure 64.2). Axial physeal fracture commonly involves the lateral aspect of the physis, which may be widened. Triplane fractures are further classified based on the number of the fracture fragments (two, three, or four fragments) and the location of epiphyseal fractures. CT (Figure 64.3) is commonly indicated to evaluate the surgical indication and pre-operative planning.

Importance

Triplane fracture does not fit into the Salter–Harris classification of physeal fractures because of its complexity. Prompt diagnosis and accurate assessment of the fracture extension and displacement are important as they change the management and likely the prognosis. Non-displaced fractures and extra-articular fractures can be managed conservatively. Displaced fractures are surgically treated. Intra-articular reduction to within 2 mm is required for optimal treatment of triplane fractures. The presence of a fibular fracture appears to be associated with an increased incidence of unsuccessful closed reductions. Complications include premature physeal closure, angular deformities, and joint incongruity with subsequent degenerative arthritis.

Typical clinical scenario

Triplane fracture typically occurs in children age 12–15 years old. This injury is related to characteristic asymmetric closure of the distal tibial physis, which starts from the Kump's bump, anteromedial physeal undulation. This fracture is more common in males than in females. The patients typically present with a history of twisting injury of the ankle with varying degrees of severity. Two-part and non-displaced fractures are common and managed non-operatively. Most patients have good short-term prognosis and generally return to pre-injury activity levels without complications.

Differential diagnosis

Other physeal injuries should be differentiated from triplane fractures. Triplane fracture has a radiographic appearance of a Salter–Harris type II fracture on lateral view and of a Salter–Harris type III fracture on AP or mortise view. Juvenile Tillaux fracture is an avulsion fracture from the anterior tibiofibular ligament involving the anterolateral aspect of the distal tibial epiphysis, which is associated with an external rotation injury.

> ### Teaching point
>
> Familiarity of characteristic patterns of three plane fractures facilitates prompt radiographic diagnosis and/or evaluation by CT. CT is generally recommended to assess surgical indication and pre-operative planning.

READING LIST

El-Karef E, Sadek HI, Nairn DS, Aldam CH, Allen PW. Triplane fracture of the distal tibia. *Injury* 2000;**31**:729–736.

Jones S, Phillips N, Ali F *et al.* Triplane fractures of the distal tibia requiring open reduction and internal fixation. Pre-operative planning using computed tomography. *Injury* 2003;**34**:293–298 .

Schnetzler KA, Hoernschemeyer D. The pediatric triplane ankle fracture. *J Am Acad Orthop Surg* 2007;**15**:738–747.

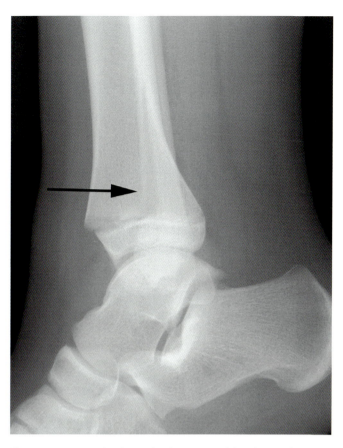

Figure 64.1 Lateral radiograph of a 14-year-old male reveals physeal fracture of the distal tibia involving the metaphysis in a coronal plane (arrow).

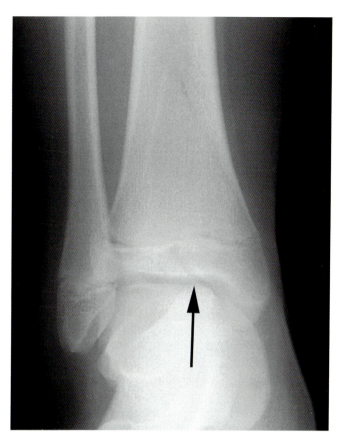

Figure 64.2 Anteroposterior radiograph of the same patient shows the fracture involving the epiphysis of the distal tibia in a sagittal plane (arrow).

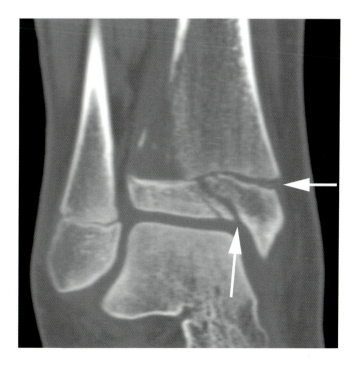

Figure 64.3 Coronal reformatted CT image of the ankle of the same patient shows the extent and displacement of the triplane fracture to better advantage (arrows).

Imaging description

Peroneal tendon dislocation can be diagnosed by a characteristic avulsion fracture off the lateral aspect of the distal fibula (Figure 65.1). A small elliptic bony fragment is avulsed from the attachment site of the superior peroneal retinaculum, which keeps the peroneal tendons in place behind the retrofibular groove. Advanced imaging studies including ultrasound, CT (Figure 65.2), and MRI can demonstrate dislocation of the peroneal tendons. Ultrasound is an effective technique to dynamically detect transient peroneal tendon dislocation. Dynamic scanning of ultrasound is performed with the foot dorsiflexed and everted passively and actively from a plantarflexed and inverted position. Static cross-sectional imaging with CT and MRI is less reliable for detecting transient dislocation.

Importance

Peroneal tendon dislocation can be complicated with fractures of the ankle and foot. Calcaneal fractures are commonly associated with peroneal tendon dislocation. As CT is frequently performed for patients with calcaneal fractures to evaluate surgical indications and pre-operative planning, peroneal tendon dislocation should be sought for those patients as it may influence the treatment and prognosis.

Typical clinical scenario

Calcaneal fractures are typically produced by axial force resulting from deceleration such as a fall from a height or a motor vehicle accident. Males are more often affected than females. The fracture pattern is affected by the magnitude and direction of the impacting force, foot position, and bone mineral content. The reported incidence of peroneal tendon dislocations in patients with calcaneal fractures is between 25% and 47.5%. The incidence of peroneal tendon dislocations increases with the grade of Sander's classification, which reflects the severity of calcaneal fractures. Peroneal tendon dislocation may reduce or persist after the subtalar joint reduction and fixation of the calcaneus.

Differential diagnosis

In acute phase, symptoms of peroneal tendon dislocation are likely masked by the damage to the calcaneus and surrounding soft tissues. Occasionally, surgeons make the diagnosis of peroneal tendon dislocation by physical examination. More commonly, CT obtained in order to evaluate calcaneal fracture provides information regarding tendon pathologies such as tear and entrapment. In chronic phase, tendinosis, tenosynovitis, and tear of the peroneal tendon should be differentiated. MRI and ultrasound are suitable to assess these conditions.

Teaching point

There is a high association between calcaneal fracture and peroneal tendon dislocation. Because CT is frequently performed for evaluation of calcaneal fracture, radiologists should look for the integrity of peroneal tendon when evaluating calcaneal fracture with CT.

READING LIST

Bradley SA, Davies AM. Computed tomographic assessment of soft tissue abnormalities following calcaneal fractures. *Br J Radiol* 1992;**65**:105–111.
Neustadter J, Raikin SM, Nazarian LN. Dynamic sonographic evaluation of peroneal tendon subluxation. *AJR Am J Roentgenol* 2004;**183**:985–988.
Rosenberg ZS, Feldman F, Singson RD, Price GJ. Peroneal tendon injury associated with calcaneal fractures: CT findings. *AJR Am J Roentgenol* 1987;**149**:125–129.
Sanders R. Displaced intra-articular fractures of the calcaneus. *J Bone Joint Surg Am* 2000;**82**:225–250.

Pearls and Pitfalls in Musculoskeletal Imaging, ed. D. Lee Bennett and Georges Y. El-Khoury. Published by Cambridge University Press. © Cambridge University Press 2013.

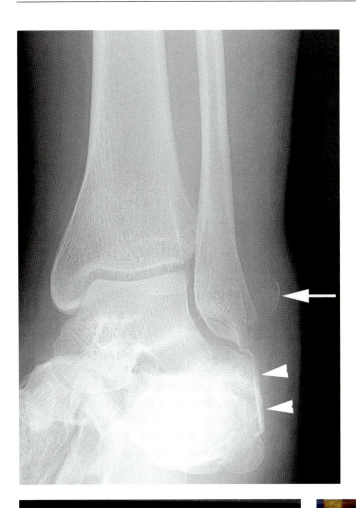

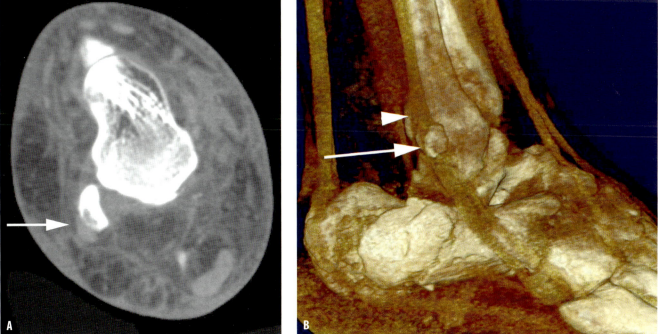

Figure 65.2 Axial CT image of the ankle (**A**) of a 46-year-old female with acute calcaneal fracture shows peroneal tendon dislocation (arrow). A three-dimensional volume-rendered image (**B**) of the ankle (view from lateral) of the same patient shows peroneal tendon dislocation (arrowhead) with an avulsion fracture of the fibula (arrow). A severe compression fracture of the calcaneus is also present. This figure is presented in color in the color plate section.

66 Anterior impingement

Imaging description

Weight bearing lateral radiographs may demonstrate bony spurs and capsular distension at the anterior aspect of the tibiotalar joint. CT can further characterize the location and size of the spurs. Soft tissue changes associated with anterior impingement such as thickening in the anterior recess can be detected with ultrasound and MRI.

Importance

Anterior impingement is considered as a common cause of chronic anterior ankle pain among athletes especially ballet dancers and soccer players. Bony spurs at the anterior ankle joint (Figure 66.1) are a component of this condition, but not all the spurs are associated with symptoms. Arthroscopic studies reveal hypertrophic synovium or scar tissue is compressed between the spurs during dorsiflexion. This compression is believed to cause pain. Therefore, these imaging findings need to be correlated with symptoms and physical findings. Anterior tibial spurs occur commonly lateral to the midline, whereas anterior talar spurs develop commonly in the medial part. Lateral radiographs can detect anterolateral osteophytes. Oblique radiographs may be necessary to detect anteromedial osteophytes (Figure 66.2).

Typical clinical scenario

The diagnosis is clinically made based on anterior ankle pain with limited and painful dorsiflexion. Soft tissue swelling and a palpable spur over the anterior ankle may be detected on physical examination. Conservative treatment is usually successful for most patients with anterior impingement. Surgical or arthroscopic resection of spurs and soft tissue lesions is effective for patients with no tibiotalar articular disease.

Differential diagnosis

Asymptomatic bony spurs in the ankle may be seen in about half of the football players and dancers. Based on the prognosis of the patients with anterior impingement following surgical and arthroscopic treatments, osteoarthritic ankle with joint space narrowing should be differentiated from this entity as these arthritic ankles require different treatment. Secondary or primary cartilage lesions of the ankle may also need to be ruled out.

Teaching point

Anterior ankle impingement is a clinical diagnosis and may be confirmed by imaging studies. Osteoarthritis with joint space narrowing should be differentiated from this entity as they may require different treatments. Role of advanced imaging studies such as CT and MRI is not clearly established. However, soft tissue changes in the anterior recess can be evaluated with ultrasound or MRI.

READING LIST

Berberian WS, Hecht PJ, Wapner KL, DiVerniero R. Morphology of tibiotalar osteophytes in anterior ankle impingement. *Foot Ankle Int* 2001;**22**:313–317.

Coull R, Raffiq T, James LE, Stephens MM. Open treatment of anterior impingement of the ankle. *J Bone Joint Surg Br* 2003;**85**:550–553.

Nihal A, Rose DJ, Trepman E. Arthroscopic treatment of anterior ankle impingement syndrome in dancers. *Foot Ankle Int* 2005;**26**:908–912.

O'Kane JW, Kadel N. Anterior impingement syndrome in dancers. *Curr Rev Musculoskelet Med* 2008;**1**:12–16.

Tol JL, Verheyen CP, van Dijk CN. Arthroscopic treatment of anterior impingement in the ankle. *J Bone Joint Surg Br* 2001;**83**:9–13.

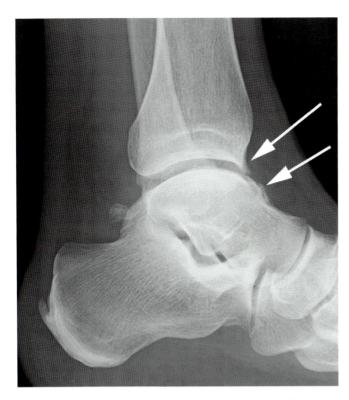

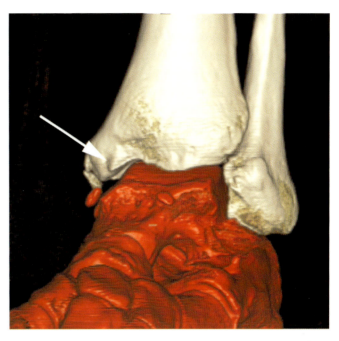

Figure 66.1 Lateral ankle radiograph of a 40-year-old male shows mild to moderate osteophytes (arrows) at the anterior aspect of the ankle joint consistent with the patient's clinical diagnosis of anterior impingement. Ankle joint space is preserved.

Figure 66.2 Volume-rendered CT image at an oblique angle of the ankle of the same patient in Figure 66.1 shows the tibial osteophyte in the anteromedial aspect of the ankle joint (arrow). This figure is presented in color in the color plate section.

143

Imaging description

Peroneocalcaneus internus (PCI) muscle is a rare accessory muscle of the posterior ankle. MRI shows an accessory muscle posterolateral to the flexor hallucis longus (FHL) tendon behind the ankle. On the axial images, the PCI is located deep to the flexor retinaculum and superficial relative to the posterior tibial neurovascular bundle behind the talus (Figure 67.1A). The PCI descends posterior and lateral to the FHL (Figure 67.1B) and inserts into the tubercle on the medial aspect of the calcaneus below the sustentaculum tali, which may be better delineated on the coronal oblique images.

Importance

Peroneocalcaneus internus muscle has been reported in one out of 100 asymptomatic volunteers. This condition is thought to be asymptomatic for most of the cases. However, a case associated with posterior impingement has been reported. With increasing popularity of endoscopic surgery, a possible risk of neurovascular injury during the procedure has been posed in patients with PCI. Because the FHL is used as the landmark for a medial boundary in the posteromedial portal, the surgeon may misidentify the PCI as the FHL and incorrectly direct the instruments toward the neurovascular bundles (Figure 67.2).

Typical clinical scenario

Symptoms related to PCI muscle are rarely reported. Because of its deep-seated location within the tarsal tunnel, it may be associated with compression neuropathy. In patients with PCI, there is a potential risk of damaging neurovascular bundles by the surgeons performing endoscopic surgery using posteromedial portal. Main indications for endoscopy in the posterior ankle include osteochondral lesions, loose bodies, posterior tibial osteophytes, synovial chondromatosis, and chronic synovitis.

Differential diagnosis

There are four anomalous muscles in the medial posterior ankle, which include the accessory soleus, flexor digitorum accessorius longus (FDAL), tibiocalcaneus internus, and PCI. The PCI as well as FDAL and tibiocalcaneus internus are located deep to the flexor retinaculum, whereas the accessory soleus is superficial to the flexor retinaculum. The PCI courses posterolateral to the FHL, whereas the accessory soleus, FDAL, and tibiocalcaneus internus are located posteromedial to the FHL.

Teaching point

The PCI is a rare, usually asymptomatic normal variation. Potential risk of damaging neurovascular bundles has been posed when the surgeon misidentifies this anomaly for FHL during ankle endoscopic procedures from posteromedial portal.

READING LIST

Mellado JM, Rosenberg ZS, Beltran J, Colon E. The peroneocalcaneus internus muscle: MR imaging features. *AJR Am J Roentgenol* 1997;**169**:585–588.

Phisitkul P, Amendola A. False FHL: a normal variant posing risks in posterior hindfoot endoscopy. *Arthroscopy* 2010;**26**:714–718.

Seipel R, Linklater J, Pitsis G, Sullivan M. The peroneocalcaneus internus muscle: an unusual cause of posterior ankle impingement. *Foot Ankle Int* 2005;**26**:890–893.

van Dijk CN, van Bergen CJ. Advancements in ankle arthroscopy. *J Am Acad Orthop Surg* 2008;**16**:635–646.

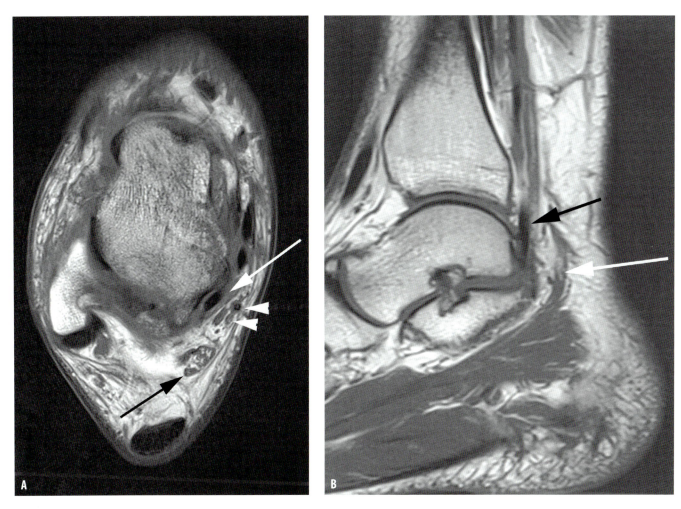

Figure 67.1 Axial T1-weighted MR image of the ankle (**A**) shows the flexor hallucis longus (FHL) tendon (white arrow), posterior tibial neurovascular bundles (arrowheads), and peroneocalcaneus internus (PCI, black arrow). Sagittal T1-weighted MR image of the ankle (**B**) reveals the peroneocalcaneus internus (PCI, white arrow) behind the flexor hallucis longus (black arrow).

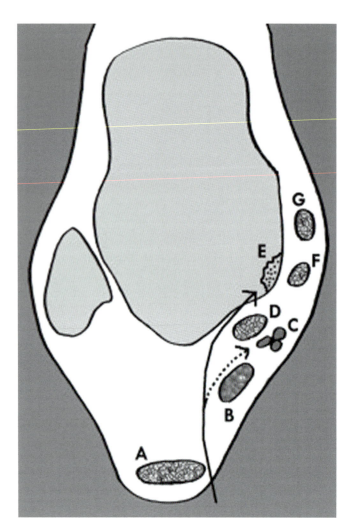

Figure 67.2 Axial diagram shows an osteochondral lesion (E) in posteromedial aspect of talar dome as an example for endoscopic indication. The solid arrow indicates the direction of the endoscopic instruments to reach the lesion, passing just lateral and deep to (D) the flexor hallucis longus muscle (FHL). The dotted arrow indicates the incorrect direction of the instruments toward (C) the neurovascular bundles when (B) the peroneocalcaneus internus is misinterpreted as the FHL. (A, Achilles tendon; F, flexor digitorum longus tendon; G, tibialis posterior tendon.) Reprinted from figure 6 of Phisitkul P, Amendola A. False FHL: a normal variant posing risks in posterior hindfoot endoscopy. *Arthroscopy* 2010;26:714–718. Copyright (2010), with permission from Elsevier.

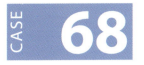

Accessory soleus muscle: a differential for posteromedial ankle mass

Imaging description

Accessory soleus can be detected on the lateral radiograph of the ankle, which shows soft tissue opacity in the pre-Achilles fat pad (Kager's triangle) (Figure 68.1). MR imaging reveals an accessory muscle between the Achilles tendon and flexor hallucis longus muscle (Figure 68.2). Normally the space is filled with fat. Accessory muscle originates from the anterior (deep) surface of the soleus from the tibia and fibula. It inserts into the Achilles tendon, superior surface of the calcaneus, or medial aspect of the calcaneus.

Importance

Accessory soleus muscle has a prevalence of 0.7–5.5% according to cadaveric studies. Real incidence of the symptomatic cases is debated. However, accessory soleus is commonly seen by musculoskeletal radiologists on radiography, CT, and MRI. Presenting symptoms include painless or painful swelling or mass on the posteromedial aspect of the ankle. Development of compartment syndrome, inadequate blood supply from the posterior tibial artery, and compression of the adjacent posterior tibial nerve have been postulated as the mechanisms of the symptomatic accessory soleus. High association with Achilles tendinopathy has been reported in patients with accessory soleus.

Typical clinical scenario

Accessory soleus is usually asymptomatic until the second decade of life. Increased muscle volume and physical activity seem to be related to the presentation of the symptoms. It is more common in males than females (2:1). A painful swelling of the posteromedial ankle is a common presenting symptom. The pain is typically exertional. Soft tissue mass is another presenting history. The patients with painful swelling are managed with avoidance of pain-producing activities and physeal therapy. Fasciotomy and excision may be indicated when conservative management has failed.

Differential diagnosis

MRI can differentiate accessory soleus from soft tissue lesions such as ganglion, lipoma, hemangioma, hematoma, and synovial sarcoma. Although accessory soleus is superficial to the flexor retinaculum, it may be associated with compression neuropathy as seen in tarsal tunnel syndrome. Three other anomalous muscles in the medial posterior ankle (flexor digitorum accessorius longus, tibiocalcaneus internus and peroneocalcaneus internus) can be differentiated on MR imaging based on the locations. (See Case 67.)

Teaching point

Accessory soleus is commonly visualized on the lateral radiograph of the ankle. Accessory soleus may become symptomatic in the second decade of life with increased muscle volume and physical activity. MR imaging is the study of choice for symptomatic cases.

READING LIST

Doda N, Peh WC, Chawla A. Symptomatic accessory soleus muscle: diagnosis and follow-up on magnetic resonance imaging. *Br J Radiol* 2006;**79**:e129–132.

Luck MD, Gordon AG, Blebea JS, Dalinka MK. High association between accessory soleus muscle and Achilles tendonopathy. *Skeletal Radiol* 2008;**37**:1129–1133.

Rossi R, Bonasia DE, Tron A, Ferro A, Castoldi F. Accessory soleus in the athletes: literature review and case report of a massive muscle in a soccer player. *Knee Surg Sports Traumatol Arthrosc* 2009;**17**:990–995.

Sookur PA, Naraghi AM, Bleakney RR *et al.* Accessory muscles: anatomy, symptoms, and radiologic evaluation. *Radiographics* 2008;**28**:481–499.

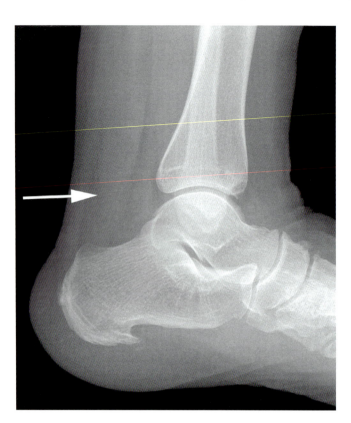

Figure 68.1 Lateral ankle radiograph shows an accessory soleus muscle (arrow) in the pre-Achilles fat pad. This was considered as an incidental finding for a 57-year-old female with chronic dorsal foot pain.

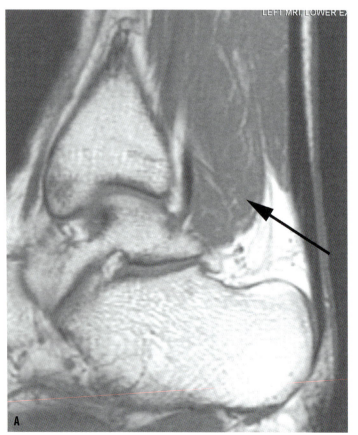

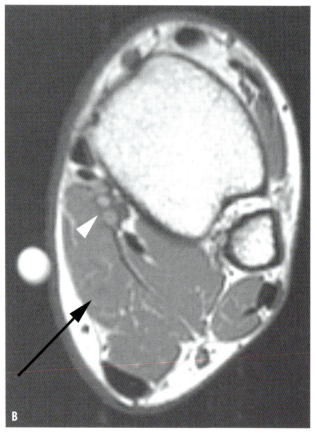

Figure 68.2 Sagittal T1-weighted MR image of the ankle (**A**) shows an accessory soleus muscle (arrow) in the pre-Achilles fat pad. MR imaging was requested to rule out mass for a 20-year-old male with aplastic anemia, who noticed posteromedial ankle fullness. Axial T1-weighted MR image of the ankle (**B**) shows an accessory soleus muscle (arrow) deep to the skin marker. Notice its close relationship to the neurovascular bundle (arrowhead).

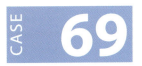
69 Xanthoma of the Achilles tendon

Imaging description

Thickening of the predominantly low-signal intensity Achilles tendon (Figure 69.1) is seen with a speckled or reticulated appearance on the axial fat-suppressed T1-weighted MR images. Sonography also shows thickening of the Achilles tendon, which reveals focal or diffuse hypoechoic lesions consistent with xanthoma. Sonographic lesions demonstrate discrete or confluent nodules with loss of normal tendon (fibrillar) architecture.

Importance

Tendon xanthoma is a hallmark of familial hypercholesterolemia (FH), an autosomal dominant disorder affecting about one in 500 in the general population. The patients with FH are at risk of premature coronary arterial disease due to an elevated low-density lipoprotein (LDL) cholesterol level. Early recognition and treatment of FH is important as effective treatment to lower cholesterol has been introduced. Familial hypercholesterolemia can be screened and diagnosed by the triad of tendon xanthoma, hypercholesterolemia (type IIa), and a family history of premature atherosclerosis. Physical examination may not detect up to 20% of the patients with FH after age 20. Imaging study can play an important role in such occasions by demonstrating xanthoma of Achilles tendon.

Typical clinical scenario

A patient who is suspected of having FH and whose physeal examination of Achilles tendon is unremarkable may be referred to sonographic study or MRI for the detection of xanthoma of Achilles tendon. A remote study showed a better detection of xanthoma of Achilles tendon by sonography compared with MRI for 10 patients with FH. Less commonly, characteristic appearance in MRI may lead to the diagnosis of FH in whom such diagnosis has not been suspected. The extensor tendons of the fingers and patellar tendons are other common sites for development of xanthoma.

Differential diagnosis

Clinical differentials for thickening of the Achilles tendon include tear (trauma), tendinosis (tendon degeneration), and systemic conditions such as rheumatoid arthritis, gout (tophus), and FH (xanthoma). Currently it is not clear if MRI findings could accurately differentiate these conditions without clinical findings.

Teaching point

Early detection and treatment of FH is clinically paramount to prevent premature atherosclerotic disease. Sonography shows a focal or diffuse hypoechoic lesion in the thickened Achilles tendon. MRI, less sensitive than sonography, may show characteristic speckled or reticulated appearance on the axial fat-suppressed T1-weighted images.

READING LIST

Bude RO, Adler RS, Bassett DR. Diagnosis of Achilles tendon xanthoma in patients with heterozygous familial hypercholesterolemia: MR vs sonography. *AJR Am J Roentgenol* 1994;**162**:913–917.

Gidding SS. Familial hypercholesterolemia: a decade of progress. *J Pediatr* 2010;**156**:176–177.

Kwiterovich PO. Primary and secondary disorders of lipid metabolism in pediatrics. *Pediatr Endocrinol Rev* 2008;**5 Suppl 2**:727–738.

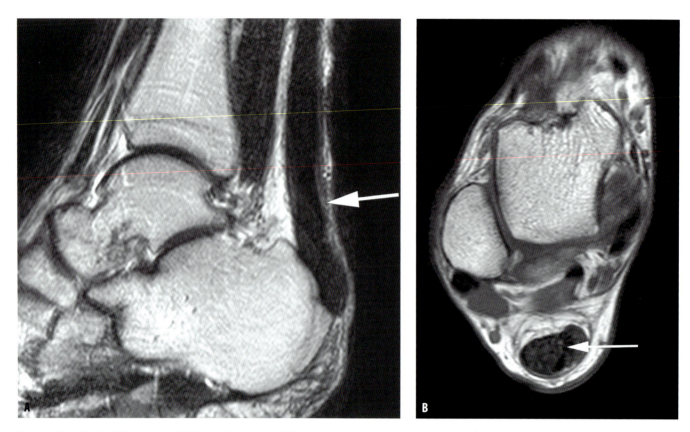

Figure 69.1 Sagittal (A) and axial (B) T1-weighted ankle MR images demonstrating a xanthoma of the Achilles tendon. The tendon thickening is associated with predominantly low signal (arrow on image A) with a superimposed speckled or reticulated appearance (arrow on image B).

Master knot of Henry

Imaging description

The master knot of Henry is best seen on coronally oriented cross-sectional imaging such as CT or MRI of the foot. After extending past the sustentaculum tali, the flexor hallucis longus (FHL) crosses from lateral to medial over the dorsal surface of the flexor digitorum longus (FDL). This cross-over is termed the master knot of Henry (Figure 70.1). At this cross-over, these two tendons are enclosed together and attached to the vault of the arch of the foot. Just distal to the master knot of Henry, there is a ligamentous attachment between the two tendons. This ligament can be proximal to distally oriented from the FHL to the FDL; it can be distal to proximally oriented from the FHL to the FDL; or it can be bifid with both distal to proximal and proximal to distal oriented ligaments as they extend from the FHL to the FDL.

Importance

Depending on the orientation of the ligament by the master knot of Henry, rupture of the FHL or FDL proximal to the master knot of Henry may not cause loss of toe flexion. When the ligament is oriented distal to proximal from the FHL to the FDL, rupture of the FHL proximal to the master knot of Henry will not cause loss of toe flexion. Conversely, when the ligament is proximal to distal from the FHL to the FDL, rupture of the FDL proximal to the knot will not cause loss of toe flexion. With a bifid ligament, then rupture of either the FHL or FDL proximal to the knot will not cause loss of toe flexion.

Typical clinical scenario

A 25-year-old dancer presents to the sports medicine clinic with history and signs of FHL rupture proximal to the level of the master knot of Henry; however, she does not have loss of toe flexion. This would indicate that the ligamentous attachment between the FHL and FDL at the master knot of Henry is bifid or extends distal to proximal from the FHL to the FDL.

Teaching point

There is a ligamentous attachment between the FHL and FDL at and immediately distal to the master knot of Henry. Depending on the orientation of this ligament, FHL rupture proximal to the master knot of Henry may not lead to loss of toe flexion.

READING LIST

Lui TH, Chow FY. "Intersection syndrome" of the foot: treated by endoscopic release of master knot of Henry. *Knee Surg Sports Traumatol Arthrosc* 2011;**19**:850–852.

O'Sullivan E, Carare-Nnadi R, Greenslade J, Bowyer G. Clinical significance of variations in the interconnections between flexor digitorum longus and flexor hallucis longus in the region of the knot of Henry. *Clin Anat* 1005;**18**:121–125.

Thakur N, Leswick DA. Case of the month #167: flexor hallucis longus tendon tear distal to the master knot of Henry. *Can Assoc Radiol J* 2011;**62**:154–157.

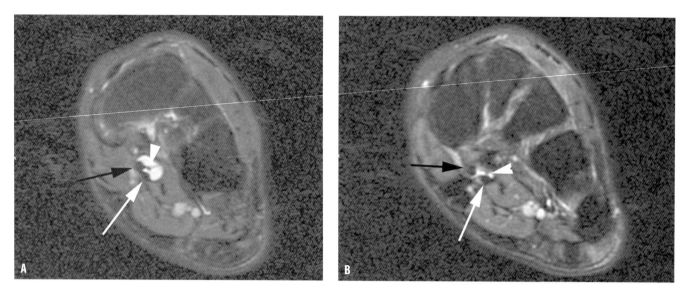

Figure 70.1 Coronal fat-suppressed T2-weighted coronal images (**A** and **B**) show the flexor hallucis longus (black arrow) and the flexor digitorum longus (white arrow) at and just distal to the master knot of Henry. These tendons are connected by a bifid ligament (arrowhead) in this patient.

Tarsal tunnel syndrome

Imaging description

The tarsal tunnel is best seen on coronal imaging with advanced cross-sectional imaging such as CT or MRI (Figure 71.1). The tarsal tunnel is superficially bounded by the flexor retinaculum. The flexor retinaculum inserts anteriorly on the medial malleolus, posteriorly on the calcaneal medial tuberosity, distally as a continuation of the plantar fascia, and proximally as a continuation of the superficial and deep aponeuroses of the leg. The deep edge of the tarsal tunnel is bounded by the medial surface of the talus and calcaneus. The tarsal tunnel contains the tibialis posterior tendon, flexor digitorum longus tendon, flexor hallucis longus tendon, and posterior tibial neurovascular bundle. Tarsal tunnel syndrome is caused by compression of the posterior tibial neurovascular bundle within the tarsal tunnel (Figure 71.2).

Importance

Typically, MRI is used to diagnose the cause of tarsal tunnel syndrome. Some of the causes that can be demonstrated by MRI are neoplasms, prominent tenosynovitis, prominent varicose veins, synovial hypertrophy, scar tissue, and ganglion cysts. The cause of the tarsal tunnel syndrome will determine whether the initial treatment of the disease is conservative or surgical. A cause of tarsal tunnel syndrome is demonstrated in approximately 50% of the cases, with the remaining 50% being idiopathic.

Typical clinical scenario

A 45-year-old female presents with pain, tingling, and a burning sensation along the plantar and medial aspect of the foot and great toe. The symptoms are exacerbated by walking and exercise. The distribution of symptoms is along that of the posterior tibial nerve and its branches. An electromyographic study is positive. MRI of the foot was ordered to evaluate for a cause of the tarsal tunnel syndrome. MRI revealed a prominent ganglion cyst in the tarsal tunnel.

Teaching point

Tarsal tunnel syndrome can be caused by mechanical nerve compression or entrapment within the tarsal tunnel in 50% of the cases. The mechanical cause can be readily demonstrated by MRI.

READING LIST

Erickson SJ, Quinn SF, Kneeland JB *et al.* MR imaging of the tarsal tunnel and related spaces: normal and abnormal findings with anatomic correlation. *AJR Am J Roentgenol* 1990;**155**:323–328.

Narváez JA, Narváez J, Ortega R *et al.* Painful heel: MR imaging findings. *Radiographics* 2000;**20**:333–352.

Rosenberg ZS, Beltran J, Bencardino JT. From the RSNA Refresher Courses. Radiological Society of North America. MR imaging of the ankle and foot. *Radiographics* 2000;**20 Spec No**:S153–S179.

Pearls and Pitfalls in Musculoskeletal Imaging, ed. D. Lee Bennett and Georges Y. El-Khoury. Published by Cambridge University Press. © Cambridge University Press 2013.

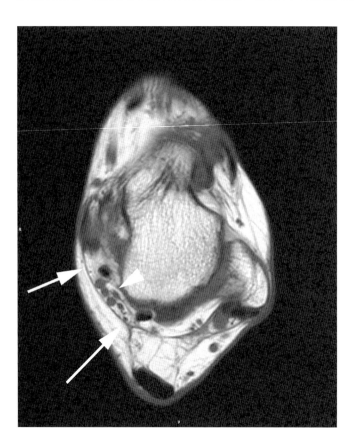

Figure 71.1 This T1-weighted oblique axial/coronal MR image readily demonstrates the flexor retinaculum (arrows) that superficially borders the tarsal tunnel. Its anterior attachment to the medial malleolus can be seen on this image. The contents of the tarsal tunnel can be seen deep to this structure, including the posterior tibial neurovascular bundle (arrowhead).

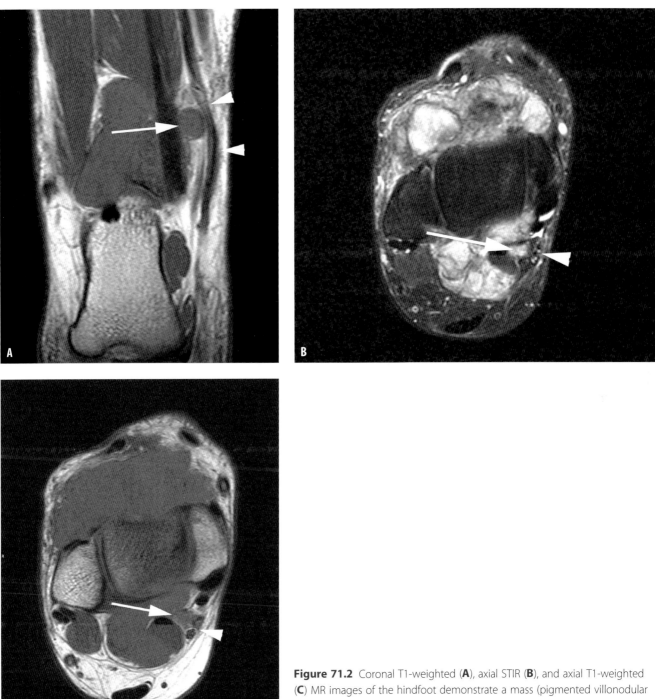

Figure 71.2 Coronal T1-weighted (**A**), axial STIR (**B**), and axial T1-weighted (**C**) MR images of the hindfoot demonstrate a mass (pigmented villonodular synovitis) within the tarsal tunnel (arrows) that is displacing the posterior tibial neurovascular bundle (arrowheads) in this patient with tarsal tunnel syndrome.

Great toe sesamoids: osteonecrosis versus stress fracture

Imaging description

Stress fractures of the great toe have been reported as occurring most commonly in the medial sesamoid. Stress fractures of the medial great toe sesamoid can be difficult to diagnose on radiographs since they are typically seen only on the AP view and can mimic a multipartite sesamoid. CT with multiplanar reconstructions can readily show the rough fracture edges of a stress fracture compared with the smooth edges of a multipartite sesamoid (Figure 72.1). If there is still confusion on CT images, MRI can be used to demonstrate abnormal bone marrow-like edema within the medial sesamoid.

Osteonecrosis of the great toe has been described as occurring primarily in the lateral sesamoid of the great toe. Osteonecrosis can be seen on axial sesamoid views of the foot as sclerosis and collapse/fragmentation of the sesamoid (Figure 72.2). It can also be seen on MRI as bone marrow-like edema within the lateral sesamoid with normal signal in the adjacent first metatarsal. It has been reported that bone marrow-like edema can be seen in the sesamoid from osteoarthritis; however, one will also see bone marrow-like edema in the subjacent first metatarsal head when osteoarthritis is the cause of the abnormal signal.

Importance

It is important to diagnose sesamoid pathology with medical imaging as it can be difficult to diagnose injuries or osteonecrosis of the great toe sesamoids based solely on history and physical exam findings. If there is clinical concern for possible great toe sesamoid pathology, the radiologist should be careful to not diagnose multiple sesamoid ossifications as a multipartite or bipartite sesamoid as both stress fractures and osteonecrosis can lead to fragmentation of the sesamoids. In these cases, CT and MRI are useful in diagnosing sesamoid stress fractures or osteonecrosis. Because of the difficulty in diagnosing these entities clinically, quick diagnosis of a multipartite sesamoid without questioning a stress fracture or osteonecrosis can lead to a delay in diagnosis.

Typical clinical scenario

The patient is usually a young adult that presents with vague pain over the plantar aspect of the first metatarsophalangeal joint. Patients with osteonecrosis of the lateral sesamoid will usually relate no history of stress or overuse of the foot; however, in the setting of a stress fracture of the medial sesamoid the patient will usually be athletically active in an endeavor that places stress on the ball of the foot.

Differential diagnosis

On radiographs, the differential would include a bipartite or multipartite sesamoid. On MRI, bone marrow-like edema in the sesamoid can also be seen with early osteoarthritis. There should usually be edema in the subjacent first metatarsal head in patients with early osteoarthritis.

Teaching point

In the setting of plantar pain over the first metatarsophalangeal joint, one should not assume that a fragmented great toe sesamoid is a bipartite or multipartite sesamoid. One should carefully consider the possibilities of stress fracture or osteonecrosis.

READING LIST

Biedert R. Which investigations are required in stress fracture of the great toe sesamoids? *Arch Orthop Trauma Surg* 1993;**112**:94–95.

Biedert R, Hintermann B. Stress fractures of the medial great toe sesamoids in athletes. *Foot Ankle Int* 2003;**24**:137–141.

Kulemann V, Mayerhoefer M, Trnka HJ, Kristen KH, Steiner E. Abnormal findings in hallucal sesamoids on MR imaging – associated with different pathologies of the forefoot? An observational study. *Eur J Radiol* 2010;**74**:226–230.

Ozkoç G, Akpinar S, Ozalay M *et al.* Hallucal sesamoid osteonecrosis: an overlooked cause of forefoot pain. *J Am Podiatr Med Assoc* 2005;**95**:277–280.

Toussirot E, Jeunet L, Michel F, Kantelip B, Wendling D. Avascular necrosis of the hallucal sesamoids update with reference to two case-reports. *Joint Bone Spine* 2003;**70**:307–309.

Pearls and Pitfalls in Musculoskeletal Imaging, ed. D. Lee Bennett and Georges Y. El-Khoury. Published by Cambridge University Press. © Cambridge University Press 2013.

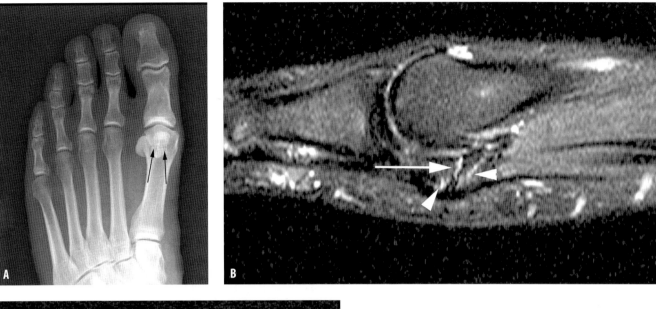

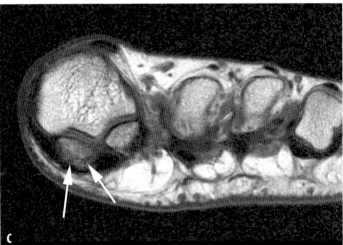

Figure 72.1 A 31-year-old runner with a great toe medial sesamoid stress fracture. The AP radiograph (**A**) of the foot demonstrates fracture in the medial sesamoid (arrows). Since this patient was a competitive athlete, an MRI was done to confirm a stress fracture rather than a bipartite sesamoid. The sagittal fat-suppressed MR image (**B**) shows the fracture line (arrow) with bone marrow-like edema in the sesamoid (arrowheads) about the fracture. A coronal T1-weighted MR image (**C**) also shows the hypointense fracture line (arrows).

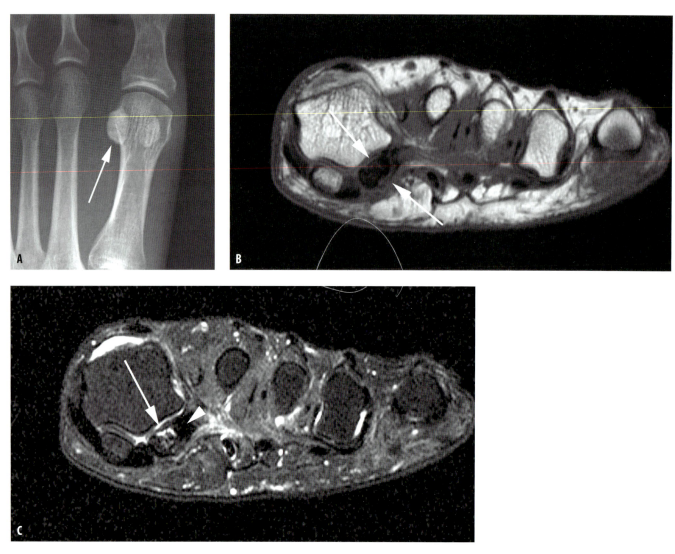

Figure 72.2 A 40-year-old female with histologically confirmed osteonecrosis of the lateral sesamoid of the great toe. An AP radiograph of the foot (**A**) shows a densely sclerotic lateral sesamoid. Coronal T1-weighted (**B**) and fat-suppressed T2-weighted (**C**) MR images show hypointensity (**B**) and patchy hyperintensity (**C**) in this sesamoid consistent with osteonecrosis. Note the normal signal characteristics in the adjacent metatarsal head.

Imaging description

The Lisfranc joint is strictly defined as the articulation between the midfoot tarsals (cuneiforms and cuboid) and the second through fifth metatarsals. A Lisfranc injury is diagnosed usually on radiographs. In particular, an unstable Lisfranc injury can be diagnosed as being present if there is misalignment at the second tarsometatarsal articulation (Figure 73.1). Specifically, the medial edge of the base of the second metatarsal should perfectly line up with the medial edge of the middle cuneiform in a normal foot. If a Lisfranc injury is clinically suspected and a non-weightbearing foot radiograph is normal, then a weightbearing AP foot radiograph must be obtained to look for any second tarsometatarsal articulation misalignment. If a weightbearing radiograph cannot be obtained or if there is still considerable clinical concern for a Lisfranc injury of the foot, then an MRI of the foot should be performed. On the coronal images of the foot, one should specifically look for a high grade sprain of the plantar Lisfranc ligament between the medial cuneiform and the bases of the second and third metatarsals (the pC1-M2M3 Lisfranc ligament). A high grade sprain of this ligament has an approximately 95% positive predictive value for an unstable Lisfranc injury; therefore, indicating surgical treatment should be considered (Figure 73.2).

Importance

Inadequate early treatment of Lisfranc joint injuries can result in substantial instability, deformity, and dysfunction of the foot. This can be especially debilitating in athletes and people that have an occupation that requires standing and/or walking.

Typical clinical scenario

A football player had their foot stepped on by a 350 lb lineman during a game and is now experiencing pain over the midfoot with any kind of ambulating or running. A radiograph demonstrated a normal exam; however, it was non-weightbearing. The patient had difficulty performing a weightbearing radiograph of the foot; therefore, an MRI of the Lisfranc joint was performed. It demonstrated rupture of the pC1-M2M3 Lisfranc ligament. At surgery the joint was found to be unstable; therefore, a reduction and internal fixation of the joint was performed.

> ## Teaching point
>
> Lisfranc injuries can usually be diagnosed by weightbearing foot radiographs. However, in the setting of clinical concern for a Lisfranc injury and a good weightbearing foot radiograph cannot be obtained or the radiographic results are equivocal, MRI can be performed to determine if an unstable Lisfranc injury is present. This is demonstrated on MRI by disruption of the pC1-M2M3 Lisfranc ligament.

READING LIST

Gupta RT, Wadhwa RP, Learch TJ, Herwick SM. Lisfranc injury: imaging findings for this important but often-missed diagnosis. *Curr Probl Diagn Radiol* 2008;**37**:115–126.

Macmahon PJ, Dheer S, Raikin SM *et al*. MRI of injuries to the first interosseous cuneometatarsal (Lisfranc) ligament. *Skeletal Radiol* 2009;**38**:255–260.

Raikin SM, Elias I, Dheer S *et al*. Prediction of midfoot instability in the subtle Lisfranc injury. Comparison of magnetic resonance imaging with intraoperative findings. *J Bone Joint Surg Am* 2009;**91**:892–899.

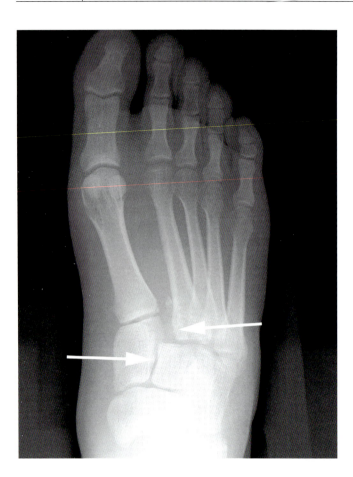

Figure 73.1 An AP radiograph of the foot in this patient reveals a divergent Lisfranc fracture/dislocation. There is obvious misalignment between the medial edges of the middle cuneiform and the second metatarsal base (arrows).

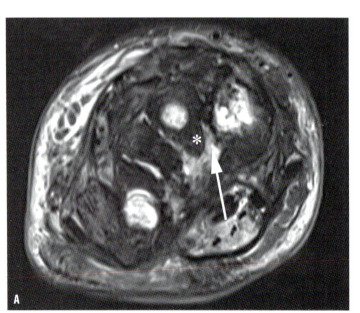 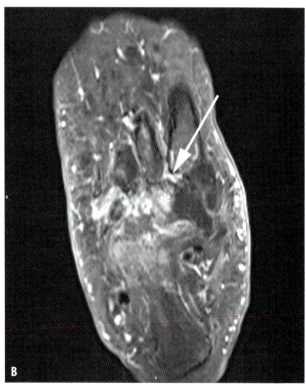

Figure 73.2 Coronal (**A**) and axial (**B**) STIR MR images of the foot. There is no visible plantar band of the Lisfranc ligament (medial cuneiform-second metatarsal ligament), and there is edema where this ligament should be (arrows); therefore, this ligament is ruptured. An asterisk identifies the base of the second metatarsal. Disruption of the plantar band is associated with an unstable Lisfranc fracture/dislocation.

Imaging description

Navicular stress fractures are seen on AP radiographs of the foot, coronal CT images, or coronal MR images as a linear or curvilinear fracture line extending longitudinally in the sagittal plane (Figure 74.1). Stress reaction of the navicular can be seen as bone marrow-like edema within the navicular on MR images. When the fracture line is curvilinear it will typically curve laterally. Stress fractures of the navicular can also be complete or incomplete. When incomplete they will be proximal in location and usually involve the proximal articular surface of the navicular bone.

Importance

Navicular stress fractures typically occur in athletes and can be difficult to diagnose on clinical exam. A high degree of suspicion must be present. Given the difficulty in diagnosing this injury clinically, the average time from onset of symptoms to diagnosis is between four to seven months. Navicular stress fractures respond well when they are treated early; however, the delay in diagnosis that usually occurs can result in suboptimal treatment. Unfortunately, misdiagnosis and delayed diagnosis resulting in inadequate treatment of these lesions can have disastrous consequences for the athlete.

Only about 20–25% of navicular stress fractures are visible on radiographs; therefore, if there is any clinical suspicion of a navicular stress fracture in an athlete, advanced imaging should be ordered so that the correct diagnosis can be made before significant damage is done.

Typical clinical scenario

A young adult female who was a long-distance runner presented with a several-week history of pain over the dorsum of the foot. Physical exam only revealed some focal tenderness to palpation over the dorsum of the foot. There were no other abnormal findings on physical exam. The initial radiographs were read as normal. Given the clinician's suspicion of a navicular stress fracture, a CT was ordered that demonstrated a navicular stress fracture (Figure 74.2). The patient was successfully treated.

Teaching point

A negative radiograph does not rule out a navicular stress fracture. If there is any clinical concern for a navicular stress fracture, advanced imaging should be ordered such as an MRI or CT.

READING LIST

de Clercq PF, Bevernage BD, Leemrijse T. Stress fracture of the navicular bone. *Acta Orthop Belg* 2008;**74**:725–734.

Jones MH, Amendola AS. Navicular stress fractures. *Clin Sports Med* 2006;**25**:151–158.

Kiss ZS, Khan KM, Fuller PJ. Stress fractures of the tarsal navicular bone: CT findings in 55 cases. *AJR Am J Roentgenol* 1993;**160**:111–115.

Sanders TG, Williams PM, Vawter KW. Stress fracture of the tarsal navicular. *Mil Med* 2004;**169**:viii–xiii.

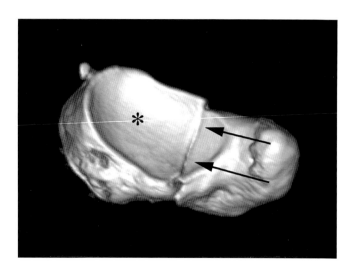

Figure 74.1 This figure shows a three-dimensional volume-rendered CT image of a navicular bone with a stress fracture (arrows). The fracture line is sagittally oriented and disrupts the proximal articular surface of the navicular (asterisk).

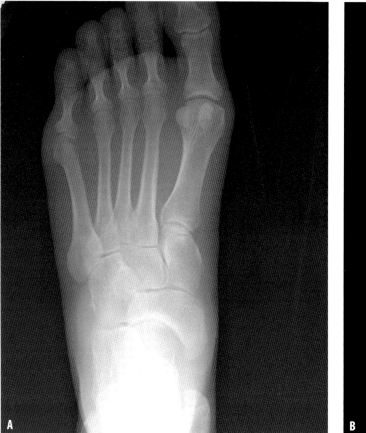

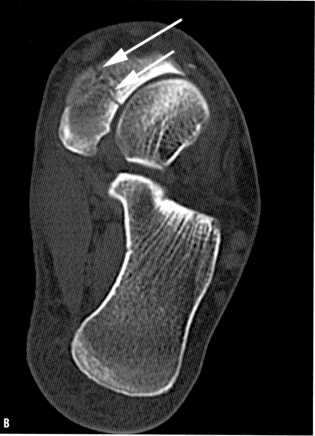

Figure 74.2 A 20-year-old female with a navicular stress fracture. The AP radiograph of the foot (**A**) was interpreted as normal. A CT (**B**) readily demonstrated the non-displaced stress fracture (arrows) of the navicular.

Intraosseous lipoma

Imaging description

Intraosseous lipomas present as solitary lesions. Radiographic features often parallel the histologic stage of the lesion. Stage 1 and 2 typically reveal geographic, lytic lesions with well-defined sclerotic margin. The lesions vary in size from 1–9 cm. In stage 3 the radiographic features of the intraosseous lipoma are non-specific. In the calcaneus and the proximal femur the radiographic pattern can be characteristic. More than half the cases show a central calcification or ossification (Figures 75.1 and 75.2). On CT the lesion shows areas of low attenuation ranging between −40 and −60 Hounsfield units (Figure 75.3). The identification of fatty area on CT is diagnostic of intraosseous lipoma. Visualizing fat within these tumors is the primary role of MRI especially in lesions without significant amounts of involution. On MRI the fatty components of the lesion are iso-intense with subcutaneous fat on all sequences. Areas of dystrophic calcification and ossification show low signal intensity on all sequences. Cysts are common within intraosseous lipomas especially in the calcaneus and they show low signal intensity on T1-weighted images and high signal intensity on T2-weighted images (Figure 75.4). On bone scan an intraosseous lipoma may show mild increase in radionuclide uptake or it may be entirely negative.

Importance

Earlier literature stressed the rarity of intraosseous lipomas but with the advent of CT and MRI the diagnosis of this lesion became fairly common. Imaging of intraosseous lipomas is very useful because it obviates the need for a biopsy or surgical excision. Intraosseous lipomas can present with varying degrees of involution resulting in areas of fat necrosis, cyst formation, and dystrophic calcifications. As a result the imaging characteristics can vary considerably depending on the degree of involution (Figure 75.1). The most common sites for intraosseous lipoma are the calcaneus, subtrochanteric region of the femur, proximal tibial metaphysis, distal femoral metaphysis, proximal and distal fibular metaphyses, spine, and pelvis. They are identified in patients between the fourth and sixth decades. Based on the histological findings Milgram classified intraosseous lipomas into three stages. In stage 1 the lesion contains viable lipocytes interspersed with fine bony trabecula. In stage 2 lesions the fatty tissue is partly necrotic and shows some calcification. Stage 3 reveals the greatest degree of involution. At this stage there is more extensive fatty necrosis with more widespread calcification and cyst formation. The stage 3 is the most difficult to diagnose even with MRI. Histologically it resembles a bone infarct.

Typical clinical scenario

Although soft tissue lipomas are more common in females, intraosseous lipomas have almost equal distribution between males and females. In the literature some intraosseous lipomas are asymptomatic and are discovered incidentally on imaging studies; more than half the patients present with symptoms. These symptoms include pain tenderness and swelling. Pathologic fractures in intraosseous lipomas are extremely rare. No treatment is required for asymptomatic lesions, however curettage and bone grafting is needed for symptomatic intraosseous lipomas.

Differential diagnosis

Stage 1 and 2 lesions can often be diagnosed on plane radiographs, however, the diagnosis with stage 3 lesions is more difficult. The differential diagnosis includes non-ossifying fibroma, simple bone cyst, aneurysmal bone cyst, fibrous dysplasia, bone infarct, chondroid tumors, and liposclerosing myxofibrous tumor. Sometimes the typical location of the lipoma and the presence of a central calcification render the diagnosis fairly straightforward. The central calcification is known as the "cockade sign" which can best be demonstrated by radiography and CT. This is particularly true of calcaneal intraosseous lipomas where the appearance is almost pathognomonic. Other lesions of the calcaneus that occur in the same location and can closely resemble an intraosseous lipoma include a simple bone cyst and a pseudo-lesion which is an area of pronounced scarcity of trabecula in the anterior calcaneus. Both of these lesions do not show a central zone of calcification or cockade sign.

Teaching point

Intraosseous lipomas are benign lesions that usually do not require any treatment. With the advent of CT and MRI the diagnosis of intraosseous lipoma has become more common and the ability to arrive at a specific diagnosis without resorting to a biopsy or surgical excision is often feasible.

READING LIST

Blacksin MF, Ende N, Benevenia J. Magnetic resonance imaging of intraosseous lipomas: a radiologic-pathologic correlation. *Skeletal Radiol* 1995;**24**:37–41.

Campbell RSD, Grainger AJ, Mangham DC *et al*. Intraosseous lipoma: report of 35 new cases and a review of the literature. *Skeletal Radiol* 2003;**32**:209–222.

Milgram JW. Intraosseous lipomas: radiologic and pathologic manifestations. *Radiology* 1988;**167**:155–160.

Propeck T, Bullard MA, Lin J *et al*. Radiologic-pathologic correlation of intraosseous lipomas. *AJR Am J Roentgenol* 2000;**185**:673–678.

Ramos A, Castello J, Sartoris DJ *et al*. Osseous lipoma: CT appearance. *Radiology* 1985;**157**:615–619.

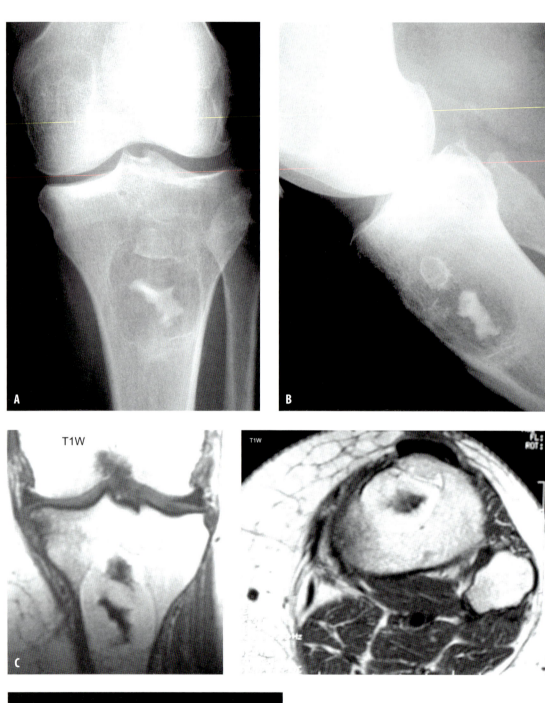

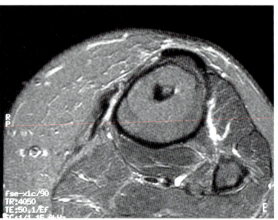

Figure 75.1 Intraosseous lipoma in the proximal left tibia. Anteroposterior (**A**) and lateral (**B**) views of the left knee show an oval lucent lesion with well-defined margin. The lesion contains two calcific densities. This radiographic appearance is highly suggestive of an intraosseous lipoma. (**C**) and (**D**) are T1-weighted coronal and axial images of the knee which show high signal intensity within the lesion along with a central low signal intensity typical of a lipoma with areas of calcification. Fat-suppressed axial T2-weighted image (**E**) through the proximal tibia shows low signal intensity throughout the lesion. The calcified center is much darker than the rest of the lesion which is made of fat.

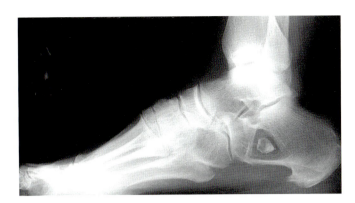

Figure 75.2 A lateral view of the right foot shows a typical location for an intraosseous lipoma. The central calcification, known as the "cockade sign" makes the appearance pathognomonic of intraosseous lipoma.

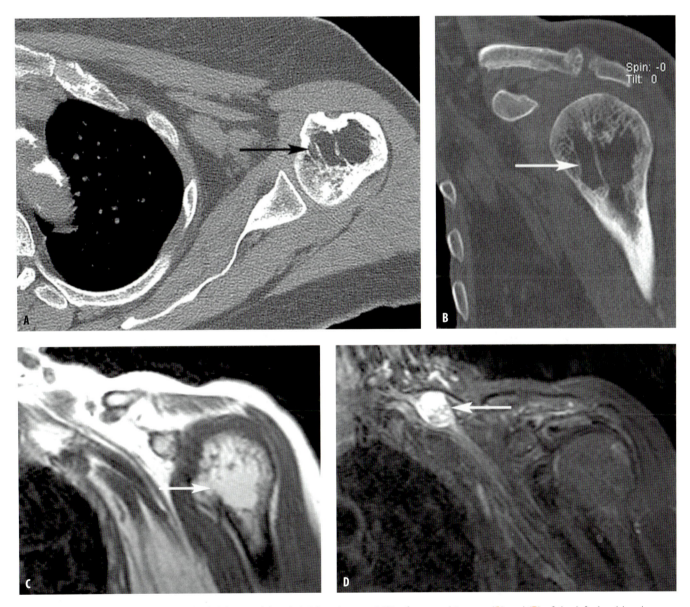

Figure 75.3 Intraosseous lipoma in the left humeral head. Axial and coronal CT reformatted images (**A**) and (**B**) of the left shoulder show a lytic lesion in the humeral head. The tissue attenuation within the lesion is similar to the subcutaneous fat. These findings alone should be diagnostic of an intraosseous lipoma (arrow). Coronal T1-weighted MR image (**C**) shows the lesion in the humeral head. It has high signal intensity typical of fat (arrow). Fat-suppressed coronal T2-weighted image (**D**) shows signal intensity within the humeral head lesion confirming that the lesion is an intraosseous lipoma. Also noted is an unrelated Schwannoma of the brachial plexus (arrow).

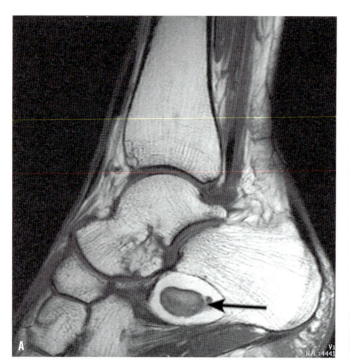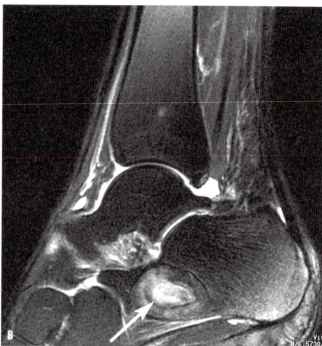

Figure 75.4 Calcaneal lipoma with cystic changes in its center. A T1-weighted sagittal image (**A**) of the ankle show a low signal-intensity oval area within the lipoma (arrow) which represents a cyst. A fat-suppressed T2-weighted sagittal (**B**) image reveals high signal intensity within the cyst.

Imaging description

Radiography shows evidence of a joint effusion, and variable degrees of osteoarthritis. Erosions have been described in about 25% of patients with lipoma arborescens but they are less common compared with pigmented villonodular synovitis. CT shows the fatty mass and the joint effusion. Attenuation measurements demonstrate the low density within the mass consistent with fat. Ultrasound is also very effective in demonstrating the joint effusion and the villous nature of the mass. In addition ultrasound demonstrates the hyperechoic appearance of the mass suggesting the presence of fat. The appearance of lipoma arborescens on MRI is believed to be pathognomonic. MRI can readily reveal the joint effusion, the mass, and the frond-like projections. The fatty components of the tumor follow the signal characteristics of the subcutaneous fat on all pulse sequences (Figure 76.1). MRI can differentiate lipoma arborescens from other intra-articular diseases like pigmented villonodular synovitis (PVNS) and synovial chondromatosis.

Importance

Lipoma arborescens is a rare intra-articular lesion where there is replacement of the subsynovial tissue with mature fat cells and the formation of proliferative villous projections. The exact etiology of lipoma arborescens is not known but it has been suggested that it represents a reactive process of the synovial membrane due to a variety of insults. Lipoma arborescens occurs in association with degenerative joint disease, rheumatoid arthritis, and trauma. The condition commonly affects men, and the knee is the most commonly involved joint although the disease has been described in the wrist, hip, glenohumeral joint, subachromal subdeltoid bursa, and tendon sheath of the peroneal tendons. In the knee, which is the most commonly involved joint, lipoma arborescens has a predilection for the suprapatellar pouch. Bilateral knee involvement has been described in about 20% of the patients. Lipoma arborescens is often associated with a joint effusion and aspiration of the effusion reveals serosanguinous fluid without crystals or microorganisms. Synovectomy is a curative treatment and recurrences are rare.

Typical clinical scenario

Clinically the disorder presents as a chronic painless swelling of the joint because of recurrent effusions. Initially the patients are asymptomatic. With time the volume of the effusion and the size of the mass increase and patients start to experience pain and limitation of motion. Physical examination confirms the existence of the joint effusion. Rarely a soft tissue mass can be palpated in the joint. Laboratory studies are normal.

Differential diagnosis

The differential diagnosis of synovial proliferative disorders should include pigmented villonodular synovitis, rheumatoid arthritis, synovial chondromatosis, synovial hemangioma, intra-articular lipoma, lipoma arborescens, and hemophilia. On MRI images PVNS usually has low signal on T1-weighted, T2-weighted, and gradient echo sequences. The fatty nature of the mass with fronds is a distinctive sign on MRI of lipoma arborescens. Lipoma arborescens typically involved the suprapatellar pouch whereas PVNS tends to extend into the semimembranosus-gastrocnemius bursa. Synovial lipoma should be differentiated from lipoma arborescens which is much more common, but this can be difficult. Synovial lipoma is a localized mass of adipose tissue with round or oval contour without synovial changes, whereas lipoma arborescens is characterized by diffuse subsynovial deposition of fat, a villous appearance, and associated joint effusion.

Teaching point

Although lipoma arborescens is a rare lesion, the imaging features on MRI are pathognomonic and radiologists should be able to make the correct diagnosis in most cases. These findings include: (1) a synovial mass with frond-like architecture; (2) fat signal intensity within the mass on all pulse sequences; (3) suppression of these signals with fat-suppression techniques; and (4) absence of hemosiderin (Figure 76.1).

READING LIST

Dawson JS, Dowling F, Preston BJ, Neumann L. Case report: lipoma arborescens of the sub-deltoid bursa. *Br J Radiol* 1995;**68**:197–199.

Feller JF, Rishi M, Hughes EC. Lipoma arborescens of the knee: MR demonstration. *AJR Am J Roentgenol* 1994;**163**:162–164.

Grieten M, Buckwalter KA, Cardinal E, Rougraff B. Case report 873. *Skeletal Radiol* 1994;**23**:652–655.

Hallel T, Lew S, Isreael K-S, Bansal M. Villous lipomatous proliferation of the synovial membrane (lipoma arborescens). *J Bone Joint Surg* 1988; **70-A**:264–270.

Laorr A, Peterfy CG, Tirman PFJ, Rabassa AE. Lipoma arborescens of the shoulder: magnetic resonance imaging findings. *Can Assoc Radiol J* 1995;**46**:311–313.

Martin S, Hernandez L, Romero J *et al*. Diagnostic imaging of lipoma arborescens. *Skeletal Radiol* 1998;**27**:325–329.

Matsumoto K, Okabe H, Ishizawa M, Hiraoka S. Intra-articular lipoma of the knee joint. *J Bone Joint Surg* 2001;**83A**:101–105.

Ryu KN, Jaovisidha S, Schweitzer M *et al*. MR imaging of lipoma arborescens of the knee joint. *AJR Am J Roentgenol* 1996;**167**:1229–1232.

Sola JB, Wright RW. Arthroscopic treatment for lipoma arborescens of the knee. *J Bone Joint Surg* 1998;**80-A**:99–102.

Vilanova JC, Barcelo J, Villalon M *et al*. MR imaging of lipoma arborescens and the associated lesions. *Skeletal Radiol* 2003;**32**:504–509.

Pearls and Pitfalls in Musculoskeletal Imaging, ed. D. Lee Bennett and Georges Y. El-Khoury. Published by Cambridge University Press. © Cambridge University Press 2013.

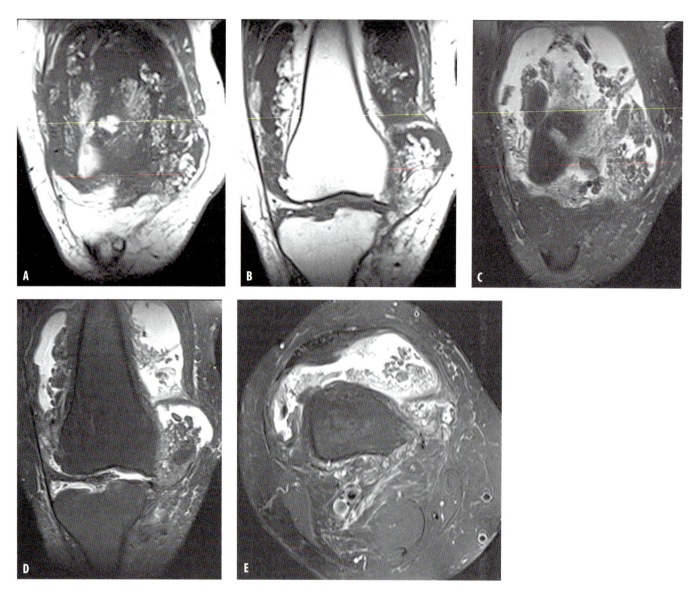

Figure 76.1 Lipoma arborescens of the knee in a 68-year-old male. Coronal T1-weighted images (**A**) and (**B**) of the right knee show a large joint effusion along with high-signal frond-like structure projecting out from the synovial lining. Fat-suppressed coronal and axial T2-weighted images (**C**, **D**, and **E**) show low signal-intensity fronds floating within the high signal-intensity synovial fluid. This is the typical MRI appearance of lipoma arborescens.

Imaging description

When a well-differentiated liposarcoma is located in the extremities it can reveal fatty densities on a radiographic examination. This is not the case with a retroperitoneal well-differentiated liposarcoma. Occasionally tumor calcifications or ossifications can be detected radiographically. CT or MRI is essential for making a definitive diagnosis. Both modalities show that the well-differentiated liposarcoma consists primarily of fatty tissue. What differentiates a well-differentiated liposarcoma from a lipoma is the presence of thick septa greater than 2 mm in thickness or nodular non-fatty tissue within the lesion (Figure 77.1). The septa and nodular structures show enhancement on gadolinium-enhanced MR images. It is important to remember that lipomas can be septated, however the septa are thin (< 2 mm). In planning a needle biopsy under CT guidance the radiologist should target areas that contain a high density of thick septa or nodularity to ensure better sampling of the tumor.

Imaging of myxoid liposarcoma is often more difficult than imaging of a well-differentiated liposarcoma. Radiography in myxoid liposarcoma is often negative or shows a non-specific soft tissue mass. CT and MRI may reveal what looks like a large lobulated cystic lesion because of its high content of myxoid tissue. The high water content of the myxoid tissue is represented on MRI with homogeneous low signal intensity on T1-weighted images and intensely high signals on T2-weighted images (Figure 77.2). In this respect a myxoid liposarcoma may be confused with a soft tissue cyst, however gadolinium enhancement will differentiate between a myxoid liposarcoma which shows enhancement following gadolinium injection compared with a cyst which does not enhance. A myxoid liposarcoma with a predominantly round cell component can reveal totally non-specific imaging features on cross-sectional imaging and therefore becomes very difficult to differentiate from other soft tissue sarcomas.

Importance

Liposarcoma is the second most common type of soft tissue sarcoma accounting for about 10–35% of all soft tissue sarcomas. It is exceeded only by malignant fibrous histiocytoma (currently known as undifferentiated high-grade pleomorphic sarcoma). Liposarcoma is divided into five histological types; they are: well-differentiated, dedifferentiated, myxoid, pleomorphic, and mixed liposarcoma. The difference in the histological characteristics of these liposarcomas is reflected in their biological behavior and imaging features. The most prevalent types are the well-differentiated and myxoid liposarcomas. Both of these tumors have fairly characteristic imaging features, but the pleomorphic and mixed type can be difficult to differentiate from other malignant soft tissue tumors. Liposarcoma arising primarily within bone is extremely rare. The well-differentiated liposarcoma is the most common type of soft tissue liposarcoma; it occurs mostly in adults between the 6th and 7th decades. The lower extremity and retroperitoneum are the commonest sites for this tumor. It is a low-grade neoplasm. Although it can locally recur, it does not metastasize; all the other liposarcomas behave aggressively and show distant metastases. Well-differentiated liposarcomas, especially those occurring in the retroperitoneum, have the tendency to dedifferentiate into a more malignant variant known as dedifferentiated liposarcoma which consists of two components – one is a well-differentiated liposarcoma and the other a non-fatty sarcoma.

The second most common liposarcoma is the myxoid liposarcoma which accounts for about 10% of all soft tissue sarcomas. It is the most common type affecting children. Histologically myxoid liposarcoma consists of two components, a myxoid component and a round cell component. Myxoid liposarcomas differ from other types of liposarcomas in their unusual pattern of metastasis. They have a high prevalence of extrapulmonary metastases. The bone and soft tissue metastases are most common followed by the lung and liver.

Typical clinical scenario

In the lower extremity a well-differentiated liposarcoma typically presents as a painless, slow-growing soft tissue mass. Retroperitoneal well-differentiated liposarcomas present with intra-abdominal symptoms. In the retroperitoneum well-differentiated liposarcomas are usually large when first discovered because retroperitoneal tumors are late to detect. The myxoid liposarcoma occurs at a younger age than other liposarcomas and it can be seen in children. The lower extremity is the most common site for this lesion, particularly the medial thigh and popliteal fossa. It presents clinically as a painless, large soft tissue mass.

Differential diagnosis

Differentiating a lipoma from a well-differentiated liposarcoma on imaging studies alone can sometimes be difficult. The key findings separating these two lesions are the presence of thick septa and non-fatty nodules or masses in the well-differentiated liposarcomas but not in lipomas. Myxoid liposarcomas in popliteal fossa can be easily confused with a Baker's cyst. MRI with gadolinium enhancement will be helpful in differentiating these two lesions.

Pearls and Pitfalls in Musculoskeletal Imaging, ed. D. Lee Bennett and Georges Y. El-Khoury. Published by Cambridge University Press. © Cambridge University Press 2013.

Teaching point

Liposarcoma is the second most common malignant soft tissue tumor. Two types constitute the majority of liposarcomas and these are the well-differentiated and the myxoid liposarcoma. Remembering the imaging features of these two lesions can be very helpful in arriving at a specific diagnosis.

READING LIST

Kransdorf MJ, Bancroft LW, Peterson JJ *et al*. Imaging of fatty tumors: distinction of lipoma and well-differentiated liposarcoma. *Radiology* 2002;**224**:99–104.

Kransdorf MJ, Meis JM, Jelinek JS. Dedifferentiated liposarcoma of the extremities: imaging findings in four patients. *AJR Am J Roentgenol* 1993;**161**:127–130.

Murphey MD, Arcara LK, Fanburg-Smith J. From the archives of the AFIP. Imaging of musculoskeletal liposarcoma with radiologic-pathologic correlation. *RadioGraphics* 2005;**25**: 1371–1395.

Sheah K, Ouellette HA, Torriani M *et al*. Metastatic myxoid liposarcomas: imaging and histopathologic findings. *Skeletal Radiol* 2008;**37**:251–258.

Sung M-S, Kang HS, Suh JS *et al*. Myxoid liposarcoma: appearance at MR imaging with histologic correlation. *RadioGraphics* 2000;**20**:1007–1019.

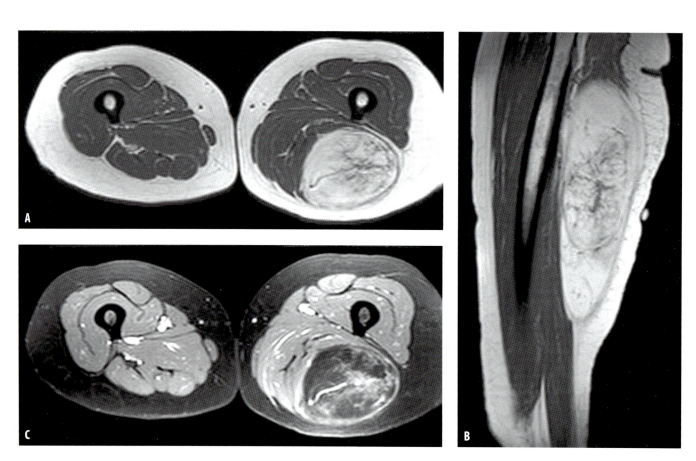

Figure 77.1 Well-differentiated liposarcoma of the posterior thigh. Axial and sagittal T1-weighted images (**A**) and (**B**) through the thigh show a posterior thigh mass with high signal intensity. The mass contains multiple thick septa which are mostly in the center of the tumor. Axial and sagittal T2-weighted images (**C**) and (**D**) showing irregular areas of increased signal intensity within the central half of the mass. Axial and sagittal fat-suppressed T1-weighted images (**E**) and (**F**) with gadolinium reveal areas of enhancement suggesting the presence of well-differentiated liposarcoma.

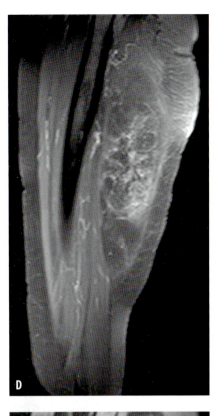

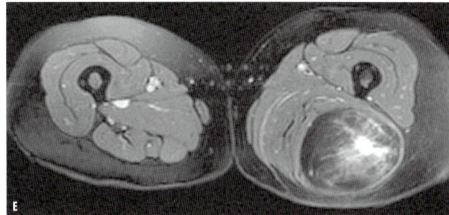

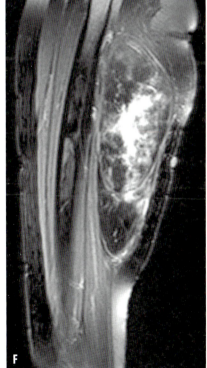

Figure 77.1 (cont.)

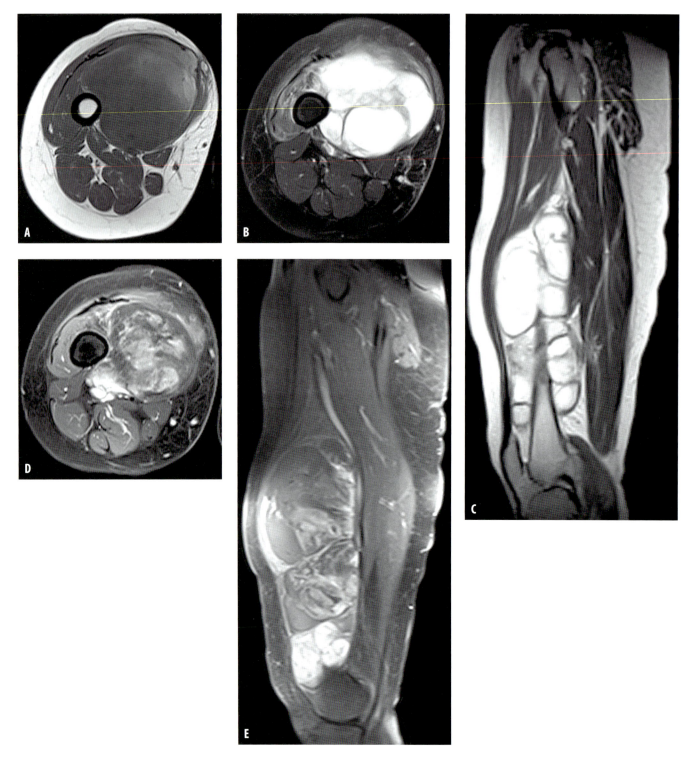

Figure 77.2 Myxoid liposarcoma. A T1-weighted axial image (**A**) through the mid-thigh shows a large mass in the muscles of the anteromedial aspect of the thigh. The mass has a well-defined edge and has low signal intensity. T2-weighted axial and sagittal images (**B**) and (**C**) of the thigh show a large intensely bright and lobulated lesion in the anteromedial muscles of the thigh. The mass resembles a large cyst but the hyperintense areas suggest myxoid tissue. Fat-suppressed axial and sagittal T1-weighted images (**D**) and (**E**) show multiple areas of heterogeneous enhancement within the mass. These findings are highly suggestive of a malignant process.

Mazabraud syndrome

Imaging description

The diagnosis of fibrous dysplasia is usually made radiographically. It demonstrates expansile lytic lesions and cortical thinning with endosteal scalloping of the affected long bones. The expanded medullary spaces reveal a characteristic ground glass appearance. Some small lesions are surrounded by a thick sclerotic border or rind. These findings are strongly suggestive of polyostotic fibrous dysplasia and no further imaging is necessary (Figure 78.1).

The diagnosis of a myxoma is best made on MRI where the signal characteristics of the lesion are determined by its high water content. Myxomas have markedly low signal intensity on T1-weighted images compared with adjacent muscles and high signal intensity on T2-weighted images. The gadolinium-enhanced T1-weighted images reflect its solid consistency because it shows internal enhancement. The degree of enhancement is mild to moderate and it is almost always heterogeneous. In more than half the patients the myxoma is multifocal (Figure 78.2).

Ultrasound is useful in differentiating a cyst from a solid lesion such as a myxoma. It shows small areas of internal echoes in myxomas.

Importance

The association of intramuscular myxoma with fibrous dysplasia is well established and it is known as the Mazabraud syndrome. This association was first described by Henschen in 1926. In the English literature it was first described in 1971 by Wirth *et al.* In Mazabraud syndrome the myxoma(s) is most frequently associated with polyostotic fibrous dysplasia although several cases have been reported with the monostotic form of the disease. The reason for the association between these two entities is not clear but one explanation is the common origin and histiogenesis of fibrous dysplasia and myxoma. The intramuscular myxoma in Mazabraud syndrome is often multifocal, but it can also be a solitary lesion. The myxoma in this syndrome is typically located in the vicinity of the most severely affected bones and it often occurs in the thigh (Figure 78.1). Mazabraud syndrome also has a predilection for occurring on the right side of the body. Typically the diagnosis of fibrous dysplasia antedates the discovery of the intramuscular myxoma. Myxoma is a mesenchymal neoplasm composed of undifferentiated stellate cells in an abundant myxoid stroma.

Typical clinical scenario

Most myxomas in Mazabraud syndrome develop in patients with known history of polyostotic fibrous dysplasia and much less frequently in patients with monostotic disease. The bone changes almost always pre-date the development of myxomas but occasionally the two diseases present at the same time. In the same patient there can be multiple myxomas (Figure 78.2). The myxoma can clinically present as a slowly growing painless mass. At surgery, most of the myxomas are typically found to be located with skeletal muscles. Some patients clinically present with precocious puberty (Albright syndrome).

Differential diagnosis

Cystic masses such as synovial cysts, ganglion cysts, and seromas can mimic the appearance of intramuscular myxoma on MRI because of its high water content, but these lesions are truly cystic and usually do not occur within skeletal muscles. Intramuscular myxomas must also be differentiated from myxoid tumors of the extremities like peripheral nerve sheath tumors, extraskeletal myxoid chondrosarcoma, myxoid liposarcoma, and myxoid leiomyosarcoma. When in doubt these lesions can be definitively differentiated from an intramuscular myxoma by using a core needle biopsy.

Teaching point

The association of fibrous dysplasia with soft tissue myxoma is well entrenched in the literature so that radiologists need to be aware of it. The key to the diagnosis lies in the detection and characterization of the soft tissue and bone lesions. A biopsy of the soft tissue mass is required to confirm the diagnosis of a myxoma; however a biopsy of the bone lesions in most cases is not required.

READING LIST

Iwasko N, Steinbach LS, Disler D *et al.* Imaging findings in Mazabraud's syndrome: seven new cases. *Skeletal Radiol* 2002;**31**:81–87.

Kransdorf MJ, Murphy MD. Case 12: Mazabraud syndrome. *Radiology* 1999;**212**:129–132.

Luna A, Martinez S, Bossen E. Magnetic resonance imaging of intramuscular myxoma with histological comparison and a review of the literature. *Skeletal Radiol* 2005;**34**:19–28.

Murphey MD, McRae GA, Fanburg-Smith JC *et al.* Imaging of soft-tissue myxoma with emphasis on CT and MR and comparison of radiologic and pathologic findings. *Radiology* 2002;**225**:215–224.

Sundaram M, McDonald DJ, Merenda G. Intramuscular myxoma: a rare but important association with fibrous dysplasia of bone. *AJR Am J Roentgenol* 1989;**153**:107–108.

Wirth WA, Leavitt D, Enzinger FM. Multiple intramuscular myxomas. *Cancer* 1971;**27**:1167–1173.

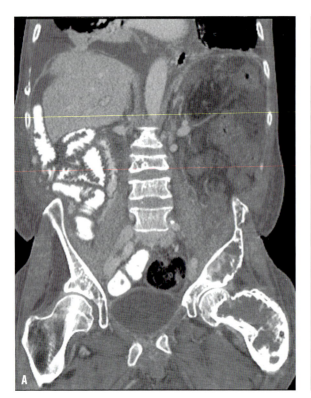

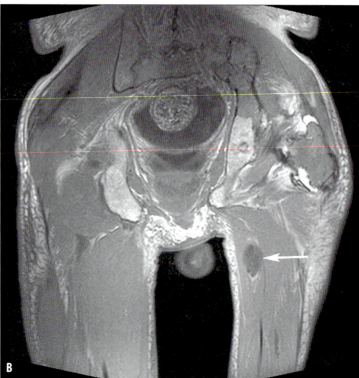

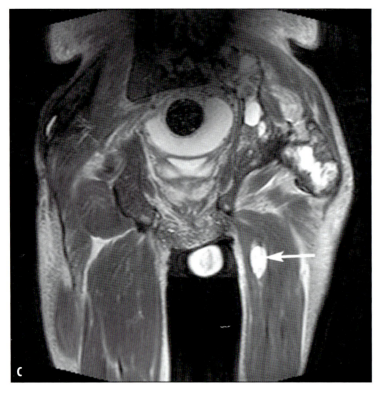

Figure 78.1 Mazabraud syndrome in a patient with polyostotic fibrous dysplasia. Coronal reformatted CT image (**A**) showing polyostotic fibrous dysplasia on the left side. The left proximal femur has a shepherd's crook deformity. Coronal T1- and T2-weighted images (**B**) and (**C**) through the posterior thigh reveal an oval mass (arrow) which is dark on T1-weighted and bright on T2-weighted images. These findings are characteristic of Mazabraud syndrome.

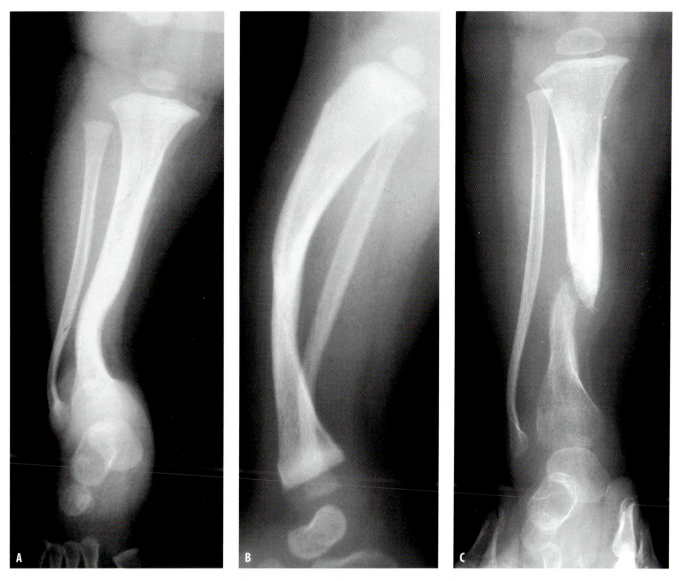

Figure 79.2 Progressive pseudoarthrosis in neurofibromatosis type I (NF I). Radiographs (**A** and **B**) showing anterolateral bowing of the tibia due to early pseudoarthrosis. The distal fibula is also bowed and thin (or dysplastic). Typical radiographic (**C**) appearance of congenital pseudoarthrosis of the tibia.

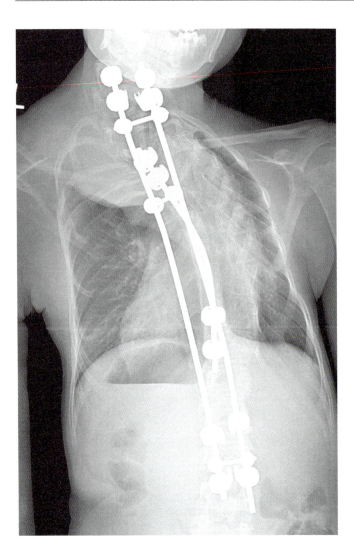

Figure 79.3 A young patient with neurofibromatosis type I (NF I) treated with spinal fusion for scoliosis. Anteroposterior view of the spine shows a left paraspinal density which represents a lateral meningocele. The ribs posterior to the lateral meningocele are thin and dysplastic.

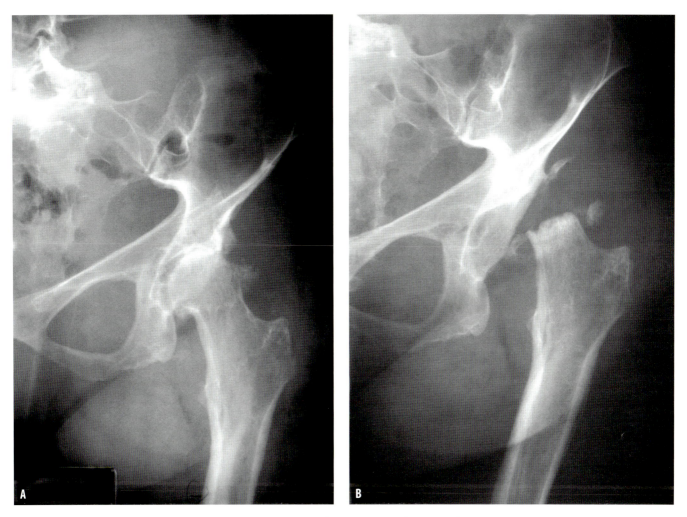

Figure 79.4 A middle-aged female with a longstanding history of NF I and a plexiform neurofibroma in the left lumbar paraspinal region. Anteroposterior views of the left hip taken 2 years apart (**A**) and (**B**) show the development of atrophic Charcot joint in the left hip.

Imaging description

Like all other soft tissue tumors, peripheral nerve sheath tumors are best imaged by MRI (Figure 80.1). There is a considerable overlap in the imaging features of schwannoma and neurofibroma. These tumors are located along nerve trunks and it is often helpful to identify the nerve of origin for these tumors. On MRI normal nerves appear as tubular structures with low signal intensity on all pulse sequences. Generally, peripheral nerve sheath tumors typically have low signal intensity on T1-weighted sequences and marked signal hyperintensity on T2-weighted images (Figure 80.2). According to Suh *et al.* the presumptive diagnosis of a peripheral nerve sheath tumor can be made if a soft tissue mass is found either along a peripheral nerve distribution or if it is connected to a nerve bundle at its proximal and distal end. A plexiform neurofibroma may have characteristic features on CT; it shows diffuse fusiform enlargement of a peripheral nerve and/or multiple masses along the course of a peripheral nerve. It has low attenuation compared with muscle with values ranging from 15 to 20 Hounsfield units on non-enhanced scans.

Differentiation of schwannoma from a neurofibroma is of relevance to the surgeon since during resection of a schwannoma the tumor can be separated from the parent nerve, but this is not possible with a neurofibroma. Some authors attempted to identify imaging criteria that can distinguish a schwannoma from a neurofibroma. MRI can show helpful features for the differentiation of schwannoma from neurofibroma, however no single imaging sign or combination of signs allow definitive differentiation between these two tumors. MRI signs that are described more commonly in schwannomas include: (1) fascicular appearance on T2-weighted images; (2) a thin hyperintense rim on T2-weighted images; (3) schwannomas are typically encapsulated showing a hyperintense mass on T2-weighted images surrounded with a low signal capsule; (4) schwannomas often demonstrate diffuse enhancement of the lesion on fat-suppressed T1-weighted images following gadolinium injection. Neurofibromas are frequently characterized by: (1) target sign seen on T2-weighted images due to a fibrous acellular area within the center of the lesion (Figure 80.3); (2) central enhancement on fat-suppressed T1-weighted images following gadolinium injection; (3) the "dumbbell" tumor causing intervertebral foramen enlargement is characteristic of neurofibroma (Figure 80.4).

Importance

Benign peripheral nerve sheath tumors are composed primarily of Schwann cells. They may occur sporadically or in the context of neurofibromatosis. The sporadic lesions rarely if ever become malignant. Peripheral nerve sheath tumors are divided into two types: schwannoma (or neurilemoma) and neurofibroma. The pathologist sometimes finds it difficult to differentiate between these two benign tumors. Most series report schwannomas to be more common than neurofibromas.

Schwannoma is a benign encapsulated tumor presenting as a solitary painless mass ranging in size from several millimeters to 20 cm or greater. Most schwannomas are not associated with neurofibromatosis but when they do they may be multiple. They occur in patients between the ages of 20 and 50 years of age and the most common locations are the spine, sympathetic nerve roots, neck and the flexor surfaces of the upper and lower extremities. The posterior mediastinum and retroperitoneum can also be involved. Most are attached to large nerve trunks in extremities, especially peroneal and ulnar nerves. They typically arise on the surface of the involved nerve and therefore can be dissected surgically off the nerve without causing any damage to the nerve. Large schwannomas can undergo degeneration with cyst formation, calcification, ossification, hemorrhage, and fibrosis within the lesion. Such schwannomas are known in the literature as ancient schwannomas.

Neurofibromas can occur sporadically or in association with neurofibromatosis. There are three types of neurofibromas: (1) localized neurofibroma which is not associated with neurofibromatosis; it is the most common type accounting for about 90% of all neurofibromas; it is a slow-growing painless lesion and it is less than 5 cm in size. Unlike the schwannoma a localized neurofibroma develops within the affected nerve. It is not possible to isolate this tumor surgically from the involved nerve without causing damage to the nerve. Malignant transformation of localized neurofibroma is extremely rare; (2) the diffuse neurofibroma is a rare ill-defined infiltrative subcutaneous lesion; and (3) plexiform neurofibroma which is always associated with neurofibromatosis I. The presence of a plexiform neurofibroma is regarded as evidence of neurofibromatosis even when it seems to be a solitary lesion. It presents as a mass of nerves resembling a "bag of worms" (Figure 80.1).

Typical clinical scenario

Schwannomas and neurofibromas both present as slow-growing painless masses. Occasionally they may cause pain and neurological symptoms. Neurofibroma tends to present at a younger age group than a schwannoma.

Differential diagnosis

On MRI schwannomas and neurofibromas are similar in appearance to other soft tissue tumors. However the target sign and hyperintensity on T2-weighted images as well as the location of the tumor in relationship to a nerve or nerve plexus are important clues for the diagnosis of a peripheral nerve sheath tumor. Occasionally an enlarged lymph node due to cat scratch disease, in the axilla or above the elbow, can resemble a peripheral nerve sheath tumor. A useful MRI sign in such cases is the presence of edema around the inflamed lymph node, which can differentiate cat scratch disease from a benign peripheral nerve sheath tumor.

Teaching point

Benign peripheral nerve sheath tumors are fairly common soft tissue neoplasms. These are schwannoma and neurofibroma. Certain imaging signs have been used to distinguish between a schwannoma and neurofibroma, however these signs are not definitive.

READING LIST

Beggs I. Pictorial review: imaging of peripheral nerve tumours. *Clin Radiol* 1997;**52**:8–17.

Bourgouin PM, Shepard J-A O, Moore EH, McLoud TC. Plexiform neurofibromatosis of the mediastinum: CT appearance. *AJR Am J Roentgenol* 1988;**151**;461–463.

Cerofolini E, Landi A, DeSantis G et al. MR of benign peripheral nerve sheath tumors. *J Comput Assist Tomogr* 1991;**15(4)**:593–597.

Jee W-H, Oh S-N, McCauley T et al. Extraaxial neurofibromas versus neurilemmomas: discrimination with MRI. *AJR Am J Roentgenol* 2004;**183**:629–633.

Lin J, Martel W. Cross-sectional imaging of peripheral nerve sheath tumors: characteristic signs on CT, MR imaging and sonography. *AJR Am J Roentgenol* 2001;**176**:75–82.

Murphey MD, Smith WS, Smith SE et al. From the archives of the AFIP. Imaging of musculoskeletal neurogenic tumors: radiologic-pathologic correlation. *RadioGraphics* 1999;**19**:1253–1280.

Suh J-S, Abenoza P, Galloway HR et al. Peripheral (extracranial) nerve tumors: correlation of MR imaging and histologic findings. *Radiology* 1992;**183**:341–346.

Varma DGK, Moulopoulos A, Sara AS et al. MR imaging of extracranial nerve sheath tumors. *J Comput Assist Tomogr* 1992; **16(3)**:448–453.

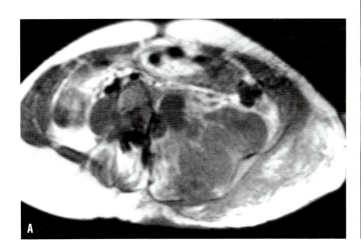
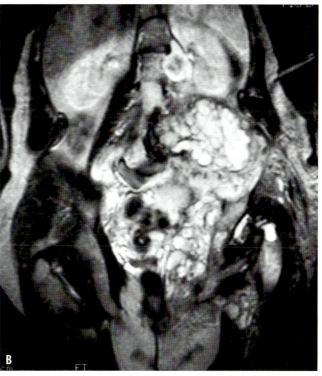

Figure 80.1 Plexiform neurofibroma in a patient with neurofibromatosis type I (NF I). T1-weighted axial and T2-weighted coronal images (**A**) and (**B**) show a large retroperitoneal plexiform neurofibroma. The "bag of worms" appearance is best demonstrated on the T2-weighted image (**B**).

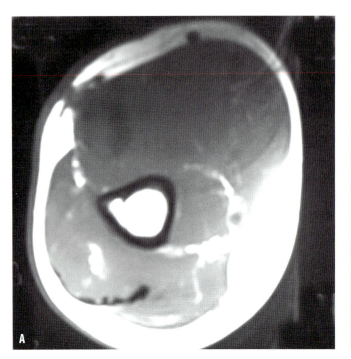

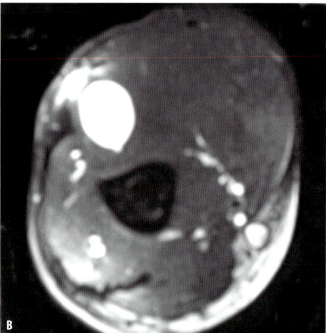

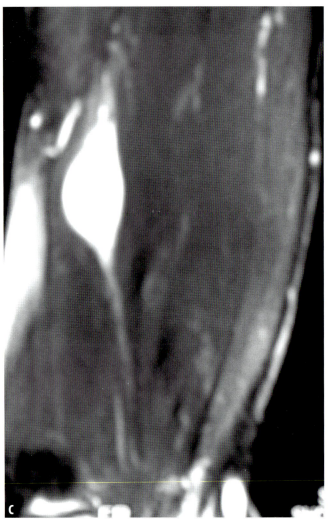

Figure 80.2 Typical MR appearance of a peripheral nerve sheath tumor in the arm. T1- and T2-weighted axial images (**A** and **B**) show a mass within the lateral aspect of the biceps muscle. Coronal fat-suppressed T2-weighted image (**C**) shows the peripheral nerve sheath tumor arising within the radial nerve.

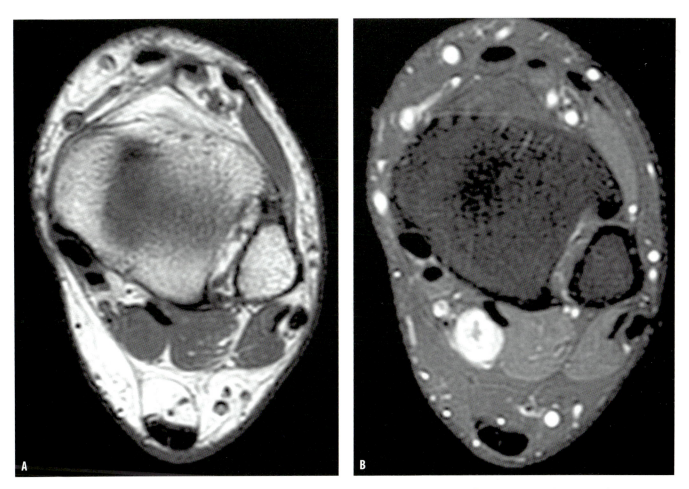

Figure 80.3 The target sign typical of a peripheral nerve sheath tumor. Axial T1-weighted image (**A**) showing a small low signal intensity mass medial to the flexor hallucis longus tendon. On the T2-weighted image (**B**), the mass reveals the target sign.

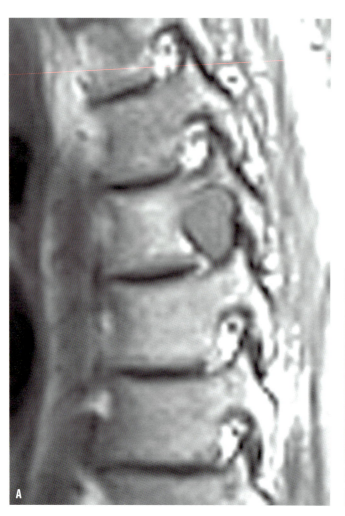

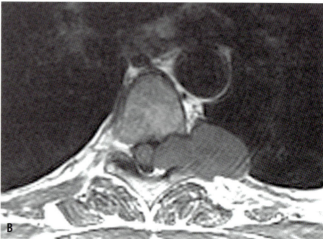

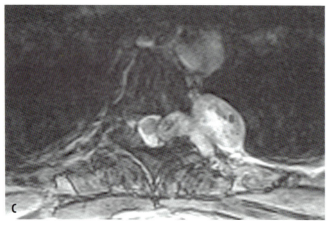

Figure 80.4 A "dumbbell" neurofibroma in the mid-thoracic spine. Sagittal (**A**) and axial (**B**) T1-weighted images along with an axial T2-weighted image (**C**) show a "dumbbell" neurofibroma.

Malignant peripheral nerve sheath tumors (MPNSTs)

Imaging description

Radiography is often negative or it shows a non-specific soft tissue mass. As with other soft tissue tumors MRI is the diagnostic modality of choice for imaging malignant peripheral nerve sheath tumors (MPNSTs). The location of the mass in relationship to a deep large nerve trunk is helpful in diagnosing a neurogenic tumor. The tumor may appear fusiform in shape and may also be noted to enter and exit a nerve (Figure 81.1). The signal intensity of a MPNST on both T1- and T2-weighted images is non-specific. MPNSTs show low signal intensity similar to muscle on T1-weighted images and heterogeneous increase in signal intensity on T2-weighted images. On gadolinium-enhanced images MPNSTs can show central necrosis (Figure 81.2). Malignant and benign peripheral nerve sheath tumors cannot be reliably distinguished on the basis of imaging criteria alone; however certain findings should raise the suspicion that the tumor is malignant. MPNSTs tend to be larger tumors, typically more than 5 cm. They may exhibit ill-defined margins due to infiltration of adjacent soft tissues and are often associated with soft tissue edema. An infiltrative tumor border on CT or MR suggests malignancy, but may be present also in benign plexiform neurofibromas. Conversely a malignant neoplasm may have a smooth, non-infiltrating margin. Bone erosions may occur with both benign and malignant neoplasm, but are more irregular with malignant lesions.

Fluorodeoxyglucose positron emission tomography (FDG PET) is a sensitive technique in detecting MPNSTs in patients with neurofibromatosis I (NF I). PET may improve preoperative tumor staging by detecting metastases or second primary tumors, which often are present in patients with NF I.

Importance

Most MPNSTs are considered to be high-grade sarcoma; it is the malignant counterpart of the benign peripheral nerve sheath tumor. It is also known as malignant schwannoma, neurogenic sarcoma, and neurofibrosarcoma. MPNSTs arise either from a neurofibroma or *de novo* from the nerve sheath. Origin from a schwannoma is exceedingly rare. This tumor is believed to originate from multiple nerve sheath cells including Schwann cells, perineural cells, and fibroblasts. MPNST accounts for 5–10% of all soft tissue sarcomas. It occurs in patients between the ages of 20 and 50 years. About half the patients with MPNST have pre-existing neurofibromatosis and conversely 2–29% of neurofibromatosis patients develop MPNST, resulting in decreased longevity for patients with neurofibromatosis. In neurofibromatosis patients MPNST occurs at an early age, tends to be high grade, large, and arises from a plexiform neurofibroma. Sudden increase in size of a previously stable neurofibroma should be suspected of malignant transformation and therefore warrants an immediate biopsy. Intraosseous MPNST is exceedingly rare. About 10% of MPNSTs occur at previously irradiated sites after a long latency period.

Typical clinical scenario

Most patients present with pain and enlarging mass. Like benign PNST, MPNST tends to arise along major nerve trunks. Common locations for MPNST are the proximal portion of the extremities along the sciatic nerve, brachial and sacral plexuses. Clinical indicators of malignancy are persistent pain, increasing size, and neurological deficits. Patients with MPNST often have poor prognosis because the tumor can metastasize at an early stage. Early detection and thorough surgical resection with microscopically tumor-free margins can improve the prognosis. Despite aggressive treatment, local recurrence and distant metastasis are common. Bad prognosis is observed with older patient age, larger tumor size, more central location of the tumor, and positive margin at resection. Paraspinal MPNSTs have more aggressive behavior than peripheral tumors because they are difficult to resect completely. Metastases most frequently involve the lungs, bone, pleura, and retroperitoneum.

Differential diagnosis

Unfortunately imaging alone does not reliably differentiate between benign and malignant nerve sheath tumors. On T2-weighted images, heterogeneity, central necrosis, large size >5 cm, and indistinct infiltrating margins are more common in MPNST. The fascicular and target signs are more common in benign PNSTs than in MPNSTs. It is also often difficult to differentiate MPNSTs from other soft tissue sarcomas but this is rarely a problem because in both cases the treatment is similar, consisting of wide surgical excision with tumor-free margins.

Teaching point

MPNSTs are relatively common soft tissue sarcomas. They are especially prevalent in patients with neurofibromatosis type 1. In such patients, rapid change in size of a plexiform neurofibroma should be suspicious for malignant transformation.

READING LIST

Bredella MA, Torriani M, Hornicek F *et al*. Value of PET in the assessment of patients with neurofibromatosis type 1. *AJR Am J Roentgenol* 2007;**189**:928–935.

Kourea HP, Bilsky MH, Leung DHY *et al*. Subdiaphragmatic and intrathoracic paraspinal malignant peripheral nerve sheath tumors. A clinicopathologic study of 25 patients and 26 tumors. *Cancer* 1998; **82(11)**: 2191–2203.

Levine E, Huntrakoon M, Wetzel LH. Malignant nerve-sheath neoplasms in neurofibromatosis: distinction from benign tumors by using imaging techniques. *AJR Am J Roentgenol* 1987;**149**: 1059–1064.

Lin J, Martel W. Pictorial essay. Cross-sectional imaging of peripheral nerve sheath tumors: characteristic signs on CT, MR imaging, and sonography. *AJR Am J Roentgenol* 2001;**176**:75–82.

Mautner VF, Friedrich RE, von Deimling A *et al*. Malignant peripheral nerve sheath tumours in neurofibromatosis type 1: MRI supports the diagnosis of malignant plexiform neurofibroma. *Neuroradiology* 2003;**45**:618–625.

Murphey MD, Smith WS, Smith SE *et al*. From the archives of the AFIP. Imaging of musculoskeletal neurogenic tumors: radiologic-pathologic correlation. *RadioGraphics* 1999;**19**:1253–1280.

Stull MA, Moser RP, Kransdorf MJ *et al*. Magnetic resonance appearance of peripheral nerve sheath tumors. *Skeletal Radiol* 1991;**20**:9–14.

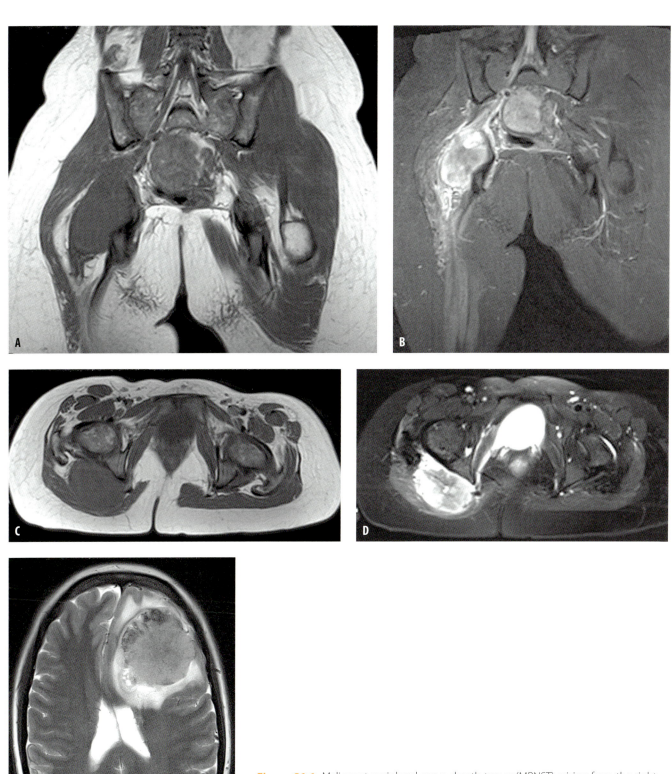

Figure 81.1 Malignant peripheral nerve sheath tumor (MPNST) arising from the right sciatic nerve treated with hemipelvectomy. Coronal T1- and T2-weighted images (A) and (B) of the pelvis show a large mass within the greater sciatic notch. It is dark on T1 and non-homogeneously bright on the T2-weighted image. Axial T1- and T2-weighted images (C) and (D) again show the mass. Fourteen months after the hemipelvectomy, the patient presented with neurological symptoms. T2-weighted image (E) from a brain scan reveals a large metastatic lesion in the frontal lobe.

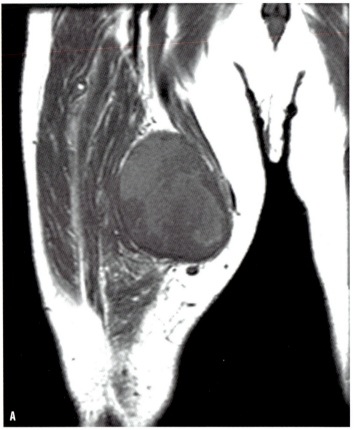

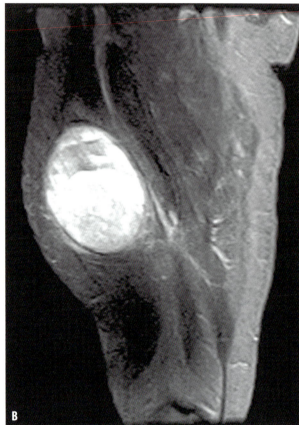

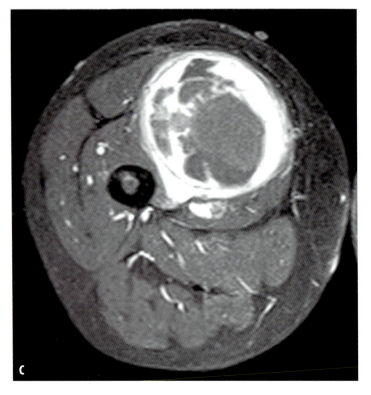

Figure 81.2 Malignant peripheral nerve sheath tumor (MPNST) arising from the right femoral nerve. Coronal T1-weighted image (**A**) of the right thigh shows a large soft tissue mass with non-homogeneously bright signal intensity. Sagittal T2-weighted image (**B**) shows the mass with non-homogeneously bright signal intensity. (**C**) is a fat-suppressed T1-weighted image after an IV gadolinium injection; the lesion shows areas of central necrosis.

Imaging description

Radiography in the majority of synovial sarcomas is either negative or shows a non-specific soft tissue mass. In about 30% of the cases calcifications can be identified (Figure 82.1). CT can identify small or ill-defined calcifications in anatomically complex areas. Usually the calcifications are eccentric or peripheral but rarely they can be extensive and involve the entire lesion. Some authors believe that an extensively calcified synovial sarcoma is associated with better prognosis. Most soft tissue sarcomas do not involve bone, however synovial sarcoma is an exception to this rule. Bone involvement by synovial sarcoma can present with different radiographic patterns, for example, extrinsic pressure infiltration with significant bone destruction.

As with other soft tissue sarcomas, synovial sarcoma is best studied by MRI. T1-weighted images reveal heterogeneous low signal intensity which is similar or slightly higher than muscle. T2-weighted images are described as showing prominent heterogeneity with predominant high signal intensity intermixed with areas of low and intermediate signal; this was described by Jones *et al.* as the triple sign. Although this sign is common with synovial sarcoma it is however not specific and other soft tissue tumors can show similar MR imaging characteristics. Fluid-fluid levels have been described in 10–25% of synovial sarcomas as resembling a bowl of grapes. Neurovascular encasement is also reported as a common finding with synovial sarcoma. A synovial sarcoma that invades an adjacent joint is more frequent than an intra-articular lesion; this invasion most commonly occurs in the anterior aspect of the knee in the Hoffa's fat pad (Figure 82.2).

Importance

Synovial sarcoma is a relatively rare malignant soft tissue sarcoma contributing to about 5–10% of all malignant soft tissue tumors. Despite the name the lesion occurs close to a joint but not within the joint, except when there is secondary invasion. The majority of synovial sarcomas occur in patients between the ages of 20 and 40 years, however there is a wide age range at presentation. The median age at presentation is in the mid-thirties. In the pediatric age group, synovial sarcoma is the most common soft tissue sarcoma after rhabdomyosarcoma. Most synovial sarcomas occur in the lower extremity with some concentration around the knee. The presenting complaint is a palpable mass with or without pain. The duration of symptoms are often longlasting for a few years before a diagnosis is made.

Histologically the distinguishing feature of this lesion is in its biphasic nature where two types of neoplastic cells coexist, the epithelial and the spindle cell components. Histologically synovial sarcomas are divided into three subtypes; these are the monophasic, biphasic, and poorly differentiated. Monophasic synovial sarcoma is the most common type representing 50–60% of all cases. In the monophasic type the mesenchymal spindle cell is the predominant cell. The biphasic synovial sarcoma represents 20–30% of lesions and this subtype consists of both spindle cells and epithelial cells which can form gland-like structures and therefore may resemble an adenocarcinoma. Poorly differentiated synovial sarcoma has epithelial morphology in addition to high mitotic activity. This subtype constitutes 15–25% of all synovial sarcomas. Histologically the poorly differentiated synovial sarcoma can be confused with round cell tumors such as Ewing's sarcoma. When the diagnosis is histologically in doubt, cytogenetic testing demonstrates reciprocal translocation between chromosome X and 18 t(X;18) confirming the diagnosis of synovial sarcoma. This test can be helpful since the genetic abnormality is highly specific for synovial sarcoma.

Synovial sarcoma is considered an aggressive malignant neoplasm; it spreads by direct extension along the myofascial planes. The development of metastasis, commonly to the lungs, may occur several years after the initial treatment. Tumor size greater than 5 cm has a great impact on prognosis. Like all intermediate- and high-grade sarcomas, synovial sarcoma is an aggressive lesion which is treated with wide local excision along with the removal of a normal cuff of surrounding tissue. The most frequent metastatic site is the lungs followed by lymph nodes.

Typical clinical presentation

Patients with synovial sarcoma usually present with a palpable soft tissue mass. Associated pain and tenderness are fairly common in patients with synovial sarcoma; this is in contradistinction with other soft tissue sarcomas which typically present as painless soft tissue masses. Initially synovial sarcomas grow slowly and present as a small mass giving the false impression of a benign lesion. In young patients synovial sarcoma is the most common soft tissue tumor in the deep soft tissues of the foot and ankle. Younger age and smaller tumor size, < than 5 cm, are associated with better long-term prognosis. The poorly differentiated subtype is associated with bad prognosis.

Differential diagnosis

Like most malignant soft tissue tumors, it is difficult to come up with a specific diagnosis for synovial sarcoma. There are however clinical and imaging features, which in some cases

Pearls and Pitfalls in Musculoskeletal Imaging, ed. D. Lee Bennett and Georges Y. El-Khoury. Published by Cambridge University Press. © Cambridge University Press 2013.

can suggest the correct diagnosis. The majority of synovial sarcomas occur in adolescents and young adults between the ages of 15 and 40 years. Synovial sarcomas most often occur in the extremities especially the popliteal fossa. It is often associated with pain and tenderness which are typically not present with other soft tissue sarcomas. The presence of soft tissue calcifications and bone erosions on imaging studies are highly suggestive of synovial sarcoma.

Teaching points

Synovial sarcoma is an intermediate- to high-grade lesion. It is the fourth most common malignant soft tissue neoplasm. Although the imaging features are not pathognomonic there are a few clinical and imaging signs that, in some patients, can help in arriving at a specific diagnosis. There are two features of synovial sarcoma that may lead to the mistaken diagnosis of a benign lesion. These are the slow growth in early synovial sarcoma and the small size (<5 cm).

READING LIST

Blacksin MF, Siegel JR, Benevenia J, Aisner SC. Synovial sarcoma: frequency of nonaggressive MR characteristics. *J Comput Assist Tomogr* 1997;**21**(**5**):785–789.

Israels SJ, Chan HSL, Daneman A, Weitzman SS. Synovial sarcoma in childhood. *AJR Am J Roentgenol* 1984;**142**:803–806.

Jones BC, Sundaram M, Kransdorf MJ. Synovial sarcoma: MR imaging findings in 34 patients. *AJR Am J Roentgenol* 1993;**161**:827–830.

Maxwell JR, Yao L, Eckardt JJ, Doberneck SA. Case report 878. *Skeletal Radiol* 1994;**23**:673–675.

McCarville B, Spunt SL, Skapek SX, Pappo AS. Synovial sarcoma in pediatric patients. *AJR Am J Roentgenol* 2002;**179**:797–801.

Murphey MD, Gibson MS, Jennings BT *et al*. From the archives of the AFIP. Imaging of synovial sarcoma with radiologic-pathologic correlation. *RadioGraphics* 2006;**26**:1543–1565.

Murray JA. Synovial sarcoma. *Ortho Clin North Am* 1977;**8**(**4**):963–972.

Sanchez Reyes JM, Mexia MA, Tapia DQ, Aramburu JA. Extensively calcified synovial sarcoma. *Skeletal Radiol* 1997;**26**:671–673.

Spielmann A, Janzen DL, O'Connell JX, Munk PL. Intraneural synovial sarcoma. *Skeletal Radiol* 1997;**26**:677–681.

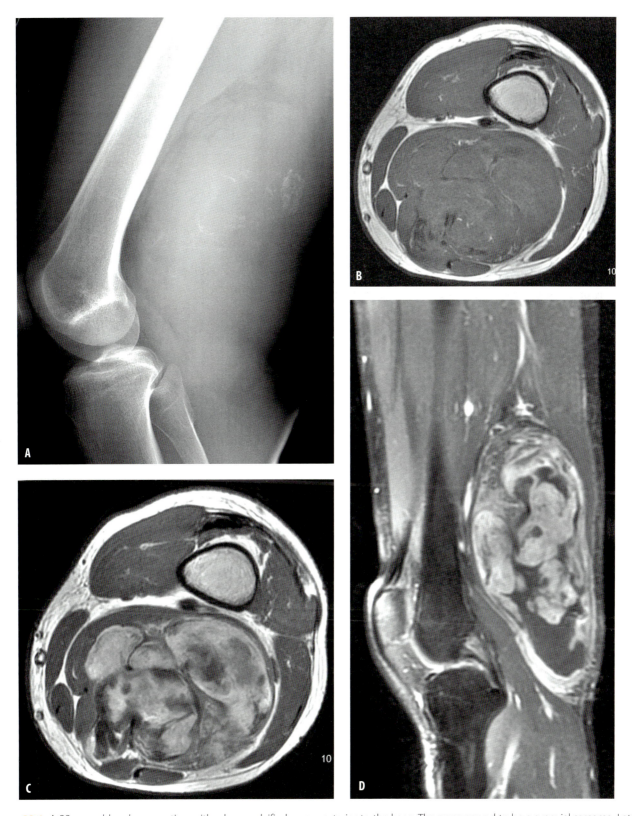

Figure 82.1 A 28-year-old male presenting with a large calcified mass posterior to the knee. The mass proved to be a synovial sarcoma. Lateral radiograph (**A**) reveals a large soft tissue mass with multiple punctate calcifications within it. T1-weighted axial image (**B**) shows a low signal-intensity mass. The darker areas within the mass are believed to represent calcifications with the tumor. T2-weighted axial image (**C**) shows non-homogeneously high signal-intensity mass posterior to the distal femur. Fat-suppressed sagittal T1-weighted image following an IV gadolinium injection (**D**) shows non-homogeneous enhancement. The diffusely dark areas are likely due to tumor necrosis.

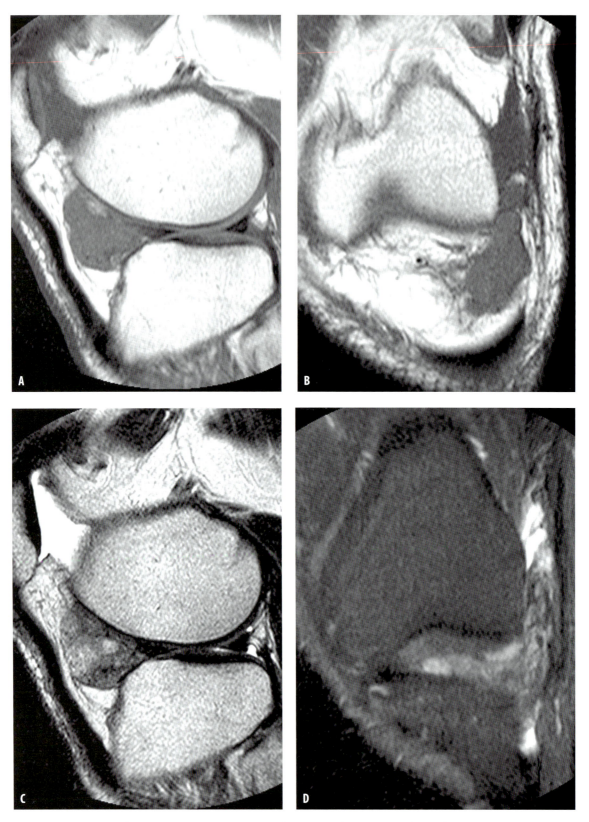

Figure 82.2 Intra-articular synovial sarcoma. Sagittal (**A**) and coronal (**B**) T1-weighted images of the left knee show a mass invading Hoffa's fat pad and the soft tissue adjacent to the lateral femoral condyle. T2-weighted sagittal image (**C**) of the knee reveal non-homogeneously increased signal within the mass. On the fat-suppressed coronal sequence after an IV gadolinium injection (**D**), the mass shows mild enhancement.

83 Aggressive fibromatosis (desmoid tumor)

Imaging description

The principal role of imaging is in the management of aggressive fibromatosis, as well as staging in pre-operative planning and for the follow-up of progression in patients who are treated non-operatively. In post-operative follow-up imaging plays a key role in detecting recurrence. On conventional radiographs, aggressive fibromatosis is either undetectable or identified as an amorphous soft tissue mass. Calcification within the mass is uncommon. On rare occasions radiography may show bony infiltration or destruction of adjacent bones (Figure 83.1). As with most soft tissue tumors, MR is the best imaging modality for assessing aggressive fibromatosis. The majority of lesions appear iso- to mildly hyperintense relative to muscle on T1-weighted image. The T1 signal intensity is usually homogeneous. On T2-weighted images the majority of lesions are hyperintense relative to muscle (Figure 83.1). In about one third of the patients aggressive fibromatosis displays lower signal intensity than muscle on T2-weighted images (Figure 83.2). These lesions have less cellularity and more collagen than tumors with high signal-intensity T2-weighted images. The hyperintense lesions on T2-weighted images are typically heterogeneously hyperintense. Bands of low signal intensity within the lesion on all sequences are reported to occur in about two thirds of cases. This is in concordance with previously published data. After injection of IV gadolinium, these tumors show either avid or moderate enhancement.

Importance

Aggressive fibromatosis is a subdivision of adult fibromatosis; it is a benign infiltrating fibroblastic process. It occurs within the deep soft tissues and mimics low-grade fibrosarcoma. This tumor is also known by other names such as extra-abdominal desmoid tumor and musculo-aponeurotic fibromatosis. The lesion is a mesenchymal non-metastasizing tumor which locally invades surrounding tissues and frequently recurs following surgical excision. The term desmoid is derived from the Greek word "desmos" which means band or tendon. Most cases are sporadic, but there is a clear association with familial adenomatous polyposis (Gardner's syndrome), suggesting a link with mutation of APC gene on chromosome 5q22. Histologically aggressive fibromatosis consists of moderately cellular proliferation of spindle-shaped fibroblasts arranged as interlacing bundles. These cells are bland and are noted to invade and extend between fascicles of skeletal muscle. Malignant features such as pleomorphism are absent and mitotic figures are rare. When the tumor infiltrates muscle tissue, the entrapped muscle fibers undergo

atrophy. Microscopically the differential diagnosis of aggressive fibromatosis includes low-grade fibrosarcoma and reactive fibrosis. Local invasion of adjacent bones is rare although some cases have been reported in the literature. Aggressive fibromatosis can grow into a large size and on rare occasions patients present with multicentric lesions. It is important to note that after a period of rapid alarming growth of either primary or recurrent disease, spontaneous growth arrest may take place and this phase can persist indefinitely. Aggressive fibromatosis often starts as a painless, deep soft tissue mass in the extremities or head and neck. It is locally invasive and commonly recurs locally but does not metastasize. MR imaging findings are those of an intramuscular soft tissue mass with low signal intensity on T1-weighted images and heterogeneously high signal intensity on T2-weighted images, with low signal-intensity band-like areas. Histologic confirmation of the imaging diagnosis is often needed prior to any treatment.

Typical clinical presentation

Aggressive fibromatosis can occur at any age, with a peak incidence between the ages of 25 and 35 years. Females are more likely to be affected than males and some authors believe that this tumor is more aggressive in young patients below the age of 30 years.

Patients present with firm, deeply seated masses that grow slowly and cause little or no focal symptoms until late in their course. Tumor distribution includes the shoulders, supraclavicular region, thighs, arms, posterior part of the thorax, and buttocks. Despite their benign histology the tumors frequently behave in a locally aggressive manner. Reported recurrence is 25–65%. The approach to the treatment has recently changed as the natural history of the disease became better understood. There have been several reports showing growth arrest or spontaneous regression of aggressive fibromatosis. This lesion is believed to display a self-limiting behavior, even in recurrent cases. Therefore a conservative strategy of observation and avoidance of unnecessary surgery is found to provide satisfactory results.

Differential diagnosis

The main differential diagnosis of aggressive fibromatosis on imaging is malignant soft tissue sarcoma. As a general rule most soft tissue sarcomas form a pseudocapsule, grow within a single muscle compartment, and respect fascial boundaries. As they grow, sarcomas outgrow their blood supply and develop central necrosis. Aggressive fibromatosis typically shows an infiltrative growth pattern; it crosses fascial boundaries and

Pearls and Pitfalls in Musculoskeletal Imaging, ed. D. Lee Bennett and Georges Y. El-Khoury. Published by Cambridge University Press. © Cambridge University Press 2013.

does not show central necrosis. Low signal intensity on all pulse sequences is said to be characteristic of, but not specific for, aggressive fibromatosis.

Teaching points

MRI provides the optimum method to tumor evaluation at all stages of this disease including recurrence. The relationship of the tumor to nerves, vessels, deep viscera, and bone can be accurately assessed with MRI. A core biopsy under imaging guidance is sufficient for histologic characterization.

READING LIST

Casillas J, Sais GJ, Greve JL et al. Imaging of intra-and extraabdominal desmoid tumors. *RadioGraphics* 1991;**11**:959–968.

Griffiths HJ, Robinson K, Bonfiglio TA. Aggressive fibromatosis. *Skeletal Radiol* 1983;**9**:179–184.

Lee JC, Thomas JM, Phillips S et al. Aggressive fibromatosis: MRI features with pathologic correlation. *AJR Am J Roentgenol* 2006;**186**:247–254.

Nakayama T, Tsuboyama T, Toguchida J et al. Natural course of desmoid-type fibromatosis. *J Orthop Sci* 2008;**13**:51–55.

O'Keefe F, Kim EE, Wallace S. Magnetic resonance imaging in aggressive fibromatosis. *Clin Radiol* 1990;**42**:170–173.

Rock MG, Pritchard DJ, Reiman HM et al. Extra-abdominal desmoid tumors. *J Bone Joint Surg* 1984;**66-A**;1369–1374.

Sundaram M, Duffrin H, McGuire MH, Vas W. Synchronous multicentric desmoid tumors (aggressive fibromatosis) of the extremities. *Skeletal Radiol* 1988;**17**:16–19.

Sundaram M, McGuire MH, Schajowicz F. Soft-tissue masses: histologic basis for decreased signal (short T2) on T2-weighted MR images. *AJR Am J Roentgenol* 1987;**148**:1247–1250.

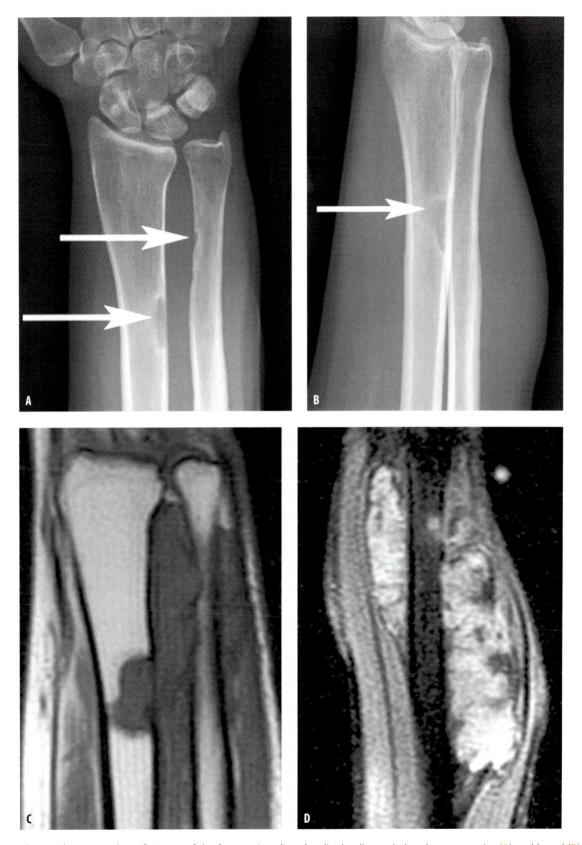

Figure 83.1 Desmoid tumor in the soft tissues of the forearm invading the distal radius and ulna. Anteroposterior (**A**) and lateral (**B**) views of the forearm show the desmoid tumor occupying the dorsum of the distal forearm. The radius and ulna are both invaded by the tumor (arrows). T1-weighted coronal image (**C**) of the forearm shows the desmoid tumor infiltrating the marrow space of the distal radius and ulna. The tumor has low signal intensity on this T1-weighted image. T2-weighted sagittal image (**D**) reveals the tumor to be heterogeneously bright, suggesting high cellularity.

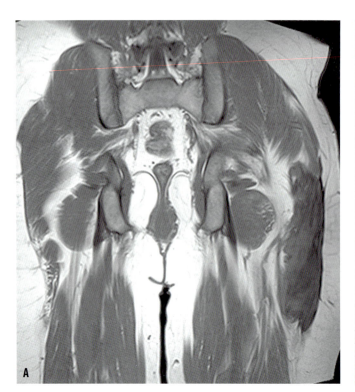
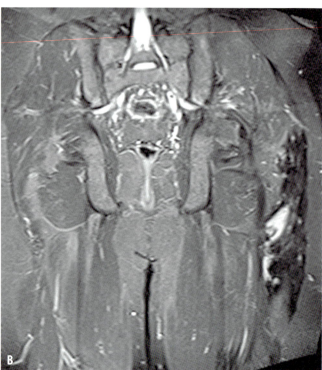

Figure 83.2 Desmoid tumor in the left proximal thigh. The signal intensity in both T1- and T2-weighted images is low (dark) suggesting the lesion contains mainly collagen. Coronal T1- and T2-weighted images (**A** and **B**) show the lesion as having dark signals on both sequences.

Imaging description

On radiography conventional chondrosarcomas typically show a lytic, lobulated, expansile lesion with scattered sclerotic areas which represent mineralized chondroid matrix (Figure 84.2). Characteristically a mineralized chondroid matrix reveals a punctate or popcorn pattern of calcifications. Higher-grade chondrosarcoma (grade 3) often contain less extensive areas of matrix mineralization. When these calcifications are tiny or faintly visualized, CT can show them better than radiography. The lesion appears to be slow growing and somewhat expansile causing some cortical thickening. With continued tumor growth endosteal scalloping develops and cortical disruption with invasion of the soft tissues can be detected. Murphey *et al.* stressed the importance of the extent of the endosteal scalloping (Figure 84.2). They believe that endosteal scalloping greater than two thirds the normal thickness of the long bone cortex is a strong evidence of chondrosarcoma rather than an enchondroma. They add that longitudinal endosteal scalloping in long bone lesions greater than two thirds of the lesion length is also more suggestive of chondrosarcoma than enchondroma.

MRI is the ideal method for demonstrating the extent of the marrow involvement as well as the soft tissue extension. The tumor reveals low to intermediate signal on T1-weighted sequence. The non-mineralized cartilaginous or myxoid component of the tumor shows high signal intensity on T2-weighted images. The mineralized cartilage shows low signal intensity on all MR pulse sequences. Conventional chondrosarcoma shows peripheral and septal enhancement following the IV injection of gadolinium (Figure 84.1).

Importance

Chondrosarcoma is the second most common primary bone tumor after osteosarcoma; it represents 10–15% of all malignant bone tumors. It is typically a disease of middle-aged individuals and the elderly, and it is more common in males. About 16% of chondrosarcomas occur in patients below the age of 21 years, and in one third of these patients the chondrosarcomas arise in benign pre-existing solitary or multiple cartilaginous lesions. In young patients chondrosarcomas generally tend to be more aggressive and have worse prognosis than those in adults.

Chondrosarcoma consists of a family of malignant tumors which can be classified into conventional (central), or intramedullary, and juxtacortical or periosteal. There are some other rare varieties and they include clear cell, mesenchymal, myxoid, and dedifferentiated chondrosarcomas. The mesenchymal and myxoid chondrosarcomas can occur within bone or in the soft tissues. Soft tissue chondrosarcomas are much less common than those arising in bone and they contribute to only 1.7% of all chondrosarcomas. By definition tumors arising from soft tissues are not attached to bone, cartilage, or periosteum. Chondrosarcomas may also be primary, arising *de novo*, or secondary arising from a pre-existing enchondroma or osteochondroma.

Histological grading of chondrosarcomas is classified into three grades, 1, 2, and 3 or low, intermediate, and high grade. Sometimes a fourth grade is added which is reserved for a highly malignant tumor, the dedifferentiated chondrosarcoma. The grading system is widely used because it determines management of these tumors and directly influences prognosis. Tumor grade seems to correlate with the incidence of metastasis and the survival rate. Grade 1 is a low-grade tumor consisting of chondrocytes with small dense nuclei and a few binucleated cells. The stroma is predominantly chondroid. The grade 1 chondrosarcoma is often difficult to differentiate from an enchondroma. Grade 2 chondrosarcoma is an intermediate-grade tumor. It has less chondroid and more myxoid matrix. The lesion is more cellular than grade 1 and the chondrocyte nuclei are large and hyperchromatic. The chondrocytes can be binucleated or multinucleated. Grade 3 shows greater cellularity and nuclear pleomorphism than grade 2. (Pleomorphism denotes variations in size and shape of the nucleus.) Nuclei are also much larger than normal and chondroid matrix is sparse to absent.

Clinically the most common primary chondrosarcoma is the conventional (intramedullary) chondrosarcoma accounting for about 45% of all chondrosarcomas. It has a predilection for males and it occurs most commonly in the 4th and 5th decades of life. The most common location for conventional chondrosarcoma is the long tubular bones, which are also a common site for enchondromas. The femur followed by the tibia and the proximal humerus are common locations. The flat bones such as the pelvis, especially the acetabular region, and the ribs are also common sites for this tumor. The spine, scapula, sternum, and fibula are less frequently involved.

Juxtacortical or surface chondrosarcoma arises on the surface of the bone and it is of two types. The first one develops from the cartilage cap of a pre-existing osteochondroma and the other arises on the periosteal surface of the cortical bone (Figure 84.1).

Dedifferentiated chondrosarcoma is characterized by conventional low-grade chondrosarcoma with microscopically abrupt transition into a higher-grade non-cartilaginous aggressive sarcoma. This aggressive sarcoma component is

Pearls and Pitfalls in Musculoskeletal Imaging, ed. D. Lee Bennett and Georges Y. El-Khoury. Published by Cambridge University Press. © Cambridge University Press 2013.

usually due to a malignant fibrous histiocytoma, osteosarcoma, or fibrosarcoma. Chondrosarcomatous dedifferentiation occurs in approximately 10% of patients with chondrosarcoma. The tumor behaves in an aggressive manner and metastasizes as a high-grade sarcoma. The prognosis of the dedifferentiated chondrosarcoma is much worse than that of a low-grade chondrosarcoma. The dedifferentiated chondrosarcoma is sometimes referred to as a grade 4 lesion.

Clear cell chondrosarcoma is a low-grade neoplasm with better prognosis than conventional chondrosarcoma. It comprises about 2% of all chondrosarcomas. It is more common in males and the age ranges between 25 and 45 years. It occurs in the subchondral regions of long bones such as the proximal femur and proximal humerus. Radiographically it resembles a chondroblastoma except that age is typically older and the matrix in this tumor rarely calcifies.

Mesenchymal chondrosarcoma is a rare type of chondrosarcoma. It is a high-grade tumor consisting of undifferentiated round cells and islands of well-differentiated hyaline cartilage. The tumor commonly arises in bone but 30–49% of cases arise in soft tissues. It presents as a well-demarcated soft tissue mass with densely granular calcification. Shapeero *et al.* reported that the prognosis in adults with extraskeletal mesenchymal chondrosarcoma is poor but children with this tumor have a good prognosis.

Myxoid chondrosarcoma is also a rare tumor that occurs in both bone and soft tissue and is considered as an intermediate grade tumor. It typically affects patients aged 50–60 years, but it is also known to occur at a younger age. Patients with soft tissue myxoid chondrosarcoma present with a tender palpable mass. The tumor has high water content due to abundant myxoid stroma and hyaline cartilage.

Typical clinical scenario

Most chondrosarcomas arise in patients older than 40 years of age. There are some benign conditions that predispose patients to develop the chondrosarcoma; these include: enchondroma, osteochondroma, multiple familial exostoses, Ollier's disease, and Maffucci syndrome. The most common symptom at presentation is pain and local swelling. The tumor occasionally presents with a pathologic fracture.

Differential diagnosis

In clinical practice the distinction between an enchondroma versus a chondrosarcoma is a fairly common problem. The presence of deep or extensive endosteal scalloping should favor a chondrosarcoma. If an intramedullary cartilage lesion erodes more than two-thirds of the cortex or breaks through

into the soft tissues the diagnosis of chondrosarcoma becomes a primary consideration. The hands and feet are common sites for enchondroma but not for chondrosarcomas. Enchondromas in the hands and feet can produce endosteal scalloping without transforming into a chondrosarcoma. It is important to remember that a cartilage lesion in the spine is very unlikely to represent an enchondroma. Chondrosarcoma is the most common malignant tumor of the spine after chordoma. A cartilage cap in an osteochondroma thicker than 2 cm should raise the possibility of malignant degeneration into a chondrosarcoma.

> ## Teaching point
>
> Chondrosarcoma is a common malignant bone tumor. It is divided into multiple types and different pathologic grades. Chondrosarcoma is predominantly located in the pelvis, femur, humerus, ribs, sternum, and spine. In the long bones a chondrosarcoma typically starts in metaphysis or proximal diaphysis. Chondrosarcomas are rare in the hands and feet.

READING LIST

Boriani S, DeLure F, Bandiera S *et al*. Chondrosarcoma of the mobile spine. *Spine* 2000;**25(7)**:804–812.

Casadei R, Ricci M, Ruggieri P *et al*. Chondrosarcoma of the soft tissues. *J Bone Joint Surg* 1991;**73-B**;162–168.

Hashimoto N, Ueda T, Joyama S *et al*. Extraskeletal mesenchymal chondrosarcoma: an imaging review of ten new patients. *Skeletal Radiol* 2005;**34**:785–792.

Huvos AG, Marcove RC. Chondrosarcoma in the young. A clinicopathologic analysis of 79 patients younger than 21 years of age. *Am J Surg Pathol* 1987;**11(12)**:930–942.

Kumar R, David R, Cierney G III. Clear cell chondrosarcoma. *Radiology* 1985;**154**:45–48.

Murphey MD, Walker EA, Wilson AJ *et al*. From the archives of the AFIP. Imaging of primary chondrosarcoma: radiologic pathologic correlation. *RadioGraphics* 2003;**23**:1245–1278.

Present D, Bacchini P, Pignatti G *et al*. Clear cell chondrosarcoma of bone. A report of 8 cases. *Skeletal Radiol* 1991;**20**:187–191.

Shapeero LG, Vanel D, Couanet D *et al*. Extraskeletal mesenchymal chondrosarcoma. *Radiology* 1993;**186**:819–826.

Sissons HA, Matlen JA, Lewis MM. Dedifferentiated chondrosarcoma. *J Bone Joint Surg* 1991;**73-A**:294–300.

Tateishi U, Hasegawa T, Nojima T *et al*. MRI features of extraskeletal myxoid chondrosarcoma. *Skeletal Radiol* 2006;**35**:27–33.

Weber KL, Raymond AK. Low-grade/dedifferentiated/high-grade chondrosarcoma: a case of histological and biological progression. *Iowa Orthopaed J* 2002;**22**:75–80.

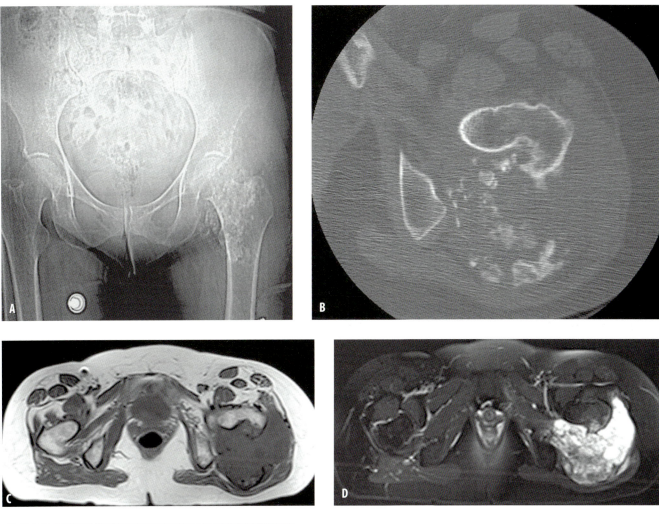

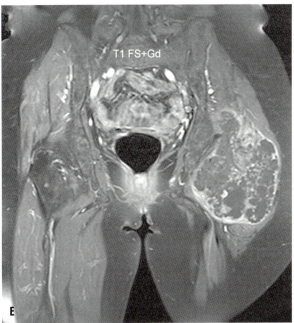

Figure 84.1 Chondrosarcoma arising from the periosteal surface of the proximal femur. Anteroposterior digital scanagram (**A**) taken prior to a CT scan of the pelvis reveals numerous punctate calcifications projecting over the left hip. Axial CT section (**B**) shows the lesion arising on posterior surface of greater trochanter. Axial T1- and T2-weighted images (**C**) and (**D**) show a low signal-intensity mass on the T1-weighted image (**C**) and bright signal of the cartilage component on the fat-suppressed T2-weighted image (**D**). The areas on T2 which are dark likely represent calcifications within the chondrosarcoma. Fat-suppressed coronal T1-weighted image (**E**) following IV gadolinium injection reveals peripheral and septal enhancement. The majority of the tumor does not enhance.

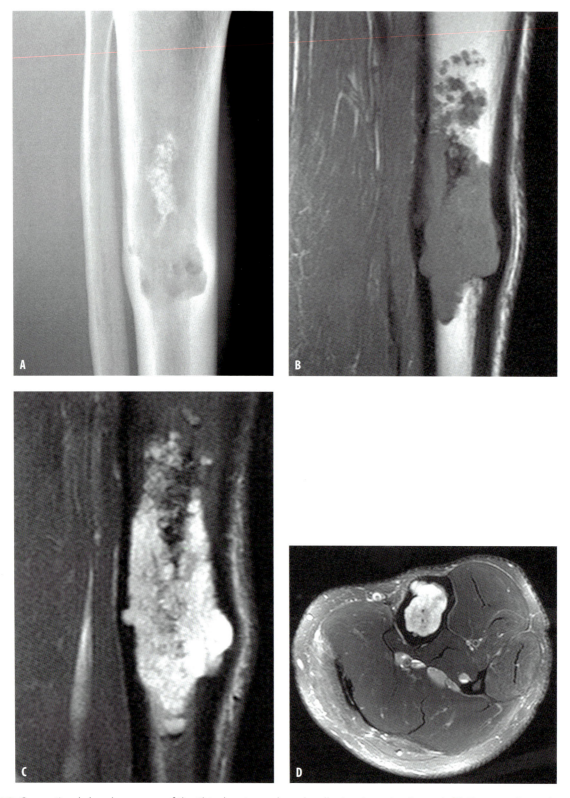

Figure 84.2 Conventional chondrosarcoma of the tibia showing endosteal scalloping. Lateral radiograph (**A**) illustrates the endosteal scalloping. The scalloping on these coronal T1-weighted (**B**) and fat-suppressed T2-weighted (**C**) images involves more than two thirds of the tibial cortex. Fat-suppressed axial T2-weighted image (**D**) also reveals extensive endosteal scalloping.

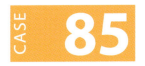

Pigmented villonodular synovitis (PVNS)

Imaging description

The radiographic changes vary with the type of pigmented villonodular synovitis (PVNS), and whether the disease is localized or diffuse, and also on the joint involved (Figures 85.1 and 85.2). Giant cell tumor of the tendon sheath presents radiographically as a soft tissue mass, with or without a well-marginated erosion in the underlying bone. Giant cell tumor of the tendon sheath is rarely imaged with CT or MRI because the diagnosis is often made clinically. In the localized intra-articular type of PVNS the radiographic examination is usually normal. Radiographs of patients with diffuse PVNS may appear normal early in the disease but more commonly they show a large joint effusion. A joint aspiration typically reveals bloody fluid. Bone erosions are more common in joints with a tight capsule such as the hip or elbow (Figure 85.3). In the knee joint, which is the most commonly involved joint with diffuse PVNS, erosions develop late in the disease because the joint capsule is fairly distensible. Bone erosions are most frequently seen in the hip where about 90% of patients have erosions. Erosions are best delineated with CT. CT can sometimes show a lobulated high-attenuation mass surrounding the involved joint. This is attributed to the high hemosiderin content in the abnormal synovium. Periarticular osteopenia and joint space narrowing in diffuse PVNS are rare findings.

MRI is the diagnostic test of choice for all types of PVNS. In the diffuse type MRI demonstrates the joint effusion as well as the heterogeneous villous and nodular synovial proliferation; bony and soft tissue infiltration is also well demonstrated by MRI. The signal intensity of the abnormal synovium is intermediate to low on T1-weighted images and low on the T2-weighted images because of the high concentration of hemosiderin in the synovium (Figure 85.4). Gradient echo sequences are used to show "blooming" of the low signal intensity due to magnetic susceptibility artifacts produced by the hemosiderin (Figure 85.5).

Importance

PVNS is a monoarticular proliferative process affecting the synovium of large joints, tendon sheath, or bursae. It presents as a nodule, a villous, or villonodular lesions. Three types are described: (1) an extra-articular localized lesion in a tendon sheath which is also known as a giant cell tumor of the tendon sheath. This type most commonly involves the hand and wrist, especially the index and long fingers; (2) a localized intra-articular nodule, which is the least common presentation of PVNS and occurs almost exclusively in the knee (Figure 85.1); (3) a diffuse villous type which presents as pigmented proliferation of the entire synovium in a large joint. In this type there is synovial hypertrophy consisting of irregular papillary and villonodular projections. All three types of PVNS have similar histological appearance characterized by neoplastic proliferation of the synovial fibroblasts and histiocytes. PVNS is currently recognized as a benign neoplasm that does not metastasize but the diffuse form can locally infiltrate bone and surrounding soft tissues. PVNS is a rare synovial disease which affects relatively young individuals. Fortunately the disease has specific imaging findings. Early diagnosis is important especially in the diffuse type where advanced disease can produce irreversible joint damage.

Typical clinical presentation

Patients commonly seek medical attention between the 3rd and the 5th decade of life. The localized extra-articular type of PVNS (giant cell tumor of the tendon sheath) is the most common type. Patients present with pain and a soft tissue mass. Patients with the localized intra-articular PVNS typically complain of joint swelling, pain, and decreased range of motion. Diffuse PVNS involves mainly the knee (66–80% of cases), followed by the hip, ankle, shoulder, and elbow. Patients complain of joint pain, and chronic joint effusion. The treatment for the localized types is surgical excision while for the diffuse type it is total synovectomy; however, because total synovectomy is not always possible and the recurrence rate is high, irradiation has been used to arrest the disease.

Differential diagnosis

The differential diagnosis for PVNS should include amyloid arthropathy, hemophilic arthropathy, and synovial chondromatosis. Amyloid deposits have low signals on T1- and T2-weighted images. Amyloid arthropathy manifests as intra-articular and periarticular clumps of low signal intensity without villous or nodular proliferation of the synovium. The deposits do not bloom on gradient echo sequences since they do not contain hemosiderin. Amyloid is typically polyarticular while PVNS is monoarticular. The clinical picture should be very helpful in differentiating hemophilic arthropathy from PVNS. The majority of synovial chondromatosis cases show calcified loose bodies on the radiographic examination. On the rare occasions when the loose bodies are not calcified, MRI shows small hyperintense round or oval structures within the joint which are typical of cartilaginous loose bodies.

Pearls and Pitfalls in Musculoskeletal Imaging, ed. D. Lee Bennett and Georges Y. El-Khoury. Published by Cambridge University Press. © Cambridge University Press 2013.

Teaching points

When imaging reveals a soft tissue mass of the finger or toe associated with a well-circumscribed bone erosion, one should consider the diagnosis of extra-articular PVNS (or giant cell tumor of tendon sheath). If a large joint reveals diffuse proliferative synovitis with prominent synovial villi and nodules along with a sizable joint effusion one should consider diffuse PVNS. This is particularly true if the synovium is dark on T1- and T2-weighted images and shows dark blooming nodules on gradient echo images.

READING LIST
Cotton A, Flipo R-M, Mestdagh H, Chastanet P. Diffuse pigmented villonodular synovitis of the shoulder. *Skeletal Radiol* 1995;**24**:311–313.

Garner HW, Ortiguera CJ, Nakhleh RE. Best cases from the AFIP. Pigmented villonodular synovitis. *RadioGraphics* 2008;**28**:1519–1523.

Lin J, Jacobson JA, Jamadar DA, Ellis JH. Pigmented villonodular synovitis and related lesions: the spectrum of imaging findings. *AJR Am J Roentgenol* 1999;**172**:191–197.

Llauger J, Palmer J, Roson N *et al.* Pigmented villonodular synovitis and giant cell tumors of the tendon sheath: radiologic and pathologic features. *AJR Am J Roentgenol* 1999;**172**:1087–1091.

Murphey MD, Rhee JH, Lewis RB *et al.* From the archives of the AFIP. Pigmented villonodular synovitis: radiologic-pathologic correlation. *RadioGraphics* 2008;**28**:1493–1518.

Srinivasa A, Vigorita VJ. Pigmented villonodular synovitis (giant-cell tumor of the tendon sheath and synovial membrane). *J Bone Joint Surg* 1984;**66-A**:76–94.

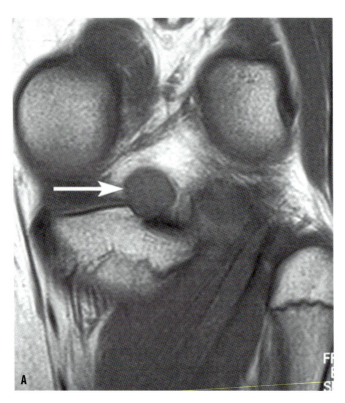
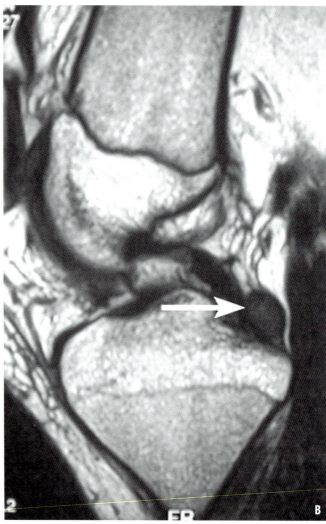

Figure 85.1 Localized pigmented villonodular synovitis (PVNS). Coronal T1-weighted (**A**) and sagittal T2-weighted (**B**) images reveal a small low signal-intensity mass at the insertion of the PCL to the tibia (arrows).

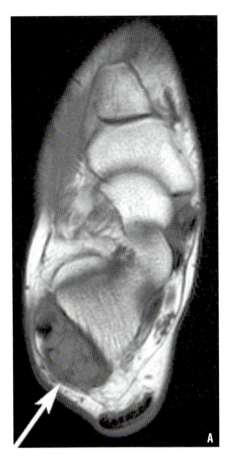
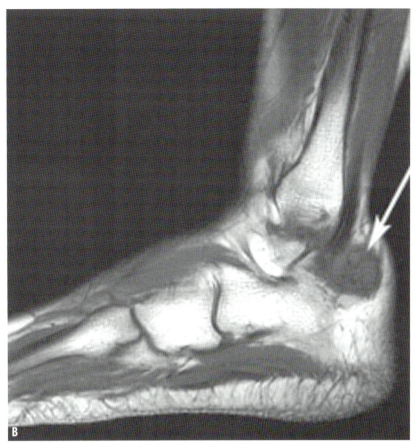
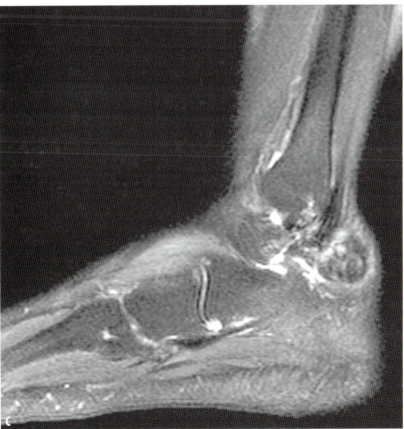

Figure 85.2 Giant cell tumor of the tendon sheath. Axial (**A**) and sagittal T1-weighted (**B**) images show mass associated with peroneal tendon sheath (arrows). On T2-weighted sagittal image (**C**) the mass has low signal intensity.

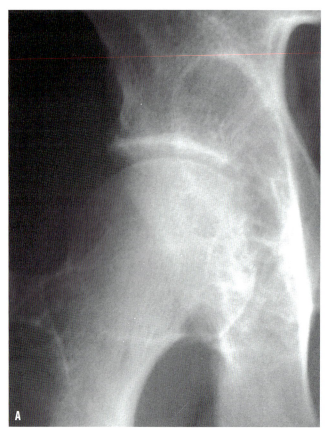

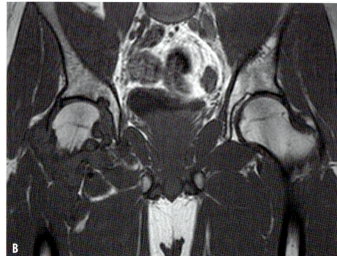

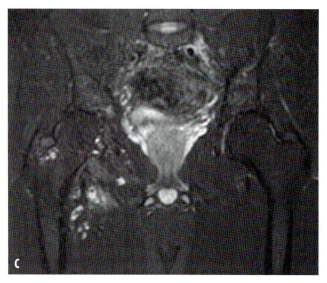

Figure 85.3 Diffuse pigmented villonodular synovitis (PVNS) of the right hip with bone erosions. Anteroposterior radiograph of the right hip (**A**) shows lucent areas on both sides of the joint which represent erosions. Coronal T1-weighted (**B**) and STIR (**C**) images of the pelvis show invasion of the bone and soft tissues around the right hip joint with PVNS.

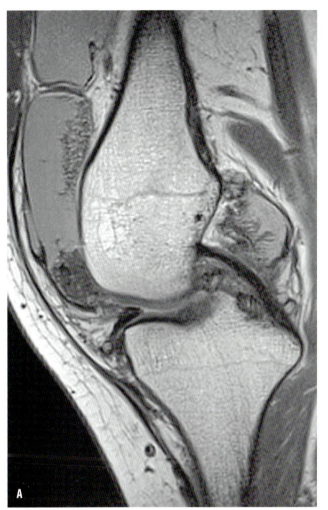

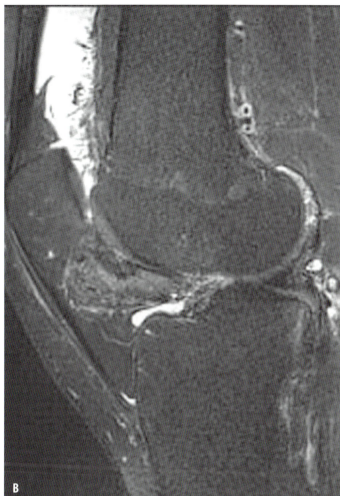

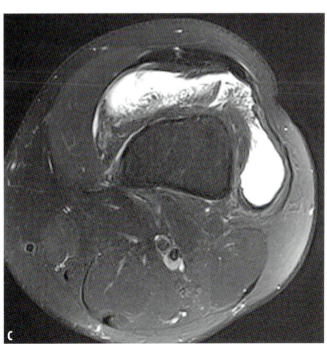

Figure 85.4 Diffuse pigmented villonodular synovitis (PVNS) in the knee. Proton density sagittal (A), fat-suppressed T2-weighted sagittal (B), and axial fat-suppressed T2-weighted (C) images show the typical villous proliferation of the synovium.

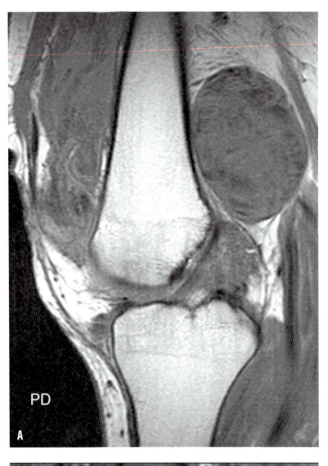

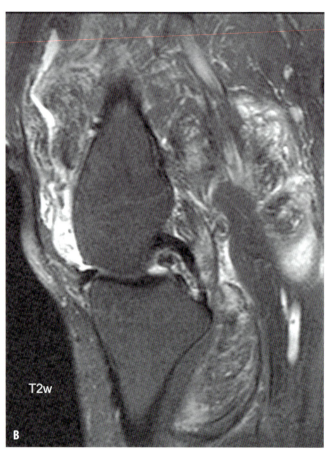

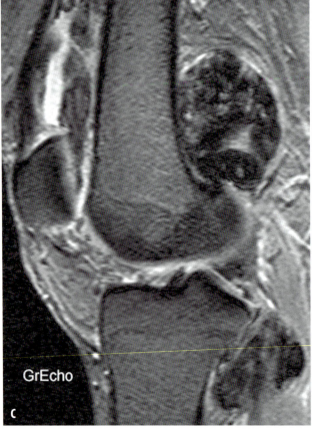

Figure 85.5 Pigmented villonodular synovitis (PVNS) in the knee. Proton density (**A**), fat-suppressed T2-weighted (**B**), and gradient echo (**C**) sagittal images demonstrating PVNS in the knee. The gradient echo MR image reveals the intensely dark signals within the PVNS lesion due to the presence of hemosiderin.

Synovial chondromatosis (osteochondromatosis)

Imaging description

The radiographic appearance of primary synovial chondromatosis is that of multiple round or oval calcified loose bodies, usually of similar size, and without underlying diseases that can be associated with loose body formation (Figure 86.1). In about one third of patients the loose bodies are not mineralized and radiographs may be normal or reveal only soft tissue swelling of the affected joint (Figure 86.2). In tight joints such as the hip, elbow, and ankle deep bony erosions are common (Figure 86.2). The extra-articular form of synovial chondromatosis is particularly rare. The hands, feet, and wrists are most commonly affected (Figure 86.3). In the hip joint both intra- and extra-articular involvement has been described; the extra-articular synovial chondromatosis in the hip often involves the iliopsoas bursa (Figure 86.4).

Secondary synovial osteochondromatosis is much more common than the primary type and it is seen in older patients. It typically occurs in conjunction with underlying osteoarthritis. The calcified loose bodies tend to be larger than those seen with the primary type, less in number, and more varied in size (Figure 86.5).

Importance

Primary or idiopathic synovial chondromatosis is a rare monoarticular disease characterized by the formation of multiple cartilaginous or osteocartilaginous loose bodies. The disease is commonly intra-articular but occasionally it can be extra-articular involving a tendon sheath or bursa. Secondary synovial chondromatosis is the more common type and it is seen as a result of other joint diseases such as osteoarthritis, osteochondritis dissecans, osteochondral fractures, and neuroarthropathy. In the literature different names have been used to describe this condition but currently the most frequently used terms are synovial chondromatosis or synovial osteochondromatosis when the loose bodies are ossified. Loose bodies can only become ossified if they have a blood supply and therefore are attached to the synovium. Cartilaginous loose bodies are typically free to move within the joint and they get their nourishment from the synovial fluid. The etiology of primary synovial osteochondromatosis is not known but many authors believe that the synovium undergoes cartilaginous metaplasia and becomes able to produce cartilaginous nodules, which later detach and become cartilaginous loose bodies. Microscopically these nodules consist of hyaline cartilage with mineralized chondroid matrix. Hypercellularity with atypical nuclei is common and has been misinterpreted as malignancy.

The disease is most common between the 3rd and 5th decade; males are about twice as commonly involved than females. Synovial chondromatosis has been reported occasionally in children where there may be fewer and less opaque calcifications. Any joint can be affected but the most commonly involved joints are the knee, hip, shoulder, elbow, and ankle. Malignant transformation of synovial chondromatosis to a chondrosarcoma has been described but it is very rare.

The disease is easily diagnosable radiographically when the cartilaginous loose bodies are calcified, however in up to 30% of cases the loose bodies are not calcified rendering the diagnosis of synovial chondromatosis difficult, especially early in the disease. Delayed diagnosis and treatment can lead to joint damage and secondary osteoarthritis. Synovial chondromatosis can produce deep and circumferential bony erosions especially in tight joints like the hip where these erosions can make the femoral neck weak and at risk for a pathologic fracture.

Typical clinical scenario

Primary synovial osteochondromatosis is a monoarticular disease which in the majority of the patients affects the knee. The most common clinical presentation is pain, swelling, giving way, and decreased range of motion. Patients typically present with joint effusion, crepitus, and locking. When the cartilaginous masses are large they can be palpated on physical examination.

Differential diagnosis

Fewer numbers of loose bodies along with underlying osteoarthritis are expected in the secondary type of osteoarthritis. The extra-articular type of osteochondromatosis which typically occurs in the hands and feet should be differentiated from periosteal chondroma. When the intra-articular cartilaginous loose bodies are not calcified early diffuse PVNS can simulate synovial chondromatosis on MRI. Massive cortical erosions with invasion of the medullary canal should raise the possibility of a malignancy; the most critical entity to exclude in such a scenario is a chondrosarcoma.

Teaching point

Secondary synovial chondromatosis or osteochondromatosis is a common disease and it should be differentiated from primary synovial chondromatosis. The secondary type often occurs in elderly patients with underlying osteoarthritis. Radiographically the loose bodies are few in number and they vary in size.

Pearls and Pitfalls in Musculoskeletal Imaging, ed. D. Lee Bennett and Georges Y. El-Khoury. Published by Cambridge University Press. © Cambridge University Press 2013.

READING LIST

Abdelwahab IF, Contractor D, Bianchi S *et al.* Synovial chondromatosis of the lumbar spine with compressive myelopathy: a case report with review of the literature. *Skeletal Radiol* 2008;**37**:863–867.

Azouz EM, Kozlowski K, Marsel J. Soft tissue tumors of the hand and wrist of children. *Can Assoc Radiol* 1989;**40**:251–255.

Coolican MR, Dandy DJ. Arthroscopic management of synovial chondromatosis of the knee. *J Bone Joint Surg* 1989;**71-B**:498–500.

DeBenedetti MJ, Schwinn CP. Tenosynovial chondromatosis in the hand. *J Bone Joint Surg* 1979;**61-A**:898–902.

Ginai AZ. Case report 607. *Skeletal Radiol* 1990;**19**:227–231.

Kaiser TE, Ivins JC, Unni KK. Malignant transformation of extra-articular synovial chondromatosis: report of a case. *Skeletal Radiol* 1980;**5**:223–226.

Karlin CA, DeSmet AA, Neff J *et al.* The variable manifestations of extraarticular synovial chondromatosis. *AJR Am J Roentgenol* 1981;**137**:731–735.

Lazarus E, Song JH, Lambiase RE, Tung GA. Case of the day. General case of the day. *RadioGraphics* 1996;**16**:709–712.

Norman A, Steiner GC. Bone erosion in synovial chondromatosis. *Radiology* 1986;**161**:749–752.

Pope TL Jr, Keats TE, de Lange EE *et al.* Idiopathic synovial chondromatosis in two unusual sites: inferior radioulnar joint and ischial bursa. *Skeletal Radiol* 1987;**16**:205–208.

Sim FH, Dahlin DC, Ivins JC. Extra-articular synovial chondromatosis. *J Bone Joint Surg* 1977;**59-A**:492–495.

Trias A, Quintana O. Synovial chondrometaplasia: review of world literature and a study of 18 Canadian cases. *Can J Surg* 1976;**19**:151–158.

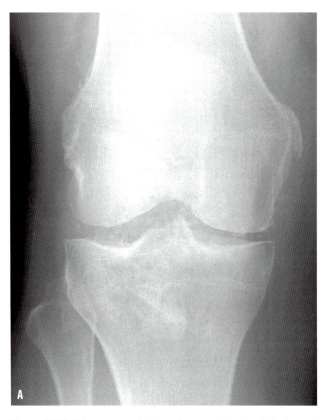 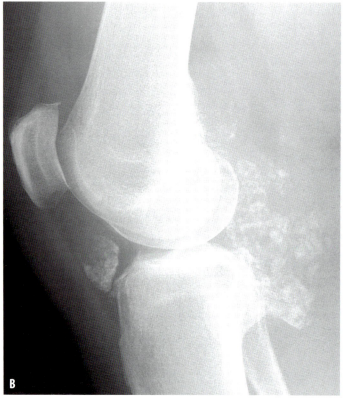

Figure 86.1 Primary synovial chondromatosis in the right knee. Anteroposterior (**A**) and lateral (**B**) views of the right knee show multiple tiny cartilaginous loose bodies with calcifications. Radiography alone is diagnostic in this case.

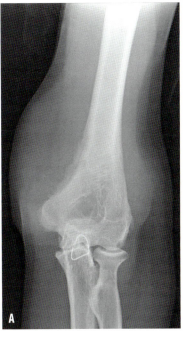
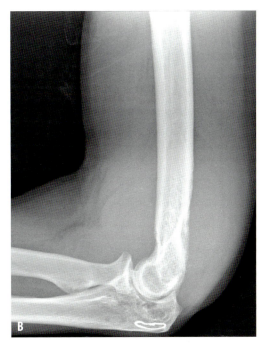
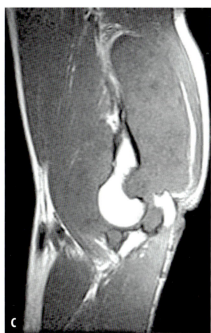

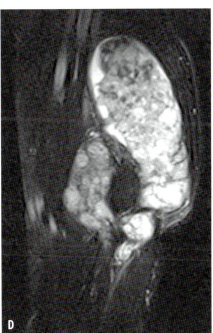
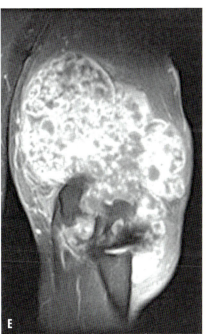

Figure 86.2 Primary synovial chondromatosis; the loose bodies here are not mineralized. Anteroposterior (**A**) and lateral (**B**) radiographs of the left elbow reveal soft tissue masses around the elbow joint. Note also the large erosion in the olecranon process. T1-weighted (**C**), fat-suppressed T2-weighted (**D**), and post-contrast fat-suppressed T1-weighted (**E**) images of the elbow confirm the presence of cartilaginous loose bodies within the joint.

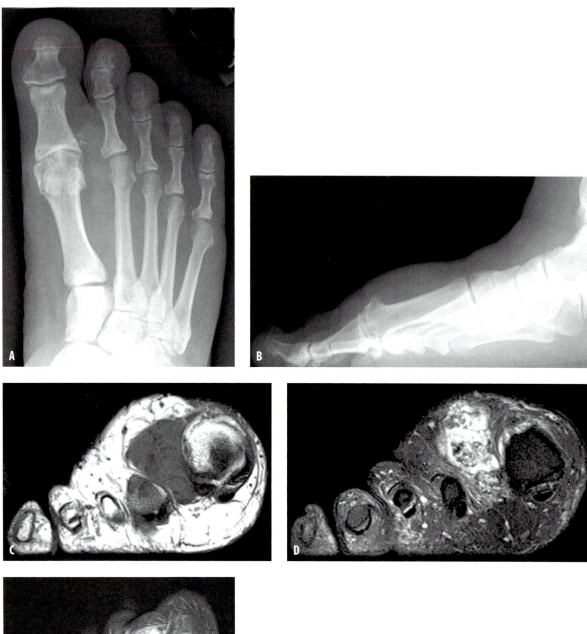

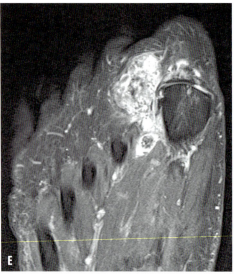

Figure 86.3 Extra-articular synovial chondromatosis. Anteroposterior (**A**) and lateral (**B**) views of the forefoot demonstrate the presence of a faintly calcified mass between the first and second metacarpo-phalangeal joints. Axial T1-weighted (**C**), axial fat-suppressed T2-weighted (**D**), and coronal fat-suppressed T2-weighted (**E**) images confirm the presence of a collection of cartilaginous loose bodies within the soft tissues of the forefoot.

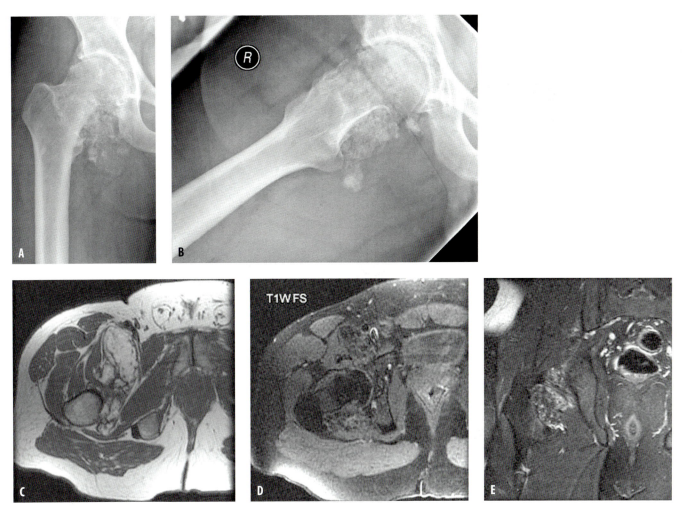

Figure 86.4 Primary synovial chondromatosis of the right hip showing calcified cartilaginous loose bodies within the joint and in the soft tissues around the joint. Anteroposterior (**A**) and lateral (**B**) views of the hip show numerous calcified loose bodies around the hip joint. Axial T1-weighted (**C**), axial fat-suppressed T2-weighted (**D**), and post-contrast coronal T1-weighted fat-suppressed (**E**) images show cartilaginous loose bodies within the hip joint and in the soft tissues around the joint.

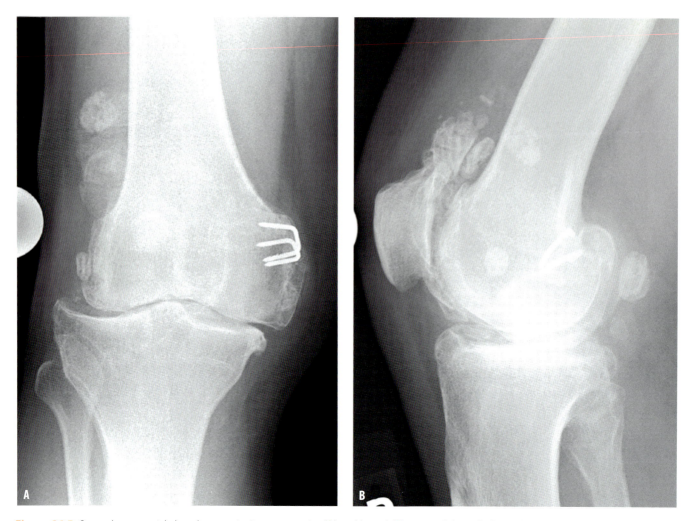

Figure 86.5 Secondary synovial chondromatosis. Anteroposterior (**A**) and lateral (**B**) views of the right knee show several calcified loose bodies of different sizes and shapes. The knee joint reveals severe changes of osteoarthritis.

Myositis ossificans

Imaging description

Despite the advances in imaging techniques diagnosing myositis ossificans remains a challenging problem, especially in early stages. It is important to remember that no one set of imaging findings obtained at one time can characterize all the stages of myositis ossificans. In fact the imaging findings rapidly change depending on the degree of maturation of the lesion. Initially radiographs can be entirely normal. Within 2 weeks after the injury radiography may show a soft tissue mass along with thin uninterrupted periosteal reaction in the adjacent bone. The periosteal reaction is more often seen in children where it can sometimes be thick and lamellated. At this stage the best indication that the lesion is not a neoplasm is the fact that the periosteal reaction is uninterrupted. Biopsies of the soft tissue mass, at this early stage, reveal rapidly proliferating mesenchyme that may be mistaken for a sarcoma. By 3–4 weeks the lesion starts to form osteoid which in the following weeks begins to mineralize. At this stage radiographs show clumps of calcifications within the soft tissue mass. By 5–8 weeks a zoning pattern appears which represents the most important diagnostic feature of myositis ossificans (Figures 87.1 and 87.2). This presents radiographically as peripheral calcifications followed by ossifications which surround the lesion. At 2 months the ossifications become thicker and denser, and later on the lesion starts to appear essentially similar to mature trabecular bone. By 3–5 months the lesion becomes diffusely ossified, smaller, and may eventually adhere to the adjacent bone (Figure 87.1, G and H).

Computed tomography plays a key role in making an early and definitive diagnosis of myositis ossificans. By 4–6 weeks after the soft tissue mass is discovered, CT is capable of demonstrating a zoning pattern which represents a rim of calcifications with a central lucency.

Currently MRI is the modality of choice for most soft tissue lesions, but in the case of myositis ossificans the early use of MRI can be confusing because it reveals non-specific findings that resemble soft tissue infection or neoplasm. MRI findings depend on the maturity of the lesion. In the early stages of the disease MRI shows a soft tissue mass surrounded by extensive edema. The mass is difficult to separate from the edema and both present with low signal intensity on T1-weighted images and high signal intensity on T2-weighted images. Histologically the mass corresponds to a central collection of proliferating fibroblasts and myofibroblasts within a myxoid stroma. The extensive muscle edema is typical of myositis ossificans but is an unusual finding with most primary soft tissue neoplasms. After 4–5 weeks the MRI findings become more specific revealing a rim of low signal intensity, on both T1- and T2-weighted images, indicating the presence of peripheral calcifications (Figure 87.1, E and F). On MRI, mature or chronic myositis ossificans resembles normal bone. The lesion at this stage demonstrates a central area of high signal intensity representing fatty marrow and peripheral low signal intensity representing bony cortex.

A radionuclide bone scan is rarely used except for assessing the maturity of the lesion in cases where resection is planned to release contractions around large joints in patients with severe burns.

Importance

Myositis ossificans is a non-neoplastic disease characterized by heterotopic bone formation in skeletal muscles. Two types of myositis ossificans are described: (1) myositis ossificans progressiva which is also known as fibrodysplasia ossificans progressiva. This is a hereditary generalized disease and is always fatal; (2) myositis ossificans circumscripta or traumatica is a fairly common disease which is often associated, although not always, with trauma. The post-traumatic myositis ossificans results in focal heterotopic bone formation within a skeletal muscle; it is caused by either a single direct blow or repeated minor trauma although 40% of patients do not have a clear history of trauma; the heterotopic bone is usually limited to a single muscle or muscle group. The commonest locations for myositis ossificans are the quadriceps and brachialis muscles. A small percentage of cases occur in patients with paraplegia, tetanus, and severe burns. Myositis ossificans circumscripta is seen at any age, but most commonly occurs in adolescents and young adults, over half the cases occurring in the third decade. The disease is seen in children but it is rare below the age of 10 years. Myositis ossificans is a self-limiting disease and when the radiographic appearance is typical conservative management is sufficient.

Typical clinical scenario

Patients clinically present with pain, swelling, and limitation of motion in the hip, thigh, or anterior arm. On physical examination a hard painful mass is palpated. The majority of patients give a history of recent trauma to the muscle.

Differential diagnosis

When no clear history of trauma is available the correct diagnosis of myositis ossificans may be difficult to make especially in early phases. Before the development of the characteristic peripheral calcifications and ossification, the imaging finding may suggest a soft tissue infection or neoplasm. Later in the disease and after faint calcification start to develop

Pearls and Pitfalls in Musculoskeletal Imaging, ed. D. Lee Bennett and Georges Y. El-Khoury. Published by Cambridge University Press. © Cambridge University Press 2013.

myositis ossificans can be confused with synovial sarcoma and sometimes more mature lesions can resemble parosteal osteosarcoma or sessile osteochondroma.

Teaching point

Awareness of the imaging appearance in the different stages of myositis ossificans is important for the diagnosis and treatment of this condition.

READING LIST

Amendola MA, Glazer GM, Agha FP *et al*. Myositis ossificans circumscripta: computed tomographic diagnosis. *Radiology* 1983;**149**:775–779.

DeSmet AA, Norris MA, Fisher DR. Magnetic resonance imaging of myositis ossificans: analysis of seven cases. *Skeletal Radiol* 1992;**221**:503–507.

Gindele A, Schwamborn D, Tsironis K, Benz-Bohn G. Myositis ossificans traumatica in young children: report of three cases and review of the literature. *Pediatr Radiol* 2000;**30**:451–459.

Kransdorf MJ, Meis JM, Jelinek JS. Myositis ossificans: MR appearance with radiologic-pathologic correlation. *AJR Am J Roentgenol* 1991;**157**:1243–1248.

Nuovo MA, Norman A, Chumas J, Ackerman LV. Myositis ossificans with atypical clinical, radiographic, or pathologic findings: a review of 23 cases. *Skeletal Radiol* 1992;**21**:87–101.

Parikh J, Hyare H, Saifuddin A. The imaging features of post-traumatic myositis ossificans, with emphasis on MRI. *Clinical Radiol* 2002;**57**:1058–1066.

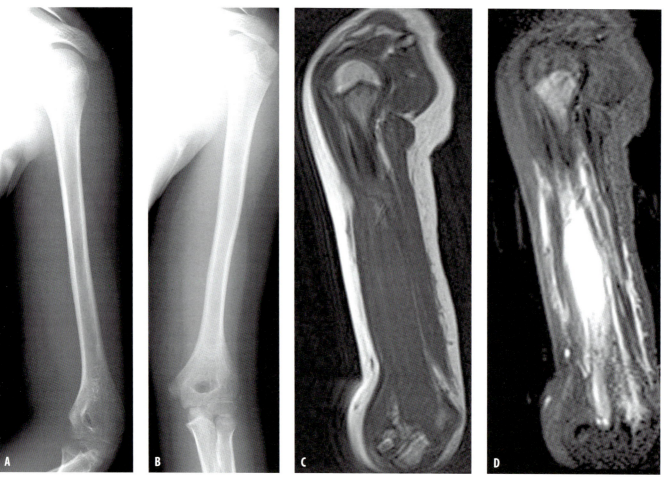

Figure 87.1 A 14-year-old male suspected of having myositis ossificans in his arm. He plays football at his school, but there was no definite history of trauma. He was followed up with radiography and MRI of the arm for 3 months. He was sent to the Orthopaedic Oncology Clinic because of a painful mass which was palpated in his arm. Anteroposterior (**B**) and lateral (**A**) radiographs of the arm 14 days after the symptoms started. They were interpreted as showing no abnormalities. T1-weighted (**C**) and fat-suppressed T2-weighted (**D**) images obtained 3 weeks after onset of symptoms show a large area of increased signal intensity, on the T2-weighted image, in the brachialis muscle. The findings are non-specific and may be due to a neoplasm, edema, muscle bleeding, or early myositis ossificans. T1-weighted (**E**) and fat-suppressed T2-weighted (**F**) images taken at 8 weeks after onset of symptoms reveal a rounded mass with a low signal intensity rim which is diagnostic for myositis ossificans (zoning phenomenon). Anteroposterior (**G**) and lateral (**H**) radiographs of the arm taken at 3 months shows the myositis ossificans to be adherent to the cortex. There is also associated uninterrupted periosteal reaction.

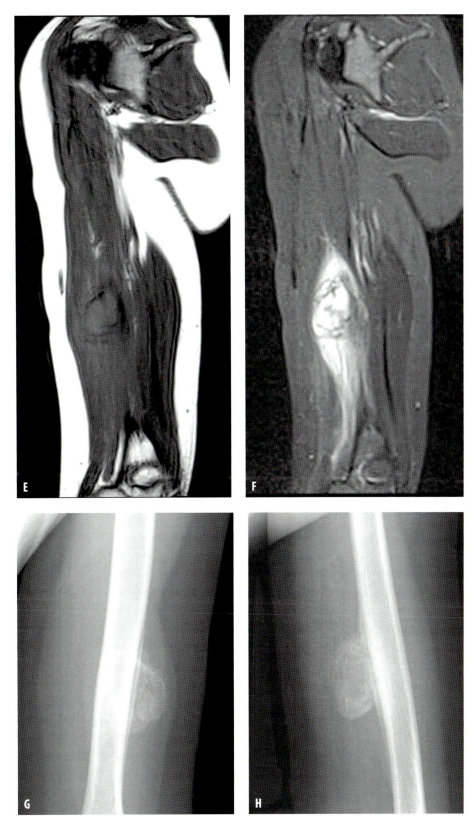

Figure 87.1 (cont.)

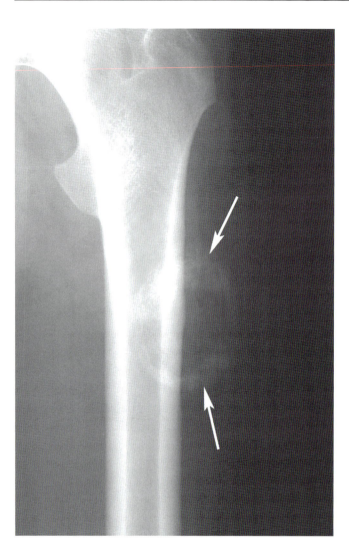

Figure 87.2 Anteroposterior radiograph of the proximal femur shows the typical zoning pattern with a thick rim of mineralization at the periphery of the lesion in the proximal thigh (arrows). Patient sustained an injury a week earlier. The zoning pattern helps in differentiating myositis ossificans from a surface osteosarcoma which lacks the zoning pattern.

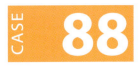

88 Aneurysmal bone cyst (ABC)

Imaging description

In the long bones, spine, and flat bones, the majority of aneurysmal bone cysts (ABCs) are eccentrically located whereas in the short tubular bones they are usually central in location. All lesions show expansion and cortical thinning (Figure 88.1). Aneurysmal bone cyst is one of the few lesions that can invade the epiphyseal plate and cross from the metaphysis to the epiphysis causing growth abnormalities. The natural history of ABC is described as evolving through four radiographic stages: initial, active, stabilization, and healing stage. In the initial stage, the lesion is characterized by a well-defined lytic area associated with periosteal reaction. This is followed by the active stage where the lesion grows rapidly and aggressively, producing a "blown-out" radiographic appearance, resembling a malignant lesion (Figure 88.2). This stage is succeeded by a stabilization period which is characterized by the "soap bubble" appearance caused by maturation of the surrounding shell and internal septa between the cystic spaces. The lesion in the healing phase or quiescent phase shows progressive ossification of the bony shell and internal septa. Radiographs typically show an eccentric lytic lesion with an expanded or "blown-out" bony contour. Cortically based lesions comprise about 12–18% of cases, whereas purely surface lesions are less common and comprise about 7–8% of cases. Rarely radiographs may show flocculent densities within the lesion which mimic chondroid matrix.

MRI reveals an expanding well-defined mass with high signal intensity on T2-weighted images and without a soft tissue component. After gadolinium administration, primary ABC shows peripheral and septal enhancement, while secondary ABC may show a nodular and a peripheral thick rind of tissue because of the coexistence of a solid component. MRI commonly shows the fluid-fluid pattern within the ABC (Figures 88.2 and 88.3). The fluid in the cysts may show high signal intensity on T1-weighted images presumably due to the methemoglobin (Figure 88.2B).

Importance

Aneurysmal bone cyst is a benign locally aggressive expansile lesion which accounts for 2% of primary bone tumors, and 75% of all ABCs occur before the age of 20 years. The etiology of this lesion is uncertain; however it is postulated to arise from an increase in the venous pressure leading to local hemorrhage. Some cases are reported to have developed at the site of previous trauma or fracture. The lesion consists of multiple cystic cavities filled with blood and separated by fibrous septa. Aneurysmal bone cysts are divided into two types: primary, where the ABC arises *de novo* and secondary, where it is associated with other benign or malignant lesions, such as giant cell tumor,

chondroblastoma, osteoblastoma, simple bone cyst, fibrous dysplasia, non-ossifying fibroma, and osteosarcoma (Figure 88.1). Among these lesions, giant cell tumor is the one most commonly associated with an ABC. About 15% of all giant cell tumors have cystic areas that resemble ABC, and in about one third of all ABCs a pre-existing lesion can be identified.

The spine is involved by ABC in about 20% of cases. Characteristically, the lesion arises within the posterior column and then extends into the vertebral body. The diagnosis can easily be made by imaging because of the characteristic appearance of ABC on CT and MRI (Figure 88.1). Embolization can be used as an adjunct to surgery in order to reduce the bleeding during the operation, or as a definitive treatment. In the spine an ABC arising within one vertebra can cross to an adjacent vertebra.

Histological examination of ABCs shows cavernous spaces lined by endothelium and filled with unclotted blood. The walls or septa between the spaces are fibrous and contain benign giant cells. A solid variant of ABC has been described; it is similar clinically and radiographically to the cystic form of ABC, but lacks the cavernous spaces. A soft-tissue ABC has been recently described; it is a rare entity which is identical to ABC of bone, except for its extraosseous location.

Typical clinical scenario

The majority of patients are fairly young, presenting before the age of 20 years; the lesion is however rare in children below 5 years of age. Symptoms include mild pain and swelling. More than half of all ABCs occur in the metaphysis of long bones, such as the proximal humerus, distal femur, and proximal tibia. Pathological fractures are however rare. The pelvis accounts for half of all flat bone lesions. The posterior column of the vertebrae is the site for 12–30% of ABC cases. Spinal lesions can present with neurological symptoms due to spinal cord or nerve root compression.

Differential diagnosis

Although ABC is a benign lesion it sometimes grows rapidly, mimicking aggressive malignant tumors. Fluid-fluid levels are most often seen with an ABC, however this finding is not pathognomonic. Giant cell tumor is the lesion that occasionally reveals cystic spaces with fluid-fluid levels on MRI and therefore resembles an ABC. Clinically however giant cell tumors present after closure of the physeal plate whereas an ABC presents in patients below the age of 20 years. A lesion that is easily confused with an ABC, on imaging studies, is telangiectatic osteosarcoma. Telangiectatic osteosarcoma however shows enhancing soft tissue or nodular components after

Pearls and Pitfalls in Musculoskeletal Imaging, ed. D. Lee Bennett and Georges Y. El-Khoury. Published by Cambridge University Press. © Cambridge University Press 2013.

Gd administration whereas the cystic cavities in ABC enhance at the cyst walls and septa.

Teaching point

In patients below the age of 20 years, ABC is a relatively common benign, lytic expansile lesion. The majority of lesions occur in the metaphysis of long bone, flat bones, especially in the pelvis and in the posterior column of vertebrae. An ABC can be a primary lesion where it arises alone in bone, or it can start in association with another benign or malignant lesion. Such lesions are called secondary ABC. Aneurysmal bone cyst develops in stages and in the active phase it can grow rapidly assuming a "blown out" appearance on imaging. At this stage an ABC can resemble an aggressive malignant lesion.

READING LIST

Ajilogba KA, Kaur H, Ducan R et al. Extraosseus aneurysmal bone cyst in a 12-year-old girl. Pediatr Radiology 2005;35:1240–1242.

Bonakdarpour A, Levy WM, Aegerter E. Primary and secondary aneurysmal bone cyst: a radiological study of 75 cases. Radiology 1978;126:75–83.

Capanna R, Springfield DS, Biagini R et al. Juxtaepiphyseal aneurysmal bone cyst. Skeletal Radiol 1985;13:21–25.

Dabezies EJ, D'Ambrosia RD, Chuinard RG, Ferguson AB Jr. Aneurysmal bone cyst after fracture. J Bone Joint Surg 1982;64-A:617–621.

DiCaprio MR, Murphy MJ, Camp RL. Aneurysmal bone cyst of the spine with familial incidence. Spine 2000;25(12):1589–1592.

Kransdorf MJ, Sweet DE. Aneurysmal bone cyst: concept, controversy, clinical presentation, and imaging. AJR Am J Roentgenol 1995;164:573–580.

McGrath A, Sri-Ram K, Yeung E et al. Benign bone tumours. In Bulstrode C, Wilson-MacDonald J, Eastwood D et al., eds. Oxford Textbook of Trauma and Orthopaedics. 2nd edn. New York, NY: Oxford University Press, 2011;141–143.

Sanerkin NG, Mott MG, Roylance J. An unusual intraosseous lesion with fibroblastic, osteoclastic, osteoblastic, aneurysmal and fibromyxoid elements. Cancer 1983;51:2278–2286.

Scully SP, Temple HT, O'Keefe RJ, Gebbardt MC. Case report 830. Skeletal Radiol 1994;23:157–160.

Tsai JC, Dalinka MK, Fallon MD et al. Fluid-fluid level: a nonspecific finding in tumors of bone and soft tissue. Radiology 1990;175:779–782.

Wang XL, Gielen JL, Salgado R et al. Soft tissue aneurysmal bone cyst. Skeletal Radiol 2004;33:477–480.

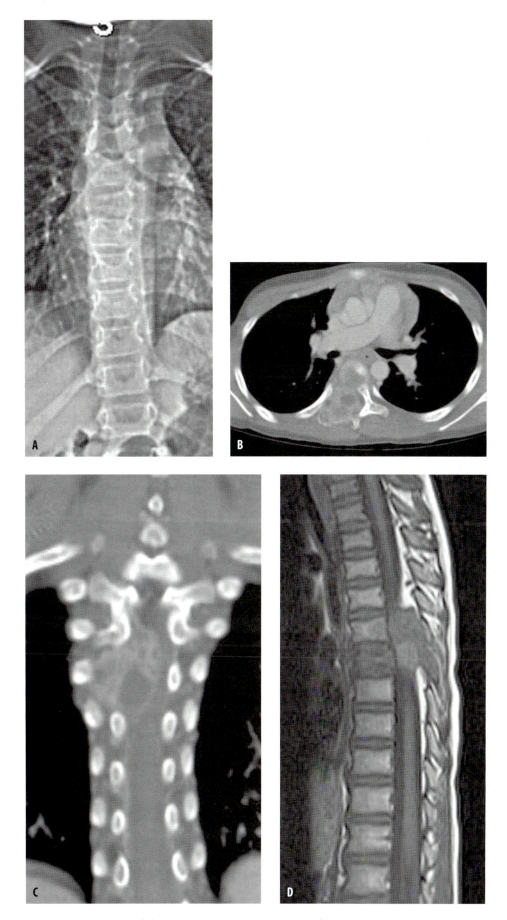

Figure 88.1 A 7-year-old male presenting with lower extremity weakness. He was diagnosed pre-operatively to have an osteoblastoma of T6 associated with a secondary aneurysmal bone cyst (ABC). Digital radiograph (**A**), axial (**B**), and coronal (**C**) CT images reveal a destructive expansile lesion of right pedicle and laminae of T6. Sagittal T1-weighted (**D**), sagittal T2-weighted (**E**), and axial T2-weighted (**F**) images reveal the fluid-fluid levels typical of ABC. A post-contrast fat-suppressed T1-weighted axial image (**G**) shows an enhancing solid component of the associated osteoblastoma.

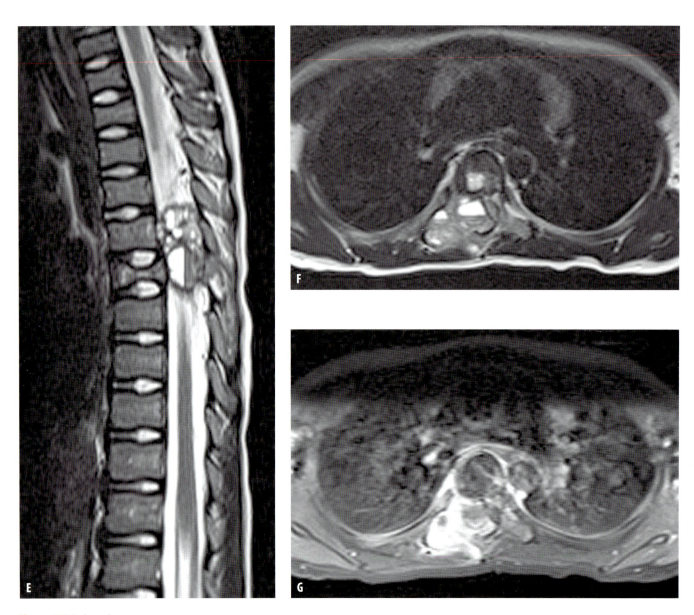

Figure 88.1 (cont.)

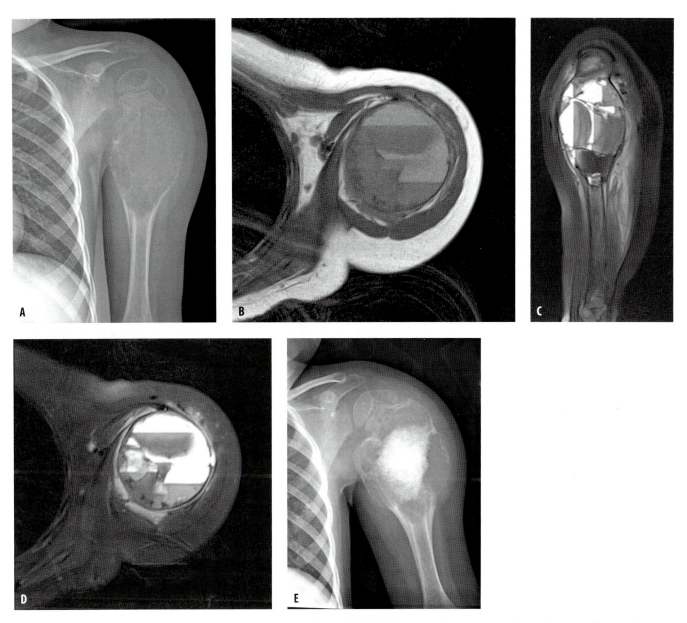

Figure 88.2 Aneurysmal bone cyst (ABC) in the proximal metaphysis of the left humerus during its active phase. Because of its rapid expansion, it was thought clinically to be a malignant tumor. Anteroposterior view (**A**) of the humerus shows a lytic expansile lesion in proximal humerus. This is associated with a Codman's triangle. Axial T1-weighted (**B**) MR image showing fluid-fluid level. The fluid at the top is more bright than muscle because of the presence of methemoglobin. Sagittal (**C**) and axial (**D**) T2-weighted fat-suppressed MR images showing multiple fluid-fluid levels. Anteroposterior radiograph (**E**) about 6 weeks after curettage and grafting. The lesion, however, continued to expand because it was still in the active phase.

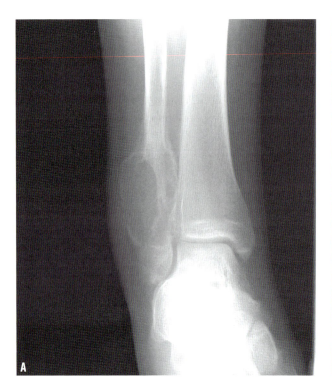
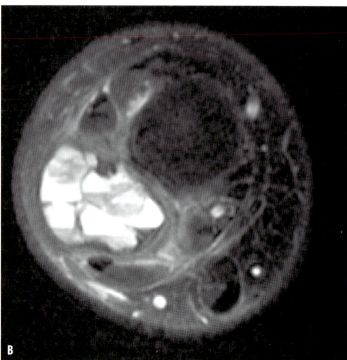

Figure 88.3 Aneurysmal bone cyst (ABC) in the distal metaphysis of the fibula. An AP radiographic view (**A**) of the ankle demonstrates an expansile lytic lesion in the distal metaphysis of the fibula. Axial fat-suppressed T2-weighted MR image (**B**) showing fluid-fluid levels within the ABC.

89 Soft tissue hemangioma

Imaging description

Cavernous hemangioma is the lesion that most commonly contains fat (Figure 89.1); so much so that portions of some cavernous hemangiomas may be indistinguishable from a lipoma. A recurrent history of pain and swelling of the knee in children and young adults is a characteristic presentation of synovial hemangioma (Figure 89.2).

On plain radiographs the presence of phleboliths (calcified thrombi) within muscles are fairly specific of an intramuscular hemangioma. Sung *et al.* described a spectrum of periosteal reactions in patients with deep soft tissue hemangiomas, including lobulated solid periosteal reaction, solid continuous periosteal reaction, elliptical cortical hyperostosis, undulating periosteal reaction, and thin solid periosteal reaction. Radiographically, the differential diagnosis of reactive bone changes in soft tissue hemangiomas includes both benign and malignant bone and soft tissue neoplasm. Solid continuous periosteal reaction is the most common periosteal response associated with deep soft tissue hemangiomas. This pattern can be easily confused with a stress fracture. An associated elliptical cortical hyperostosis can simulate an osteoid osteoma but the absence of a nidus should help in the differential diagnosis. Coarsened trabecular pattern, similar to that of an intraosseous hemangioma of the spine, can be seen in association with deep soft tissue hemangiomas of the extremities.

On MRI intermediate or slightly high signal intensity on T1-weighted images and strikingly high signals on the T2-weighted images have been described in some studies. The high signal intensity on T1-weighted images corresponds to the fatty tissue in the lesion. In a recent publication Teo *et al.* described distinguishing features on MRI which helped in differentiating hemangiomas from malignant soft tumors. On T2-weighted images hemangiomas present with multiple lobules or tubules with high-signal intensity configuration interspaced with linear and lace-like areas. The high signals on T2-weighted images reflect the pooling of blood with cavernous spaces and slow flow within dilated venous channels. On T2-weighted sequence some high signal intensity lobules have been shown to contain central low-intensity dots which represent fast blood flow (Figures 89.1 C and 89.1 D). Suh *et al.* stressed that no single feature is specific of hemangioma, but the constellation of several MRI findings may help in reaching the correct diagnosis.

Importance

Hemangiomas are common soft tissue tumors which account for 7–10% of all benign soft tissue tumors. Based on location soft tissue hemangiomas may be cutaneous, subcutaneous, intramuscular, intermuscular, or synovial. Cutaneous and superficial subcutaneous lesions are usually easy to diagnose clinically, while the deeply situated hemangiomas arising in the deep subcutaneous tissues, muscle or synovium invariably pose diagnostic difficulties. Intramuscular hemangioma represents the most common type of deep soft tissue hemangiomas. Soft tissue hemangiomas exhibit a variety of clinical and histologic patterns. There are five types that are classified based on histologic features and vessel size within the tumor; these are the capillary, cavernous, venous, arteriovenous, and mixed types. Tumors composed of small vessels are called capillary hemangiomas, whereas those with mostly larger vessels are cavernous or venous hemangiomas. The dominant pattern is the cavernous hemangioma.

All hemangiomas contain variable amounts of non-vascular tissue such as fat, smooth muscle, fibrous tissue, and bone. Cavernous hemangioma is the lesion that most commonly contains fat (Figure 89.1); so much so that portions of some cavernous hemangiomas may be indistinguishable from a lipoma.

Synovial hemangioma is a rare benign lesion that occurs most frequently in the knee where it commonly involves the suprapatellar pouch; typically patients present before the age of 16 years and almost all of them are symptomatic, presenting due to a swollen knee, pain, and limitation of motion. Synovial hemangioma is frequently misdiagnosed and the pre-operative diagnosis is made only in a small percentage of the cases. A recurrent history of pain and swelling of the knee in children and young adults is a characteristic presentation of synovial hemangioma (Figure 89.2).

Typical clinical scenario

Most intramuscular hemangiomas present during childhood and adolescence; 80–90% of patients with intramuscular hemangiomas present before the age of 30 years. The diagnosis of intramuscular hemangioma is rarely suspected clinically and when the lesion is small, it is difficult to detect it even when symptomatic. The duration of the symptoms ranges from a few months to several years. Most patients with deep-seated hemangiomas present with intermittent pain or swelling. Sometimes they complain of poorly delineated masses that become larger or smaller over time. Without imaging studies deep-seated hemangiomas are difficult to distinguish from malignant soft tissue tumors.

Differential diagnosis

There are MRI signs which characterize soft tissue hemangiomas and differentiate them from other malignant soft tissue tumors. These features include the presence of a septated

Pearls and Pitfalls in Musculoskeletal Imaging, ed. D. Lee Bennett and Georges Y. El-Khoury. Published by Cambridge University Press. © Cambridge University Press 2013.

lobulated or tubular appearance on T2-weighted images and in addition the presence of a central low intensity, the dot sign, within the lobules on T2-weighted images. An intramuscular hemangioma should be considered as a possible diagnosis in patients under the age of 30 years presenting with a soft tissue mass. A long clinical history and the presence of peripheral fat, phleboliths, or large internal vessels should alert the radiologist to the diagnosis of a benign intramuscular hemangioma.

> ## Teaching point
>
> Knowledge of the natural history and imaging appearance of intramuscular hemangiomas is important, since they may be confused with other soft tissue tumors such as liposarcoma.

READING LIST

Buetow PC, Kransdorf MJ, Moser RP Jr *et al.* Radiologic appearance of intramuscular hemangioma with emphasis on MR imaging. *AJR Am J Roentgenol* 1990;**154**:563–567.

Cotton A, Flipo R-M, Herbaux B *et al.* Synovial haemangioma of the knee: a frequently misdiagnosed lesion. *Skeletal Radiol* 1995;**24**:257–261.

Greenspan A, Azouz EM, Matthews J, Decarie J-C. Synovial hemangioma: imaging features in eight histologically proven cases, review of the literature, and differential diagnosis. *Skeletal Radiol* 1995;**24**:583–590.

Greenspan A, McGahan JP, Vogelsang P, Szabo RM. Imaging strategies in the evaluation of soft-tissue hemangiomas of the extremities: correlation of the findings of plain radiography, angiography, CT, MRI, and ultrasonography in 12 histologically proven cases. *Skeletal Radiol* 1992;**21**:11–18.

Griffin N, Khan N, Meirion J *et al.* The radiological manifestations of intramuscular haemangiomas in adults: magnetic resonance imaging, computed tomography and ultrasound appearances. *Skeletal Radiol* 2007;**36**:1051–1059.

Llauger J, Monill Jm, Palmer J, Clotet M. Synovial hemangioma of the knee: MRI findings in two cases. *Skeletal Radiol* 1995;**24**:579–581.

Suh J-S, Hwang G, Hahn S-B. Soft tissue hemangiomas: MR manifestations in 23 patients. *Skeletal Radiol* 1994;**23**:621–625.

Sung MS, Kang HS, Lee HG. Regional bone changes in deep soft tissue hemangiomas: radiographic and MR features. *Skeletal Radiol* 1998;**27**:205–210.

Teo E-L HJ, Strouse PJ, Hernandez RJ. MR imaging differentiation of soft-tissue hemangiomas from malignant soft-tissue masses. *AJR Am J Roentgenol* 2000;**174**;1623–1628.

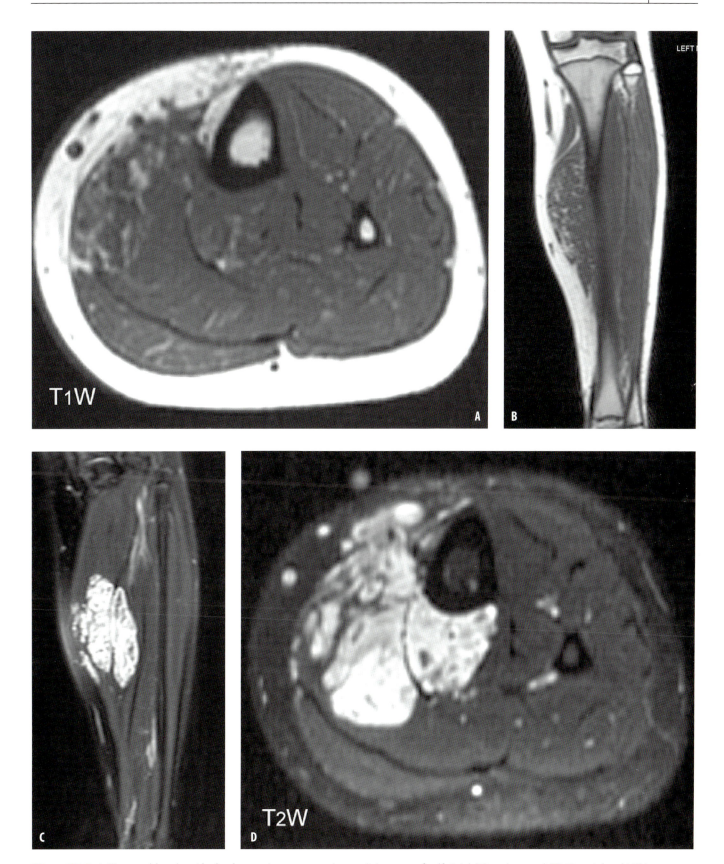

Figure 89.1 A 10-year-old male with slowly growing mass on the medial aspect of calf. Axial (**A**) and coronal (**B**) T1-weighted MR images demonstrate areas of high signal intensity within the mass. These areas represent fatty tissue. Fat-suppressed coronal (**C**) and axial (**D**) T2-weighted MR images show high signal intensity lobular and tubular structures which represent slow flow. The central low-intensity dots represent fast blood flow.

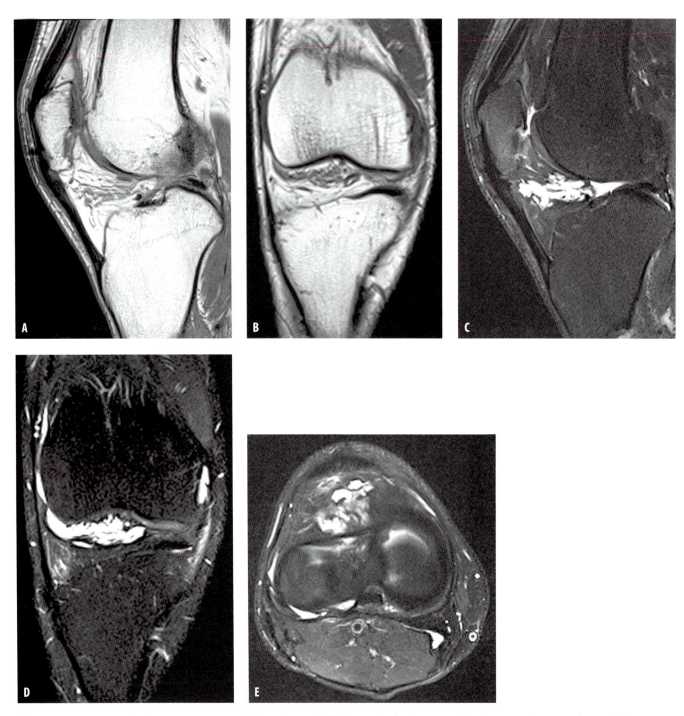

Figure 89.2 Intra-articular hemangioma. Sagittal (**A**) and coronal (**B**) T1-weighted MR images show low signal intensity linear tubular structures within Hoffa's fat pad. Fat-suppressed T2-weighted MR images (**C**, **D**, and **E**) of the knee reveal high signal intensity lobules and tubular structures in Hoffa's fat pad characteristic of a hemangioma.

90 Giant cell tumor (GCT)

Imaging description

As with most bone tumors the location and radiographic appearance are the most important features in arriving at the correct diagnosis. The vast majority of giant cell tumors (GCTs) occur in long bones at subchondral locations especially the knee. On plain radiographs, a GCT appears as an eccentric, lytic, often expansile lesion without a sclerotic margin or radiographically discernable matrix. Cortical thinning or cortical break-through is invariably present, but these findings are better visualized by CT; a secondary ABC can also be associated with a giant cell tumor (Figures 90.1 and 90.2).

Two signs on bone scintigraphy can help in narrowing down the differential diagnosis: (1) increased radionuclide uptake at the periphery of the lesion and photopenia centrally (donut sign) (2) increased radionuclide uptake in the bone across the joint from the GCT.

On MRI, the solid components of GCT demonstrate low to intermediate signal intensity on both T1- and T2-weighted images in the majority of cases (Figure 90.3). The reason for this appearance has been attributed to the hemosiderin deposition, increased cellularity, and high collagen content.

Importance

Giant cell tumor (GCT) is a fairly common bone tumor accounting for about 4–9% of all bone tumors and 21% of all benign bone tumors. Females are slightly more affected than males; however lesions in younger patients and those involving the spine demonstrate a higher female predilection. Although GCT is classified as a benign, solitary tumor, it can behave as a locally aggressive lesion with a recurrence rate of 30–50%, and less than 5% become malignant; a smaller percentage of GCT can be multicentric. Giant cell tumor typically occurs in mature young adults between the third and fourth decade. Very rarely it occurs prior to physeal fusion. Giant cell tumors arise in the subchondral region of long bone especially around the knee. In order of frequency the most common sites are: the distal femur, proximal tibia, distal radius, sacrum, and proximal humerus. Giant cell tumor occurs in the spine in about 11% of the cases with the sacrum being the most common site of involvement. Sacral lesions are associated with poorer prognosis because they are typically larger than peripheral lesions and more difficult to excise completely.

The multifocal or multicentric GCT is a variant accounting for less than 1% of all of GCTs of bone. Patients with multifocal GCT are likely to be younger than those with a solitary lesion. The number of lesions varies from two to a maximum of 20 lesions. The lesions are discovered synchronously or metachronously, and the knee is the most common location for multifocal disease.

A GCT tumor contains a large number of giant cells in a background of stromal mononuclear cells which fuse to produce the giant cells. Mitotic activity may be present in the stromal cell component of the tumor. The nuclei of the stromal cells are identical to those of the multinucleated giant cells. This is a histologic feature that can be helpful in differentiating GCT from other bone lesions which contain giant cells such as giant cell reparative granuloma, brown tumor of hyperparathyroidism, osteoblastoma, chondroblastoma, aneurysmal bone cyst (ABC), non-ossifying fibroma, and osteosarcoma. Secondary ABC is commonly associated with GCTs (Figure 90.1). Cases of GCT with prominent ABC elements present with more aggressive and more expansile radiographic appearance. Differentiating the cystic component of the ABC from the solid portion of the GCT is important because a core needle biopsy should be directed at the solid component.

Malignant GCT is a rare condition which occurs in less than 5% of cases. This term refers to a tumor where *de novo* malignant transformation occurs in a formerly benign GCT. The lesion can be divided into primary or secondary types. The primary malignant GCT is composed of a sarcomatous component adjacent to an essentially benign GCT. The secondary malignant type occurs at the site of previously irradiated benign GCT after a long latency period.

Typical clinical scenario

Clinical symptoms are non-specific and include pain, local swelling, and limitation of motion. When a GCT is in the spine it can produce neurological symptoms. Recurrence following local excision of GCT is common. Wide excision results in a lower recurrence rate, however functional and cosmetic results are not favorable. Following surgical treatment, a local soft tissue tumor with a mineralized shell at the surgical site is diagnostic of a GCT recurrence in the soft tissues.

Numerous cases of benign GCTs producing benign metastatic lung lesions have been reported in the literature. The lung lesions appear, on average, about 5 years after diagnosis of the primary tumor. At least one local recurrence of the bone lesion is detected before pulmonary metastasis appears. The lesions in the lungs are histologically indistinguishable from the primary bone tumor. The likelihood of metastasis is greater in tumors that are radiographically aggressive especially those with cortical destruction and soft tissue extension. Lesions arising in the distal radius are more likely to produce pulmonary metastatis. Complete excision of the pulmonary nodules has been successful in controlling the disease in the majority of, but not all, cases. Metastatic disease from GCT has been implicated as the cause of death in some cases.

Pearls and Pitfalls in Musculoskeletal Imaging, ed. D. Lee Bennett and Georges Y. El-Khoury. Published by Cambridge University Press. © Cambridge University Press 2013.

Differential diagnosis

Based on radiography alone other lesions can simulate GCT and these would include aneurysmal bone cyst, chondroblastoma, brown tumor of hyperparathyroidism, fibrous dysplasia, eosinophilic granuloma, and osteomyelitis. The fact that a GCT displays low to intermediate signal intensity on both T1- and T2-weighted sequences can help differentiate a GCT tumor from a large subchondral cyst, intraosseous ganglion, bone abscess, and clear cell sarcoma, all of which demonstrate high signal intensity on T2-weighted images.

Teaching point

There are a few imaging and clinical features of GCT that can be confusing. These include the benign metastasis, malignant transformation, and the multifocal or multi-centric GCT. In contradistinction to most other bone lesions GCT demonstrates low to intermediate signal intensity on both T1- and T2-weighted sequences. All these unusual manifestations of GCT are explained in this chapter and should be included in the differential diagnosis of this relatively common benign bone tumor.

READING LIST

Dahlin DC. Giant cell tumor of bone: highlights of 407 cases. *AJR Am J Roentgenol* 1985;**144**:955–960.

Hindman BW, Seeger LL, Stanley P *et al.* Multicentric giant cell tumor: report of five new cases. *Skeletal Radiol* 1994;**23**:187–190.

Lee MJ, Sallomi DF, Munk PL *et al.* Pictorial review: giant cell tumours of bone. *Clinical Radiol* 1998;**53**:481–489.

Murphey MD, Nomikos GC, Flemming DJ *et al.* From the archives of the AFIP. Imaging of giant cell tumor and giant cell reparative granuloma of bone: radiologic-pathologic correlation. *RadioGraphics* 2001;**21**:1283–1309.

Rock MG, Pritchard DJ, Unni KK. Metastases from histologically benign giant-cell tumor of bone. *J Bone Joint Surg* 1984;**66A**:269–273.

Tubbs WS, Brown LR, Beabout JW *et al.* Benign giant-cell tumor of bone with pulmonary metastases: clinical findings and radiologic appearance of metastases in 13 cases. *AJR Am J Roentgenol* 1992;**158**:331–334.

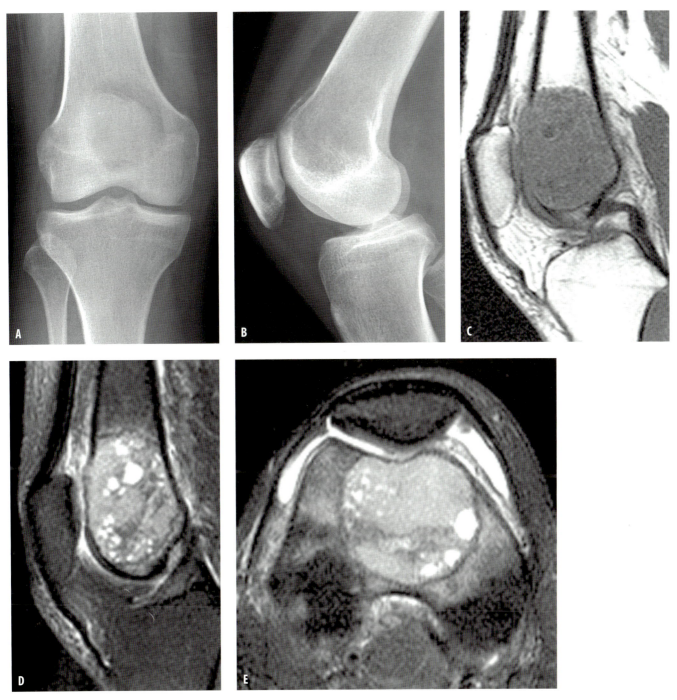

Figure 90.1 Secondary aneurysmal bone cyst (ABC) associated with a giant cell tumor (GCT) in a 32-year-old female. Anteroposterior (**A**) and lateral (**B**) radiographs demonstrating a lytic lesion in the distal femur. T1-weighted sagittal (**C**) MR image reveals the subchondral location of the lesion. The lesion has low signal intensity and it has broken through the cortex anteriorly. Sagittal (**D**) and axial (**E**) fat-suppressed T2-weighted MR images show multiple small areas of increased signal intensity within the tumor. These areas represent secondary ABC engrafted on a GCT.

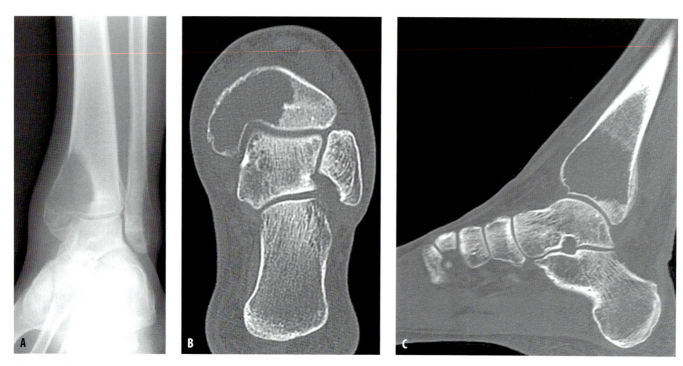

Figure 90.2 Giant cell tumor (GCT) in the distal tibia showing marked cortical thinning which is well demonstrated on CT. Mortise view (**A**) of left ankle shows a well-demarcated lytic lesion in the distal tibia. The lesion is eccentric and minimally expansile. There is no identifiable matrix within the lesion. The cortex is markedly thinned. Coronal (**B**) and sagittal (**C**) reformatted CT images show the cortical thinning caused by the tumor. The periosteal new bone formation along the posterior malleolus is not a feature of GCT; it is believed to be due to a fracture.

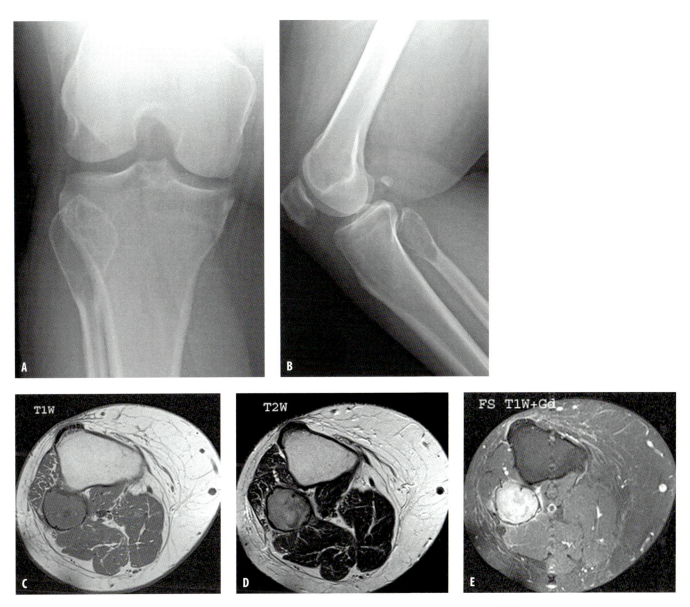

Figure 90.3 This case illustrates a fairly characteristic MRI finding in GCT. On the T2-weighted images GCT has mixed signal intensity. Anteroposterior (**A**) and lateral (**B**) radiographs of the knee show a GCT in fibular head. Axial T1-weighted (**C**), T2-weighted (**D**), and post-contrast fat-suppressed T1-weighted (**E**) MR images demonstrate heterogeneous enhancement of the tumor seen on the T1-weighted and T2-weighted sequences.

91 Ganglion cyst

Imaging description

Based on location there are two major types of ganglion cysts: intraosseous and soft tissue ganglia. Under the soft tissue variant there are a few subtypes which include dorsal wrist ganglia, periosteal or subperiosteal ganglia, intra-articular ganglia, and intraneural ganglia. The intraosseous ganglion is a relatively uncommon, benign, cyst-like, multiloculated lesion that occurs in young and middle-aged adults, usually located in the end of long bones. The most common locations for intraosseous ganglion cysts include the medial malleolus, femoral head, proximal tibia, and carpal bones (Figure 91.1).

Ganglion cyst is the most common soft tissue tumor of the hand and wrist (Figure 91.2). In the carpus ganglion cysts have been described in the capitate, lunate, pisiform, and scaphoid. Radiolucent lesions in the carpal bones are commonly encountered and they are often seen incidentally in asymptomatic patients.

With the widespread use of MRI for the study of internal derangement of the knee and shoulder, intra-articular ganglion cysts are often encountered arising from the cruciate ligaments (Figure 91.3), and within the suprascapular and spinoglenoid notches of the scapula where they are implicated in producing entrapment neuropathies.

Intraneural ganglion cysts are rare. They most commonly involve the peroneal nerve in the region of the fibular head and neck (Figure 91.4). Familiarity with this lesion can help in explaining neurological symptoms such as pain, paresthesia, and foot drop.

The etiology and pathogenesis of ganglion cysts are still unknown, but some theories have been proposed. Some of these theories include: trauma, synovial herniation, and myxoid degeneration of the periarticular connective tissues and ligaments.

Periosteal and subperiosteal ganglion cysts are rare. They have been described involving the radius, the tibia, and the iliac bone (Figure 91.5). Symptoms with this lesion are mild.

Macroscopically, there are no major differences between the intraosseous and soft tissue ganglion cysts. Ganglion cysts are typically multiloculated and filled with viscous, whitish or yellowish mucoid material. The histologic characteristics are identical regardless of location. The wall of a ganglion is made of dense collagen fibers lined with flattened cells without evidence of epithelial or synovial lining.

For intraosseous ganglion cysts conventional radiographs typically demonstrate a sharply circumscribed, lytic lesion, which is often surrounded by a sclerotic rim. The adjacent articular surface is usually preserved and shows no obvious communication between the articular surface and the ganglion cyst. The adjacent joint should appear normal and not showing any evidence of osteoarthritis, otherwise bony lucency is then more likely to be due to a degenerative cyst (or geode).

Periosteal and subperiosteal ganglion cysts can show cortical erosions and some periosteal erosions (Figure 91.5). The periosteal reaction can be speculated. For the vast majority of the other soft tissue ganglia radiographs are either entirely negative or they may show focal soft tissue swelling in the region of the ganglion cyst.

Magnetic resonance images of intraosseous ganglia show low or intermediate signals on T1-weighted images and high signal intensity on T2-weighted images. This is similar to the MRI appearance of soft tissue ganglia. Following an IV gadolinium injection a ganglion cyst shows rim enhancement but its fluid content does not enhance and it shows low signal intensity on fat-suppressed T1-weighted sequences. Ultrasound is equally effective in diagnosing soft tissue ganglia; it is fast and lower cost than MRI and should be considered for the initial imaging for patients suspected of having soft tissue ganglia (Figure 91.4E).

Importance

Ganglion cyst is the most common soft tissue tumor of the hand and wrist. Given its common occurrence, it is imperative to be familiar with its imaging appearance so that it is not misdiagnosed.

Typical clinical scenario

Intraosseous ganglia are usually encountered in middle-aged individuals and are usually asymptomatic. They are often discovered incidentally on imaging studies. Occasionally intraosseous ganglia may produce mild localized pain. The duration of symptoms can range from months to years. Dorsal carpal ganglia are an important cause of chronic wrist pain. The diagnosis of a dorsal carpal ganglion is usually made on physical examination, but some patients may not have a palpable mass because of the small size or deep location of the lesion; in such cases MRI or ultrasound may be required for the detection of occult ganglia. Intraneural ganglia most commonly involve the peroneal nerve. They typically arise in close proximity of the neck of the fibula. Patients present with pain, paresthesia, and foot drop.

Differential diagnosis

The differential diagnosis for an intraosseous ganglion is limited. It includes bone abscess, subchondral cyst due to osteoarthritis, chondroblastoma, and giant cell tumor. The

Pearls and Pitfalls in Musculoskeletal Imaging, ed. D. Lee Bennett and Georges Y. El-Khoury. Published by Cambridge University Press. © Cambridge University Press 2013.

differential diagnosis of a single lytic lesion in a carpal bone includes an enchondroma, giant cell tumor, chondroblastoma, unicameral bone cyst, osteomyelitis, and intraosseous ganglion cyst. With the widespread use of ultrasound and MRI in the evaluation of soft tissue masses, the diagnosis and differential diagnosis of soft tissue ganglion cysts has become fairly simple.

Teaching point

Intraosseous and soft tissue ganglion cysts commonly present as asymptomatic lesions, but sometimes present with symptoms. Familiarity with the various imaging manifestations of ganglion cysts can limit the confusion and spare the patient unnecessary diagnostic investigations and biopsies.

READING LIST

Bianchi S, Abdelwahab IF, Kenan S *et al.* Intramuscular ganglia arising from the superior tibiofibular joint: CT and MR evaluation. *Skeletal Radiol* 1995;**24**:253–256.

Bianchi S, Abdelwahab IF, Zwass A, Giacomello P. Ultrasonographic evaluation of wrist ganglia. *Skeletal Radiol* 1994;**23**:201–203.

Cardinal E, Buckwalter KA, Braunstein EM, Mih AD. Occult dorsal carpal ganglion: comparison of US and MR imaging. *Radiology* 1994;**193**:259–262.

Coakley FV, Finlay DB, Harper WM, Allen MJ. Direct and indirect MRI findings in ganglion cysts of the common peroneal nerve. *Clinical Radiol* 1995;**50**:168–169.

Donahue F, Turkel DH, Mnaymneh W, Mnaymneh LG. Intraosseous ganglion cyst associated with neuropathy. *Skeletal Radiol* 1996;**25**:675–678.

Heyse-Moore GH, Grange WJ. Case report 82. *Skeletal Radiol* 1979;**3**:255–256.

Kobayashi H, Kotoura Y, Hosono M *et al.* Periosteal ganglion of the tibia. *Skeletal Radiol* 1996;**25**:381–383.

Magee TH, Rowedder AM, Degnan GG. Intraosseus ganglia of the wrist. *Radiology* 1995;**195**:517–520.

Nadas S, Landry M, Duvoisin B *et al.* Subperiosteal ganglionic cyst of the iliac wing. *Skeletal Radiol* 1995;**24**:541–542.

Sundaram M. Intraosseous ganglion. In Taveras JM, Ferrucci JT, Buonocore E *et al.*, eds. *Radiology Diagnosis – Imaging – Intervention.* Philadelphia, PA: J. B. Lippincott Company, 1986;1–2.

Noel SH, Engber WD. Intraosseous carpal ganglions. *Iowa Orthopaed J* 1987;**7**:52–54.

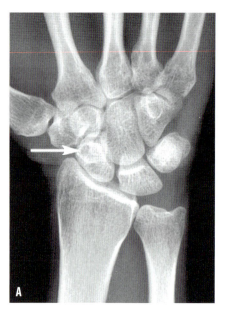
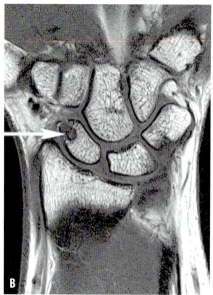
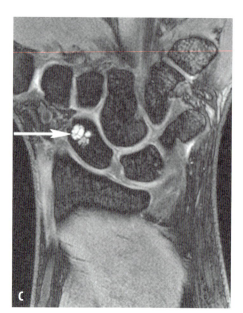
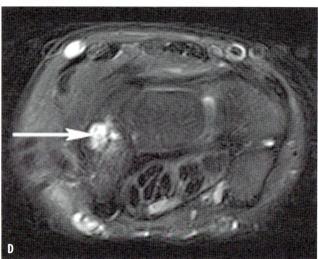

Figure 91.1 Intraosseous ganglion cyst in the scaphoid bone. Anteroposterior (**A**) radiographic view of the left wrist shows a small lucent area in the distal pole of the scaphoid (arrow). Coronal T1-weighted MR image (**B**) shows the lucent area in the distal pole of the scaphoid to be dark (arrow). On fat-suppressed T2-weighted coronal (**C**) and axial (**D**) MR images the lesion is intensely bright suggesting that it contains fluid (arrows).

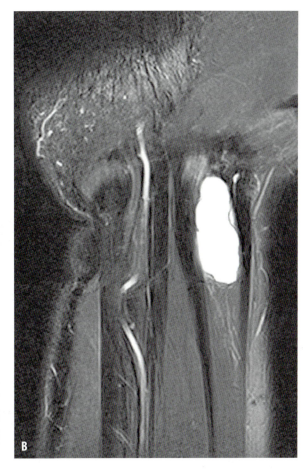

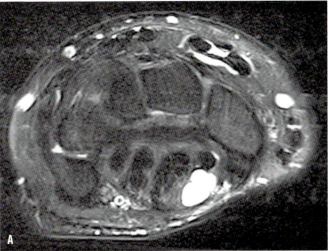

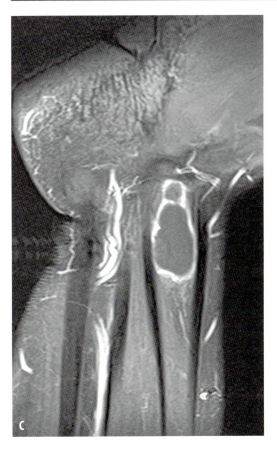

Figure 91.2 Ganglion cyst in the carpal tunnel. Axial (**A**) and coronal (**B**) fat-suppressed T2-weighted MR images show a large ganglion cyst in the carpal tunnel. Because of its fluid content, the ganglion cyst shows high signal intensity on T2-weighted MR images. Coronal post-contrast fat-suppressed T1-weighted MR image (**C**) shows enhancement of the capsule, whereas its fluid content does not enhance.

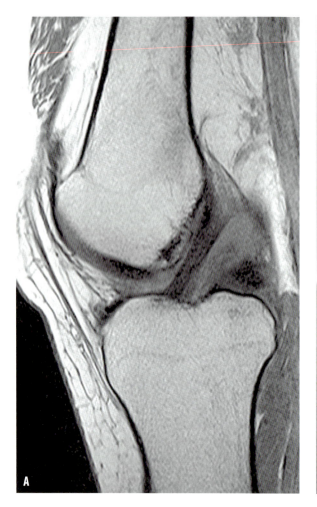

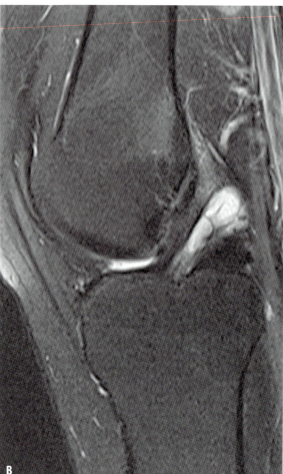

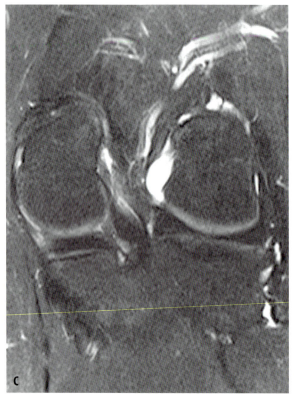

Figure 91.3 Ganglion cyst of the anterior cruciate ligament (ACL) in a 38-year-old female complaining of pain and discomfort in the knee. Sagittal proton density MR image (**A**) reveals a moderately bright structure lying along the posterior margin of the ACL. Sagittal (**B**) and coronal (**C**) fat-suppressed T2-weighted MR images show the structure associated with the ACL to be hyperintense, consistent with a ganglion cyst.

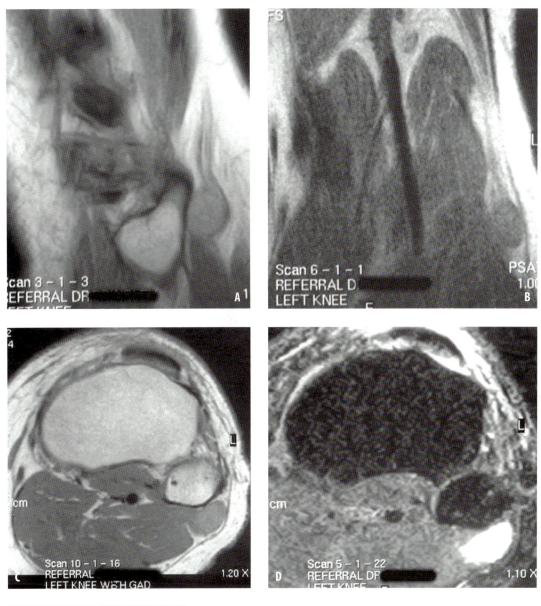

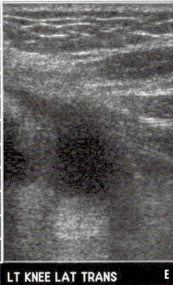

Figure 91.4 Intraneural ganglion cyst arising within the common peroneal nerve. Proton density sagittal MR image (**A**) demonstrates the peroneal nerve with a mass arising from the nerve at the level of the fibular head. Coronal T1-weighted (**B**), axial T1-weighted (**C**), and T2-weighted fat-suppressed axial (**D**) MR images show the mass to be situated posterior to the fibular head. The fact that the mass becomes hyperintense on the T2-weighted images is highly suggestive of a ganglion cyst. Ultrasound image (**E**) of the posterolateral aspect of knee revealed the mass to contain fluid and is most consistent with a ganglion cyst.

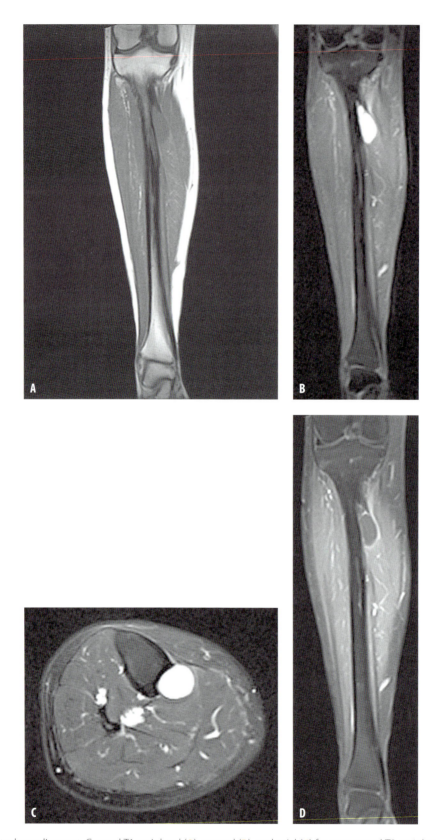

Figure 91.5 Subperiosteal ganglion cyst. Coronal T1-weighted (**A**), coronal (**B**), and axial (**C**) fat-suppressed T2-weighted MR images show a cyst eroding the posterior cortex of the tibia. Coronal post-contrast fat-suppressed T1-weighted MR image (**D**) after IV injection of gadolinium confirms the diagnosis of a ganglion cyst.

Chondroblastoma

Imaging description

In flat bones chondroblastoma is reported to occur in the acetabular region, scapula, ribs, patella, talus, and calcaneus (Figure 92.1).

The epiphyseal location for most chondroblastomas is an important diagnostic imaging feature; the lesion often traverses the epiphyseal plate into the metaphyseal region (Figure 92.2). Radiographically a chondroblastoma reveals a geographic lytic lesion measuring about 2–5 cm in diameter. The majority of chondroblastomas have a thin sclerotic border. Local thinning and expansion of the overlying cortical bone is a common finding. In a study by Brower *et al.* they observed a periosteal reaction distal to the tumor in 47% of chondroblastomas. The periosteal reaction is usually thick, solid, or layered, and its presence was helpful in distinguishing chondroblastoma from other epiphyseal lesions.

On MRI a chondroblastoma shows low to intermediate signal intensity lesion on T1-weighted images, whereas T2-weighted images show low, high, or heterogeneous signal intensity. Another imaging finding which is important in arriving at the correct diagnosis is the commonly associated bone marrow edema which presents with low signal intensity on T1-weighted images and increased signal intensity on T2-weighted images (Figure 92.3). After intravenous administration of gadolinium the edematous marrow shows enhancement on fat-suppressed T1-weighted images. Edema has also been described involving the soft tissues adjacent to the chondroblastoma. Another sign of inflammation, in addition to the edema in the bone marrow and soft tissues, is the presence of synovitis and joint effusion in the adjacent joint.

Importance

Chondroblastoma is an uncommon neoplasm representing approximately 1% of all bone tumors. It is a benign chondroid tumor that almost exclusively arises from the epiphysis or epiphysis equivalent (apophysis) of a long bone. Occasionally an epiphyseal chondroblastoma may extend into the adjoining metaphysis, especially when the growth plate is fusing or fused. Purely metaphyseal and diaphyseal chondroblastomas are exceedingly rare. Chondroblastoma can occur in any bone that develops by enchondral ossification, but the lesion has a predilection for occurring in the epiphyses of long bones especially the distal femur, proximal tibia, proximal femur, proximal humerus, and apophysis of the greater trochanter.

Chondroblastomas are most common in the second and third decade of life and males are more commonly affected than females. Although the majority of chondroblastomas behave in a benign fashion, local recurrence and distant metastasis have been described. The lung is the most common site for metastasis and the histology of the metastatic tumors are similar to the primary lesion, which is benign. Removal of the pulmonary lesions results in long-term survival.

Secondary aneurysmal bone cyst (ABC) may be associated with chondroblastoma in over one third of the cases. Most investigators however have not found any relationship between a chondroblastoma associated with secondary ABC and the rate of recurrence.

Several studies on the origin of chondroblastoma have concluded that it is derived from epiphyseal cartilage cells. Histologically chondroblastomas are highly cellular tumors consisting of uniform, round to polygonal cells with a round nucleus (chondroblasts), packed in a chondroid matrix. Characteristically, these cells are surrounded by a fine network of calcification "chicken wire."

Currently the recommended treatment consists of curettage and packing with bone grafts. This treatment results in good functional results and a local recurrence rate of about 15%. Lesions around the hip account for the majority of recurrences.

Typical clinical scenario

The mean age at presentation is about 16 years, when the tumor is located in the long bones, and 28 years when located in flat or short tubular bones. Most patients present with pain, joint effusion, or muscle wasting. The physical examination is non-specific; it may elicit signs of synovitis, swelling, tenderness, and limitation of movement in the adjacent joint.

Differential diagnosis

If the lesion is located only in the epiphysis, it can be confused with an intraosseous ganglion cyst; whereas for a lesion located both in the epiphysis and metaphysis the differential diagnosis should include a giant cell tumor, aneurysmal bone cyst, and clear cell chondrosarcoma. When a secondary aneurysmal bone cyst is associated with a chondroblastoma the radiographic findings continue to be those of a simple chondroblastoma.

Teaching point

Chondroblastoma is a benign cartilaginous tumor with distinguishing imaging features. In the long bones radiography reveals an epiphyseal lytic lesion with sharp sclerotic border. MRI clearly shows the lesion accompanied by inflammatory changes in the adjacent bone marrow and soft tissues.

READING LIST

Azorin D, Gonzalez-Mediero I, Colmenero I *et al.* Diaphyseal chondroblastoma in a long bone: first report. *Skeletal Radiol* 2006; **35**:49–52.

Bloem JL, Mulder JD. Chondroblastoma: a clinical and radiological study of 104 cases. *Skeletal Radiol* 1985;**14**:1–9.

Brower AC, Moser RP, Kransdorf MJ. The frequency and diagnostic significance of periostitis in chondroblastoma. *AJR Am J Roentgenol* 1990;**154**:309–314.

Hayes CW, Conway WF, Sundaram M. Misleading aggressive MR imaging appearance of some benign musculoskeletal lesions. *RadioGraphics* 1992;**12**:1119–1134.

Khalili K, White LM, Kandel RA, Wunder JS. Chondroblastoma with multiple distant soft tissue metastases. *Skeletal Radiol* 1997;**26**:493–496.

Kim J, Kumar R, Raymond AK, Ayala AG. Non-epiphyseal chondroblastoma arising in the iliac bone, and complicated by an aneurysmal bone cyst: a case report and review of the literature. *Skeletal Radiol* 2010;**39**:583–587.

Kyriakos M, Land VJ, Penning HL, Parker SG. Metastatic chondroblastoma report of a fatal case with a review of the literature on atypical, aggressive, and malignant chondroblastoma. *Cancer* 1985;**55**:1770–1789.

Ramappa AJ, Lee FYI, Tang P *et al.* Chondroblastoma of bone. *J Bone Joint Surg* 2000;**82-A**:1140–1145.

Yamamura S, Sato K, Sugiura H, Iwata H. Inflammatory reactive in chondroblastoma. *Skeletal Radiol* 1996;**25**:371–376.

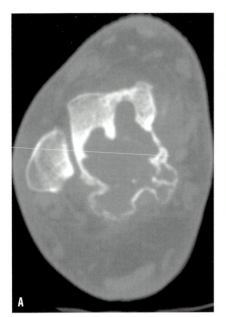
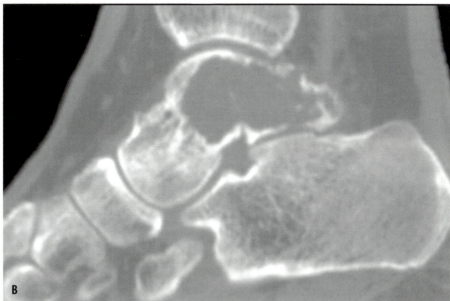
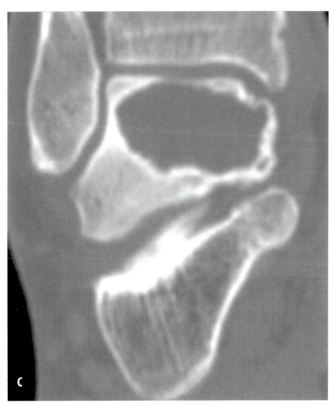

Figure 92.1 Chondroblastoma of the talus in a young male patient. Axial (**A**), sagittal (**B**), and coronal (**C**) CT images showing a well-circumscribed lytic lesion in the body of the talus; the lesion has a sclerotic margin and the location is typical for a chondroblastoma.

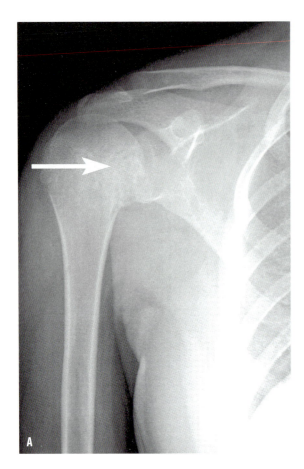

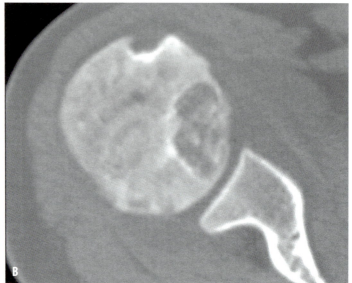

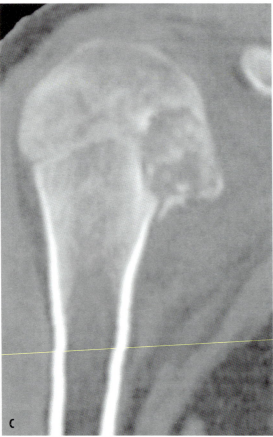

Figure 92.2 Chondroblastoma in a 16-year-old female. The lesion has crossed the epiphyseal plate. Anteroposterior radiographic view (**A**) of the right shoulder shows a lytic lesion in the medial aspect of the humeral head. The lesion is filled with punctate calcifications (arrow). Axial CT image (**B**) and coronal reformatted CT images (**C**) show the lesion crossing the physeal plate. The calcifications within the lesion are better seen by CT.

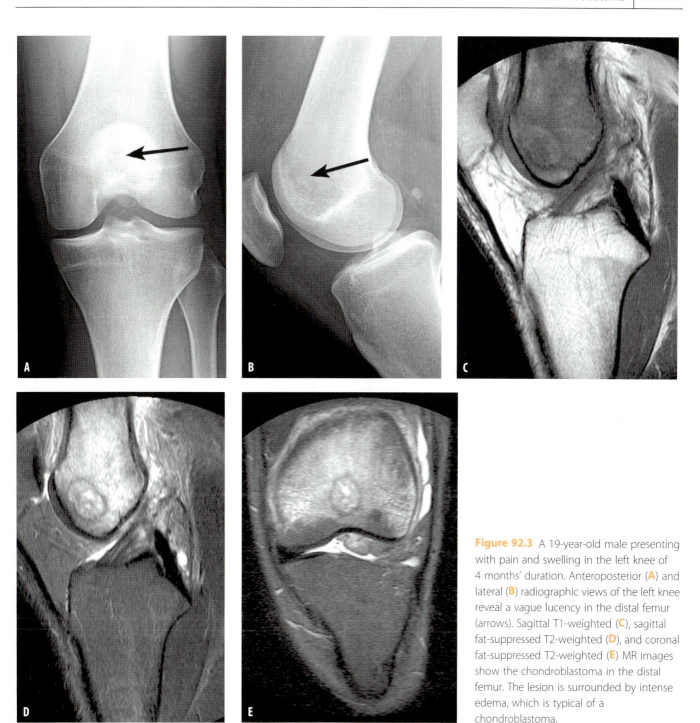

Figure 92.3 A 19-year-old male presenting with pain and swelling in the left knee of 4 months' duration. Anteroposterior (**A**) and lateral (**B**) radiographic views of the left knee reveal a vague lucency in the distal femur (arrows). Sagittal T1-weighted (**C**), sagittal fat-suppressed T2-weighted (**D**), and coronal fat-suppressed T2-weighted (**E**) MR images show the chondroblastoma in the distal femur. The lesion is surrounded by intense edema, which is typical of a chondroblastoma.

Imaging description

Imaging findings of hypertrophic osteoarthropathy (HOA) may precede the underlying condition by many months. In secondary HOA radiographs reveal symmetrical periostitis consisting of single or multiple layers of new bone formation. Periostitis occurs along the diaphyses and metaphyses of long bones in the lower and upper extremities (Figure 93.1). It is less commonly observed in the metacarpals, metatarsals, and phalanges. Rarely the periostitis can occur in the lower extremities without involvement of the upper extremities. In severe cases, the ribs, clavicles, scapulae, pelvis, and malar bones are involved. Early in HOA the periosteal reaction presents as a single layer but as the condition progresses the periosteal reaction becomes thickened and multilayered, eventually causing increased cortical thickness and an irregular cortical surface. The thickness of the periosteal reaction is time dependent; it becomes thicker and more extensive with longer disease duration (Figure 93.1). Acroosteolysis has been observed in patients with pachydermoperiostosis and with HOA.

Bone scintigraphy in HOA is characterized by symmetrical increased uptake along the cortices of the long bones. The radionuclide activity has been shown to be more intense in the lower extremities especially below the knees (Figure 93.1). Involvement of the pelvis and spine is not a feature of HOA and should suggest metastatic disease.

The experience in the literature with CT and MRI is limited. CT is reported to show the periosteal reaction surrounding the long bones, and on MRI it is seen as increased signal intensity on T2-weighted images while the elevated periosteum appears as a hypointense rim.

Importance

Hypertrophic osteoarthropathy (HOA), also known as hypertrophic pulmonary osteoarthropathy, is a syndrome characterized by the presence of periostitis, arthritis, and clubbing of the fingers and toes. The triad of periostitis, clubbing, and arthritis represent the complete form of HOA, however an incomplete form of HOA has been described consisting of periostitis and arthritis but without clubbing.

Two types of HOA are clinically recognized: (1) the primary or idiopathic type (pachydermoperiostosis) which is inherited as an autosomal dominant trait with variable expression; and (2) the secondary type, which is much more common, and an underlying disease process is typically identified.

A wide spectrum of diseases is associated with secondary HOA, most commonly pulmonary malignancies, typically non-small cell carcinomas and adenocarcinomas, which account for 80% of all cases; other intrathoracic malignancies that are known to produce secondary HOA include metastatic lung cancer, mesothelioma, and lymphoma. The incidence of HOA in patients with bronchogenic carcinoma is approximately 10%. Prompt relief of symptoms can occur with resection of the lung tumor or intrathoracic vagotomy. In addition 31% of patients with congenital heart disease and 28% of patients with liver disease are associated with HOA.

There are also malignant and benign extrathoracic conditions that can be associated with HOA and they include nasopharyngeal cancer, renal cell carcinoma, esophageal, gastric, and pancreatic cancers, intestinal lymphoma, thyroid cancer, congenital heart disease, bronchiectasis, pneumonia, cystic fibrosis, and inflammatory bowel disease. The association of HOA with childhood malignancies has been quite rare. There have also been a few cases of focal or unilateral secondary HOA in patients with infected aortofemoral grafts.

The pathogenesis of HOA is still under study although some plausible theories have been advanced. Dickinson suggested that normally megakaryocytes and large clumps of platelets are trapped by the pulmonary capillary beds. With certain disease processes such as chronic lung inflammation, bronchial malignancies, or intracardiac right to left shunts, this trapping mechanism is disrupted allowing megakaryocytes and clumps of platelets to enter the systemic circulation. From there they can reach the digits resulting in the local release of growth factors leading to fibroblast proliferation and causing clubbing.

Typical clinical scenario

Clubbing of the fingers and toes, symmetrical periosteal reaction, and arthritis are typical manifestations of HOA. Arthralgias or arthritis especially in the knees and ankles can be the first symptom. The metacarpophalangeal or proximal interphalangeal joints and wrists can be involved in a bilateral and symmetrical fashion which clinically mimics rheumatoid arthritis. The periostitis manifests with painful limbs including arthralgias and polyarthritis.

Differential diagnosis

To the non-rheumatologist, the symmetrical arthralgias and arthritis seen at presentation with HOA can closely mimic rheumatoid arthritis, a point which is repeatedly emphasized in the literature. Few other conditions may mimic the changes of periostitis in HOA. They include thyroid acropachy, leukemia, and hypervitaminosis A.

Pearls and Pitfalls in Musculoskeletal Imaging, ed. D. Lee Bennett and Georges Y. El-Khoury. Published by Cambridge University Press. © Cambridge University Press 2013.

Teaching point

An active synovitis may be the first presentation of HOA with the most commonly involved joints being the large weight-bearing joints such as the knees and ankles. It has also been reported that HOA can precede the underlying disease, such as a malignancy, by several months. Clinicians and radiologists should be aware of this possibility and they should start a thorough search for a potential pulmonary malignancy.

READING LIST

Ameri MR, Alebouyeh M, Donner MW. Hypertrophic osteoarthropathy in childhood malignancy. *AJR Am J Roentgenol* 1978;**130**:992–993.

Clarke S, Barnsley L, Peters M *et al*. Hypertrophic pulmonary osteoarthropathy without clubbing of the digits. *Skeletal Radiol* 2001;**30**:652–655.

Dickinson CJ. The aetiology of clubbing and hypertrophic osteoarthropathy. *Eur J Clin Invest* 1993;**23**:330.

Joseph B, Chacko V. Acro-osteolysis associated with hypertrophic pulmonary osteoarthropathy and pachydermoperiostosis. *Radiology* 1985;**154**:343–344.

Peck B. Hypertrophic osteoarthropathy with Hodgkin's disease in the mediastinum. *J Am Med Assoc* 1977;**238**(13):1400–1401.

Rosenthall L, Kirsh J. Observations on radionuclide imaging in hypertrophic pulmonary osteoarthropathy. *Radiology* 1976;**120**:359–362.

Spruijt S, Krijgsman AA, van den Brocek JAC *et al*. Hypertrophic osteoarthropathy of one leg – a sign of aortic graft infection. *Skeletal Radiol* 1999;**28**:224–228.

Stevens M, Helms C, El-Khoury G, Chow S. Unilateral hypertrophic osteoarthropathy associated with aortobifemoral graft infection. *AJR Am J Roentgenol* 1998;**170**:1584–1586.

Walter RD, Resnick D. Hypertrophic osteoarthropathy of a lower extremity in association with arterial graft sepsis. *AJR Am J Roentgenol* 1981;**137**:1059–1061.

Weissman BN. Imaging arthropathies associated with malignant disorders. In Weissman BN, ed. *Imaging of Arthritis and Metabolic Bone Diseases*. Philadelphia, PA: Saunders (Elsevier), 2009;290–295.

Yao Q, Altman RD, Brahn E. Periostitis and hypertrophic pulmonary osteoarthropathy: report of 2 cases and review of the literature. *Semin Arthritis Rheum* 2009;**38**:458–466.

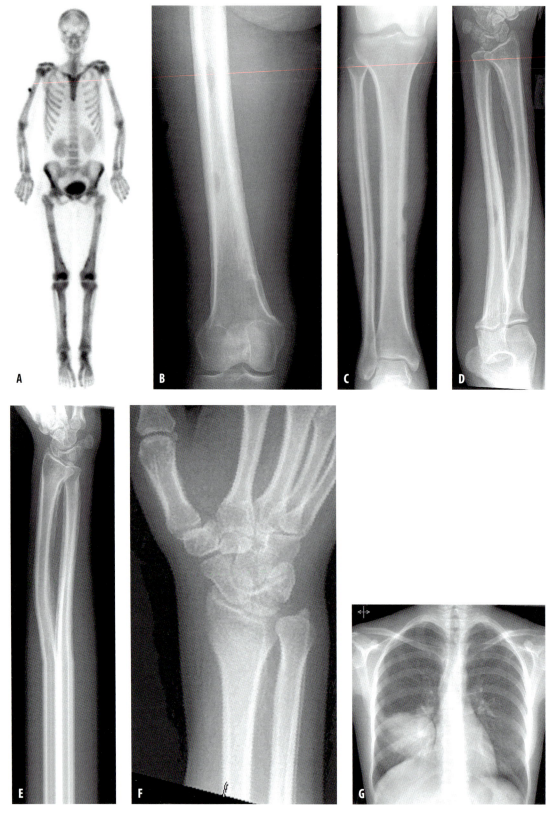

Figure 93.1 A 29-year-old female who presented to the rheumatology clinic with generalized arthralgias. After the proper imaging studies, she was diagnosed with secondary hypertrophic osteoarthropathy (HOA). A total body nuclear medicine bone scan (**A**) showed increased radionuclide uptake in the long bones, mostly in the lower extremities and to a lesser extent in the upper extremities. Anteroposterior radiographic view (**B**) of the right femur shows diffuse periosteal reaction, especially above the knee. Anteroposterior view (**C**) of the right leg shows diffuse periosteal reaction in the right tibia and fibula. The lytic lesions in the medial cortex of the tibia were thought to represent a metastatic lesion. Radiographs of both forearms (**D** and **E**) and right wrist (**F**) show extensive periosteal reaction characteristic of HOA. Anteroposterior view of the chest (**G**) demonstrated a large mass in the right lower lobe. Biopsy of this mass showed an adenocarcinoma.

Imaging description

In adults the most frequent site for the SAPHO syndrome is the sternoclavicular region (Figure 94.1). About 65–90% of patients show involvement of the sternoclavicular region. With time all the components of the anterior chest wall can become involved particularly the sternoclavicular, upper costosternal, costochondral, and manubriosternal junctions. Radiographically the most common feature is hyperostosis, characterized by chronic periosteal reaction and cortical thickening leading to bone hypertrophy (Figure 94.1). This may be associated with enthesopathy leading to ligamentous ossification, bony bridging, and joint ankylosis. Soft tissue edema and thickening may be seen adjacent to the involved bones and joint. When the disease is advanced these changes are readily identified by radiography, but early changes of sternoclavicular hyperostosis require the use of CT for a definitive diagnosis. CT and MRI may be required for detecting serious complications of sternoclavicular hyperostosis resulting from bony overgrowth which can lead to subclavian vein obstruction and superior vena cava syndrome.

On rare occasions extra-axial SAPHO can occur in the long bones (Figure 94.2), pelvis, scapula, and tarsal bones.

Bone scintigraphy is a sensitive technique for detecting SAPHO lesions throughout the skeleton in early stages of the disease (Figure 94.1 and Figure 94.2 A). The bull horn sign in the upper anterior chest wall is diagnostic of SAPHO.

Magnetic resonance imaging demonstrates the changes due to arthritis and the bone marrow edema. MRI can also be useful in the follow-up of patients to determine active from chronic inactive lesions.

In SAPHO the spine is the second most common site of involvement in adults and changes can resemble other diseases. The thoracic spine is the most frequently affected followed, in decreasing order, by the lumbar and cervical spine. Imaging findings in the spine include: (1) spondylodiscitis, which manifests on radiography and CT with irregularity and erosions in the endplates with narrowing or complete obliteration of the adjacent disc space. These endplate changes can resemble infectious spondylodiscitis. Parts of the vertebral bodies adjacent to the involved disc appear hypointense on T1-weighted images and hyperintense on T2-weighted images; however paraspinal and epidural abscesses are absent. (2) On MRI there are two patterns of abnormal marrow involving several thoracic and lumbar vertebrae. These patterns can be focal or diffuse hypointense lesions on T1- and hyperintense

on T2-weighted images. These foci are located either adjacent to the endplates or at the corners of the vertebral bodies. (3) Another finding on MRI is the presence of paravertebral soft tissue swelling which probably represents extension of the inflammatory process into the adjacent soft tissues. (4) Vertebral sclerosis which can resemble Paget's disease or blastic metastasis (Figure 94.3). (5) Paravertebral ossifications in the form of marginal syndemophytes, or more commonly non-marginal syndemophytes causing ankylosis and associated kyphosis. (6) Sacroiliitis which involves 13–52% of patients resembles a spondyloarthropathy but involvement is often unilateral. Erosions and dense sclerosis occur on the iliac side of the sacroiliac joint and is best demonstrated by CT (Figure 94.4).

Importance

For many years this syndrome was known in the literature by a variety of names but most commonly as sternoclavicular or sternocostoclavicular hyperostosis. Currently the acronym SAPHO syndrome, which was coined by Chamot et al. in 1987, is universally used to describe this syndrome which refers to synovitis, acne, palmoplantar pustulosis (PPP), hyperostosis, and osteitis. However not all the syndrome components need to be present for diagnosing this syndrome, especially the dermatologic components. The absence of skin lesions does not exclude the diagnosis of SAPHO. The skin lesion may precede, occur simultaneously with, or follow the osteoarticular manifestations. The acne in patients with SAPHO is usually of the severe forms, such as acne fulminans, acne conglobata, or hidradenitis suppurativa. Palmoplantar pustulosis, which is present in 18–55% of SAPHO patients, is considered by many dermatologists as a variant of psoriasis. In fact many consider SAPHO as one of the spondyloarthropathies. The synovitis in SAPHO occurs most commonly in the sternoclavicular and sternomanubrial joints. Extrathoracic sites of synovitis include the sacroiliac joints typically in a unilateral fashion. Occasionally peripheral synovial joints are involved with erosions and enthesopathy resembling seronegative spondyloarthropathies.

For the radiologist the most striking features of SAPHO are the hyperostosis and osteitis. Hyperostosis refers to excessive bone formation which can occur within the medullary cavity or on both surfaces (periosteal and endosteal) of the cortex. As a result the medullary canal may become stenotic and the cortical bone expanded. Osteitis refers to inflammation of the medullary and cortical bone. Clinically the bone involved with osteitis is painful and tender. Histologically the features

Pearls and Pitfalls in Musculoskeletal Imaging, ed. D. Lee Bennett and Georges Y. El-Khoury. Published by Cambridge University Press. © Cambridge University Press 2013.

of the osseous lesions in SAPHO are non-specific and variable depending on the duration of the disease. In the acute phase which lasts for about a year, there is inflammation, neutrophils, edema, and periosteal new bone formation resembling acute osteomyelitis but without infecting organisms. The intermediate phase is dominated by bone remodeling, marrow fibrosis, and chronic inflammation. In the chronic phase, SAPHO histologically resembles Paget's disease.

A variant of SAPHO which occurs in children and adolescents is known as chronic relapsing multicentric osteomyelitis (CRMO), which has a predilection for the anterior chest wall, particularly the clavicle, and the metaphysis of long bones. There is a tendency for a female preponderance in both CRMO and SAPHO.

Typical clinical scenario

Patients with SAPHO syndrome typically present between the fourth and sixth decade of life with pain, tenderness, and swelling in the upper aspect of the anterior chest wall bilaterally. Approximately two thirds of the patients will have the characteristic skin lesions associated with this syndrome. The target sites for SAPHO include most commonly the upper anterior chest wall, sacroiliac joints, spine, long bones, pelvis, and peripheral joints.

Differential diagnosis

It is important to differentiate SAPHO from other diseases that can produce similar imaging findings but have different treatment and prognosis. The differential diagnosis includes osteomyelitis, lymphoma, Ewing's sarcoma, osteosarcoma, condensing osteitis of the clavicle, POEMS, metastasis, and Paget's disease.

Teaching point

SAPHO is now considered by most authorities as belonging to the seronegative spondyloarthropathies. The radiologist plays a key role in diagnosing SAPHO because of the typical bone lesions located in characteristic target locations such as the upper anterior chest wall, spine, and sacroiliac joints. Associated skin lesions such as PPP and acne make the process of arriving at the correct diagnosis easier, however these skin lesions are not always present. Skeletal lesions may precede skin manifestations by as long as 12–20 years, although in most cases the interval is less than 2 years.

READING LIST

Boutin RD, Resnick D. The SAPHO syndrome: an evolving concept for unifying several idiopathic disorders of bone and skin. *AJR Am J Roentgenol* 1998;**170**:585–591.

Cotton A, Flipo R-M, Mentre A *et al*. SAPHO syndrome. *RadioGraphics* 1995;**15**:1147–1154.

Davies AM, Marino AJ, Evans N *et al*. SAPHO syndrome: 20-year follow-up. *Skeletal Radiol* 1999;**28**:159–162.

Earwaker JWS, Cotton A. SAPHO: syndrome or concept? Imaging findings. *Skeletal Radiol* 2003;**32**:311–327.

Kasperczyk A, Freyschmidt J. Pustulotic arthroosteitis: spectrum of bone lesions with palmoplantar pustulosis. *Radiology* 1994;**191**:207–211.

Nachtigal A, Cardinal E, Bureau NJ *et al*. Vertebral involvement in SAPHO syndrome: MRI findings. *Skeletal Radiol* 1999;**28**:163–168.

Sartoris DJ, Schreiman JS, Kerr R *et al*. Sternocostoclavicular hyperostosis: a review and report of 11 cases. *Radiology* 1986;**158**:125–128.

Suh J-S, Shin K-H, Park K-W. Hyperostotic and osteosclerotic changes of the tarsal navicular, associated with pustulosis palmaris and plantaris. *Skeletal Radiol* 1996;**25**:377–380.

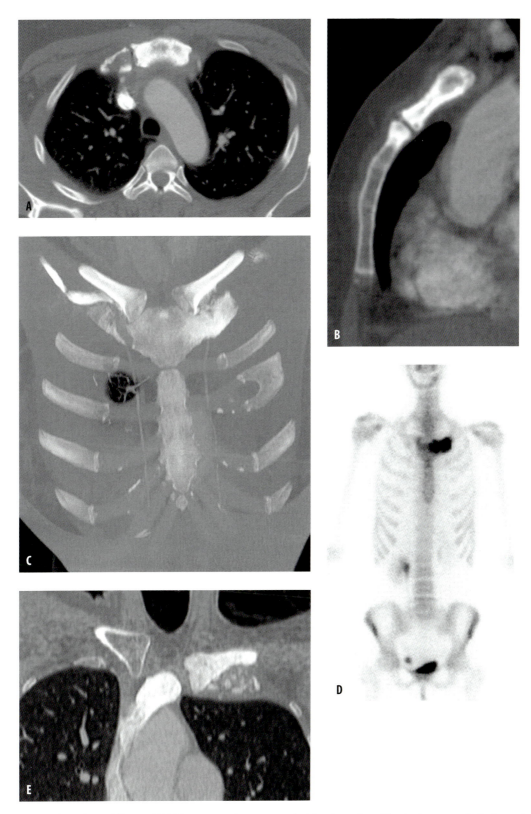

Figure 94.1 Imaging studies of two different SAPHO patients who presented with pain and swelling in the sternoclavicular region. Axial (**A**) and sagittal (**B**) CT images show hyperostosis of the manubrium and upper sternum. A coronal (**C**) CT image from another patient reveals hyperostosis of both clavicles, left first rib and adjacent portion of the manubrium. Nuclear medicine bone scan (**D**) and coronal CT image (**E**) of the anterior chest reveal increased radionuclide uptake in the left clavicle. The CT image shows hyperostosis of the left clavicle.

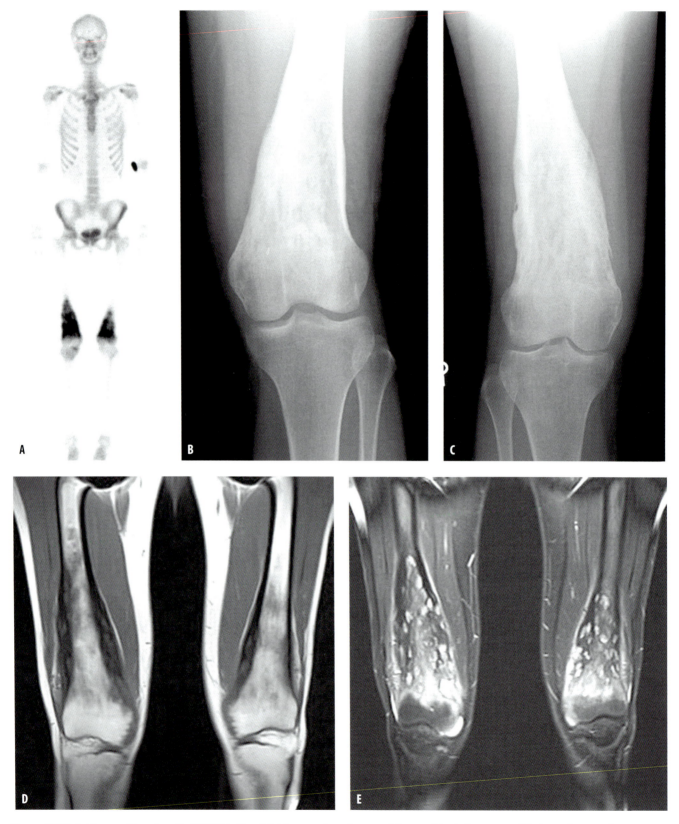

Figure 94.2 A 19-year-old male with SAPHO in the distal femora. A nuclear medicine total body bone scan (**A**) shows increased radionuclide scan in the distal femora. AP radiographs of both femora (**B** and **C**) show hyperostosis bilaterally. Coronal T1-weighted (**D**) and fat-suppressed T2-weighted (**E**) MR images again show hyperostosis and inflammation in the distal femora.

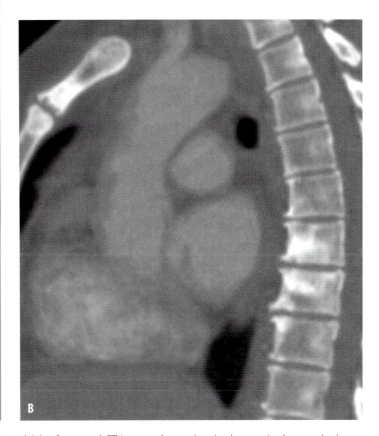

Figure 94.3 SAPHO with spine involvement. Coronal (**A**) and sagittal (**B**) reformatted CT images show sclerotic changes in the vertebral bodies of T_7 and T_8; T_9 shows mild sclerosis at its anterior superior corner. The disc spaces are relatively well preserved. There is a no paravertebral soft tissue swelling.

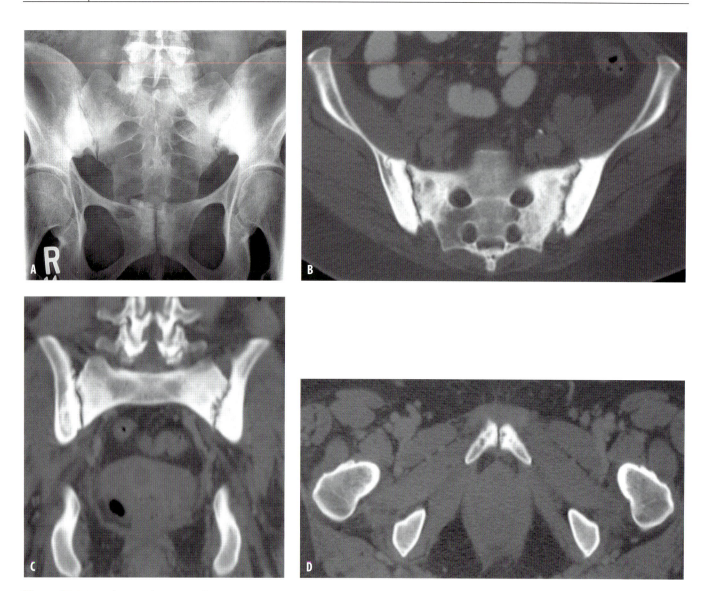

Figure 94.4 Sacroiliitis and osteitis pubis in a patient with SAPHO. A Ferguson view (**A**) radiograph of the sacroiliac joints shows bony sclerosis in both sacroiliac (SI) joints. Axial (**B**) and coronal (**C**) CT images of the SI joints show the sclerosis to be more pronounced in the left sacroiliac joint. Erosions are seen in both SI joints, but more on the left side. Axial CT section (**D**) of the pubis shows osteitis pubis.

Index